Cross Cultural Perspectives
in Medical Ethics: Readings

The Jones and Bartlett Series in Biology

The Biology of AIDS
Hung Fan, Ross F. Conner, and Luis P.Villarreal,
all of the University of California-Irvine

Basic Genetics
Daniel L. Hartl, Washington University School of Medicine;
David Freifelder, University of California, San Diego; Leon
A. Snyder, University of Minnesota, St. Paul

General Genetics
Leon A. Snyder, University of Minnesota, St. Paul; David
Freifelder, University of California, San Diego; Daniel L.
Hartl, Washington University School of Medicine

Genetics
John R. S. Fincham, University of Edinburgh

Genetics of Populations
Philip W. Hedrick, University of Kansas

Human Genetics: A New Synthesis
Gordon Edlin, University of California, Davis

Microbial Genetics
David Freifelder, University of California, San Diego

Experimental Techniques in Molecular Genetics
Stanley R. Maloy, University of Illinois-Urbana

Cells: Principles of Molecular Structure and Function
David M. Prescott, University of Colorado, Boulder

Essentials of Molecular Biology
David Freifelder, University of California, San Diego

Introduction to Biology: A Human Perspective
Donald J. Farish, California State University at Sonoma

Introduction to Human Immunology
Teresa L. Huffer, Shady Grove Adventist Hospital,
Gaithersburg, Maryland, and Frederick Community College,
Frederick, Maryland; Dorothy J. Kanapa, National
Cancer Institute, Frederick, Maryland; George W. Stevenson,
Northwestern University Medical Center, Chicago, Illinois

Molecular Biology, Second Edition
David Freifelder, University of California, San Diego

The Molecular Biology of Bacterial Growth (a symposium volume)
M. Schaechter, Tufts University Medical School; F. Neidhardt,
University of Michigan; J. Ingraham, University of California,
Davis; N.O. Kjeldgaard, University of Aarhus, Denmark, editors

Evolution
Monroe W. Strickberger, University of Missouri-St. Louis

Molecular Evolution: An Annotated Reader
Eric Terzaghi, Adam S. Wilkins, and David Penny, all
of Massey University, New Zealand

Population Biology
Philip W. Hedrick, University of Kansas

Virus Structure and Assembly
Sherwood Casjens, University of Utah College of Medicine

Cancer: A Biological and Clinical Introduction, Second Edition
Steven B. Oppenheimer
California State University, Northridge

Introduction to Human Disease, Second Edition
Leonard V. Crowley, M.D.
St. Mary's Hospital, Minneapolis

Handbook of Protoctista
Lynn Margulis, John O. Corliss, Michael Melkonian,
and David I. Chapman, editors

Living Images
Gene Shih and Richard Kessel

Early Life
Lynn Margulis, Boston University

Functional Diversity of Plants in the Sea and on Land
A.R.O. Chapman, Dalhousie University

Plant Nutrition: An Introduction to Current Concepts
A.D.M. Glass, University of British Columbia

*Methods for Molecular Cloning and Analysis of
Eukaryotic Genes*
Alfred Bothwell, Yale University School of Medicine; Fred
Alt and George Yancopoulous, both of Columbia
University

Medical Biochemistry
N.V. Bhagavan
John A. Burns School of Medicine,
University of Hawaii at Manoa

Vertebrates: A Laboratory Text, Second Edition
Norman K. Wessells, Stanford University and
Elizabeth M. Center, College of Notre Dame, editors

The Environment, Third Edition
Penelope ReVelle, Essex Community College
Charles ReVelle, The Johns Hopkins University

Medical Ethics
Robert M. Veatch, editor
The Kennedy Institute of Ethics--Georgetown University

Cross Cultural Perspectives in Medical Ethics: Readings
Robert M. Veatch, editor
The Kennedy Institute of Ethics--Georgetown University

*100 Years Exploring Life, 1888-1988, The Marine
Biological Laboratory at Woods Hole*
Jane Maienschein, Arizona State University

Writing a Successful Grant Application, Second Edition
Liane Reif-Lehrer, Tech-Write Consultants/ERIMON Associates

Cross Cultural Perspectives in Medical Ethics: Readings

Edited by

Robert M. Veatch

The Kennedy Institute of Ethics
Georgetown University

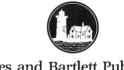

Jones and Bartlett Publishers
Boston • Portola Valley

Editorial, Sales, and Customer Service Offices
Jones and Bartlett Publishers
20 Park Plaza
Boston, MA 02116

Library of Congress Cataloging-in-Publication Data

Cross Cultural Perspectives in Medical Ethics: Readings

   Includes bibliographies.
   1.   Medical Ethics.   I.   Veatch, Robert M.
R724.R4   1989   174'.2   88-28457
ISBN   0-086720-075-8

Printed in the United States of America.

10 9 8 7 6 5 4 3 2 1

Production   Michael Bass & Associates
Cover and text design   Rafael Millán
Typesetting   The Composing Room of Michigan, Inc.

ISBN   0-086720-075-8

Preface

The renaissance in medical ethics of the past decade has provided dramatic cases involving dying patients, genetic manipulations, and allocation of scarce resources. It has also stimulated an interest in theories or systems of medical ethics. In *Medical Ethics** I attempted to provide one such systematic account. In doing so I became vividly aware of the rich and varied history of medical ethical systems and of the more systematic work on principles of normative ethics that underlie more specific and ad hoc stands taken on particular issues.

While Hippocrates, the Oath that bears his name, and the ethical principles of the American Medical Association have often been assumed to be the core of Western medical ethics, it is becoming increasingly clear that there are important alternatives to the Hippocratic system. They arise not only in the major Western religious traditions, each of which has what could be called a medical ethic of its own, but also in secular philosophical systems such as liberal political philosophy. They also arise in non-Western traditions including Marxism, Islam, and the major traditions of the East.

The foundational documents for these traditions often have existed only in obscure journals and out-of-print foreign sources. My objective here has been to gather together these documents and combine them with a selection of readings that will introduce the key ethical principles of normative ethics and provide a brief example of how they can be applied to medical ethical issues. They are intended to provide the basic readings that will introduce the student of medical ethics—whether physician, college student, or interested lay person—to the fundamental concepts, principles, and categories underlying the major issues in medical ethics today.

This collection is very different from any reader on the issue of biomedical ethics existing today. It is designed for undergraduate, graduate, and professional school courses in medical and bioethics where the objective is to provide an understanding of alternative systems of medical ethics and to introduce systematically the basic principles of normative ethics. It can be used as a companion reader to

---

*Medical Ethics, ed. Robert M. Veatch (Boston: Jones and Bartlett. Publishers, 1989).

Medical Ethics, but is designed to be a free-standing anthology. This text could not have been prepared and edited into its present form without the help of people who have provided careful and committed assistance in research and administration, including Donna Horak Mitsock, Carol Mason, Karen Y. Roberts, Denise Brooks, Michelle Lewis, and Nancy Martin. To them I express my gratitude.

Acknowledgments

The Hippocratic Oath: Text, Translation and Interpretation abridged with permission from Edelstein, Ludwig: *The Hippocratic Oath: Text, Translation and Interpretation.* Baltimore/London: The Johns Hopkins University Press, 1943, pp. 1–64.

"Declaration of Geneva," by the World Medical Association. Copyright 1986, World Medical Association. Reprinted with permission of the World Medical Association.

"Toward an Expanded Medical Ethics: The Hippocratic Ethic Revisited," by Edmund D. Pellegrino. Abridged from *Hippocrates Revisited: A Search for Meaning,* Roger J. Bulger, editor, with permission from New York: Medcom Press, 1973, pp. 133–147.

"Principles of Medical Ethics of the American Medical Association [1957]." Reprinted with permission from the *Journal of the American Medical Association* 164:1119–1120, 1957.

"Principles of Medical Ethics [1980]." Reprinted with permission of the American Medical Association, *Principles of Medical Ethics of the American Medical Association,* 1980.

"The Obligation to Heal in the Judaic Tradition," based on "Theological Considerations in the Care of Defective Newborns," by J. David Bleich. Reprinted in abridged form from Chester A. Swinyard, editor, *Decision Making and the Defective Newborn,* 1979, pp. 512–561. Courtesy of Charles C Thomas, Publisher, Springfield, Illinois.

"Ethical and Religious Directives," copyright 1975, 1971 by the United States Catholic Conference, Washington, D.C., is printed with permission. All rights reserved.

from the Johns Hopkins University Press and the *Bulletin of the History of Medicine* 13:268–277, 1943.

"The 17 Rules of Enjuin: For Disciples in Our School." *Excerpted from Western Medical Pioneers in Feudal Japan,* by John Z. Bowers, with permission from The Johns Hopkins Press, 1970, pp. 8–10.

"Medicine's Ethical Responsibilities," by Russell B. Roth. Reprinted with permission from Russell B. Roth and the *Journal of the American Medical Association* 215:1956–1958, 1971.

"Code, Covenant, Contract, or Philanthropy," by William F. May. Reprinted with permission from William F. May and the *Hastings Center Report* 5:29–38, December 1975.

"Veatch, May, Models: A Critical Review and a New View," by K. Danner Clouser. Reprinted with permission from K. Danner Clouser and D. Reidel Publishing Company, *The Clinical Encounter.* Earl Shelp, editor, 1983, pp. 89–103. Copyright 1983 by D. Reidel Publishing Company, Dordrecht, Holland.

Foundations of Bioethics, by H. Tristram Engelhardt. Excerpted with permission from H. Tristram Engelhardt and Oxford University Press, 1986, pp. 39–44.

"Do No Harm: Axiom of Medical Ethics," by Albert Jonsen. Reprinted with permission from D. Reidel Publishing Co., *Philosophical Medical Ethics: Its Nature and Significance.* Stuart F. Spicker and H. Tristram Engelhardt, Jr., editors. 1977, pp. 27–41. Copyright 1977 by D. Reidel Publishing Company, Dordrecht, Holland.

The Right and the Good, by W. D. Ross. Excerpted with permission from Oxford University Press, 1939, pp. 16–47.

"On the Supposed Right to Tell Lies from Benevolent Motives," by Immanuel Kant. Translated by Thomas Kingsmill Abbott and reprinted in Kant's *Critique of Practical Reason and Other Works on the Theory of Ethics.* London: Longmans, 1909 [1797], pp. 361–365. Reprinted with notes and references omitted.

The Methods of Ethics, by Henry Sidgwick. New York: Dover, 1966 [1874], pp. 312–319.

"Changes in Physicians' Attitudes Toward Telling the Cancer Patient," by Dennis H. Novack, Robin Plumer, Raymond L. Smith, Herbert Ochitil, Gary R. Morrow, and John M. Bennett. Reprinted with permission from Dennis H. Novack and the *Journal of the American Medical Association* 241:897–900, 2 March 1979. Copyright 1979, American Medical Association.

"Autonomy," by James Childress. Excerpted with permission from *Who Should Decide?: Paternalism in Health Care,* by James Childress. Copyright 1982 by Oxford University Press, Inc.

"Why Get Consent?", by Robert M. Veatch. Reprinted with permission from *Hospital Physician* 11:30–31, December 1975.

"The Physician's Obligation to Prolong Life: A Medical Duty Without Classical Roots," by Darrel W. Amundsen. Reprinted with references slightly abbreviated and permission from Darrel W. Amundsen and the *Hastings Center Report* 8:23–30, August 1978.

"A Reply to Rachels on Active and Passive Euthanasia," by Tom L. Beauchamp. Excerpted with permission from Tom L. Beauchamp from *Ethical Issues in Death and Dying,* edited by Tom Beauchamp and Seymour Perlin. Englewood Cliffs, N.J.: Prentice-Hall, 1978, pp. 244–258.

"Justice: A Philosophical Review," by Allen Buchanan. Reprinted with permission from D. Reidel Publishing Company, *Justice and Health Care,* edited by Earl Shelp, 1981, pp. 3–22. Copyright 1981 by D. Reidel Publishing Company, Dordrecht, Holland.

"Medical Care as a Right: A Refutation," by Robert M. Sade. Reprinted with permission from the *New England Journal of Medicine* 285:1288–1292, 1971.

"Securing Access to Health Care." Excerpted from President's Commission for the Study of Ethical Problems in Medicine and Biomedical and Behavioral Research. *Securing Access to Health Care: A Report on the Ethical Implications of Differences in the Availability of Health Services.* Washington, D.C.: Government Printing Office, 1983.

"Utilitarianism." Excerpted from *Utilitarianism,* by John Stuart Mill. *Ethical Theories: A Book of Readings,* edited by A. I. Melden. Englewood Cliffs, N.J.: Prentice-Hall, 1967, pp. 391–394.

"The Priority Problem," from *A Theory of Justice,* by John Rawls. Excerpt reprinted with permission from The Belknap Press of Harvard University Press, 1971, pp. 40–45. Copyright 1971 by the President and Fellows of Harvard College.

"Three Approaches," excerpted with permission from Joseph Fletcher, *Situation Ethics: The New Morality.* Philadelphia: Westminster Press, 1966. Copyright 1966 W. L. Jenkins. Reproduced and used by permission of the Westminster Press, Philadelphia.

"Two Concepts of Rules," excerpted with permission from John Rawls and *The Philosophical Review* 44:3–32, 1955.

Contents

Introduction

Since about 1970 there has been an explosion of interest in medical ethics. Problems of abortion, genetic engineering, human experimentation, and euthanasia have forced medical professional and lay persons alike to rethink traditional medical solutions as they apply to current ethical problems. Many of the standard discussions of the problems confronting medical ethics have proceeded to explore the alternative positions, topic by topic, and the arguments supporting them. Typical books have included chapters on these issues as well as on allocation of scarce medical resources, informed consent, psychiatric ethics, confidentiality, and the ethics of preventive medicine.

The problem with this approach is that as soon as one probes any one of these topics, one encounters more basic philosophical questions, questions that usually cut across the controversies surrounding any of these topics. For example, deciding whether to tell a dying patient the traumatic news of her impending death raises the question of whether the ethical goal is to avoid her psychological suffering or to honor her right to the truth. But that is precisely the issue underlying many conflicts over informed consent in human experimentation. Similar conflicts between choosing a course that avoids suffering and a course that honors someone's purported basic rights arise in problems of determining whether to abort a genetically afflicted fetus, choosing how to allocate scarce beds in intensive care units, and deciding whether to keep medical records confidential.

Anyone who must face these difficult questions in medical ethics is working, at least implicitly, from within a framework. What is needed is a more systematic framework from which these problems may be approached. Our preexisting ethical frameworks deal with normative questions—such as what principles or norms are relevant and whether morality can be reduced to rules. They also deal with basic issues such as the meaning of ethical terms and how moral claims are justified. When our frameworks are systematic, coherent, and consistent, they might be termed theories. Theories include answers to such questions as the relation of doing good to avoiding harm, the relation of the individual to society, and the relation of claims of rights to the production of good consequences and so forth.

Western physicians and most lay people normally think of the Hippocratic Oath as the starting point of thinking about medical ethics. The Oath and the tradition growing out of the Hippocratic ethical writings, in fact, do provide one more or less systematic approach to medical ethics. The core principle, that the physician should do what he or she thinks benefits the patient, is stated twice in the Oath, and at least until recently, has been widely accepted by physicians in the Hippocratic tradition since the time of the Oath's writing.

The Hippocratic tradition, however, is not the only more or less systematic way of thinking about problems in medical ethics. Many religious traditions have medical ethical traditions of their own, and they may differ significantly from the Hippocratic tradition. These religious traditions have developed their medical ethical positions in varying degrees.

Likewise, various philosophical traditions have implications for medical ethics. We would expect to reach different positions on problems in medical ethics depending on whether they stand in the tradition of liberal political philosophy, Marxism, existentialism, or some other philosophical school.

This volume is a collection of the most significant writings on these more systematic problems of medical ethics. Part I examines the major alternative traditions that have contributed to more or less systematic thought about medical ethics. It begins with an exploration of the Hippocratic tradition and then moves to major Western religious and philosophical alternatives. Brief explorations of non-Western traditions complete this survey and give the reader a summary of the major options for approaches to the problems of medical ethics.

Once one grasps the breadth of alternatives, it is natural to ask what might justify adoption of one of these positions. In fact, many persons may find themselves standing in more than one of these traditions simultaneously. One may be both a Jew and a physician. Another may be both a Catholic and a proponent of liberal political philosophy. The appropriate question is what it should take to justify one position or another. One soon discovers that the ancient codes such as the Hippocratic Oath differ in important details from more modern professional codifications such as the Principles of Ethics of the American Medical Association. More critically, it is not obvious that one should turn automatically to the codes of the medical profession. Particularly, if one is not a physician, one may be inclined toward some of the other traditions. What should happen, for instance, if the code of a religious group conflicts with that of a professional organization or national government? What is the ultimate standard for determining what is right conduct for health professionals and lay people in medicine? Who has the authority to articulate or establish a standard? Who should be the one to adjudicate moral disputes or discipline those who violate the accepted norms? The writings collected in Part II deal with these issues.

After these questions of the meaning and justification of ethical positions are understood, it becomes possible to examine the arguments about the principles of ethics themselves. Most contemporary approaches to medical ethics hold that there are one or more basic principles that describe the right-making characteristics of actions. These are not necessarily rigid rules that can be applied directly to case problems. Rather, they are often thought of as broad principles that help determine what tends to makes right actions right, and wrong actions wrong. Among the principles that often show up on such lists are beneficence (doing good), nonmaleficence (avoiding harm), autonomy, truth-telling, avoiding killing, and justice. Much of the current debate in ethical theory has to do with the question of which of these principles are to be included and what weight each should be given. In Part III we shall examine the writings that have been directed toward arguing for and against various principles.

The possible and variable principles that go into various medical ethical systems lead one to face the question of how such principles should be used to resolve the concrete, real-life problems of medical ethics. Two questions are critical. First, assuming one has more than one ethical principle in his or her medical ethical framework or theory, how are the various principles interrelated? Are they ranked equally so they must be "balanced" in order to determine what is right? Are they ranked in some priority order? Or is there some combination of the two approaches? Second, once one has a set of principles to work with, how are they applied to specific cases? Classical Hippocratic medical ethics is well-known for its commitment to the view that every case is unique so that general principles can only serve as guidelines. There cannot be rules derived from the principles that tell us exactly what action is right in a conflict situation. The decisionmaker (the health professional or lay person as the case may be) must move directly from general principles to case decisions on a case-by-case basis. Other theories place much greater reliance on rules. They hold that some set of rules can be derived from the broader principles and that the rules can provide more or less direct answers to the problems posed by the case—as in much Jewish thought or the philosophical position known as rule-utilitarianism. Part of the problem in approaching medical ethics is that people well-entrenched in one of these positions may not even realize that others standing in other traditions take alternative approaches seriously. Many physicians, for example, do not comprehend that there are well-developed ethical systems that grant a more significant place to rules. The writings in Chapter 8 look at the questions of the relationships among ethical principles and the role of rules in the application of principles to cases.

This outline of the kinds of problems that need to be addressed in any complete medical ethical position was first developed in my book *Medical Ethics.* In that volume I argue for a particular set of answers to the questions raised. In order to understand what the issues are and to begin to develop one's own positions on them it is important to be exposed to many different points of view. This collection of articles is designed to provide those alternative points of view. It was originally developed as readings for a course on comparative medical ethical theories. It can be used either as a free-standing collection of the most significant writings on problems in systems of medical ethics or in conjunction with *Medical Ethics* or some other systematic exploration of these issues.

Cross Cultural Perspectives in Medical Ethics: Readings

Hippocrates, the Popes, Ahimsa, and Patients' Rights:

Introduction to a History of Diversity

1

The Hippocratic Tradition

INTRODUCTION

By far the most significant tradition in the medical ethics of Western physicians is that surrounding the Hippocratic Oath. This Hippocratic tradition began as a minority movement within Greek medicine, grounded in a group or school identified with a figure called Hippocrates. The Hippocratic group articulated important and novel positions placing medicine on a more empirical footing. A large collection of writings have been brought together. They are collectively often referred to as the Hippocratic corpus. As with other ancient collections the content was not univerally agreed upon. Many writings were clearly not by the historical figure, Hippocrates. They were written over several centuries.

Some of the writings in the collection have a particularly ethical content. The Hippocratic Oath is the most famous. It shows the clear marks of a cult or school. It contains an oath of secrecy as well as a code with a set of moral imperatives. The most famous of these imperatives could be called the Hippocratic principle, the notion that the physician ought to act so as to benefit the patient and keep the patient from harm according to the physician's ability and judgment.

The Oath contains some more esoteric provisions including a prohibition on "cutting for the stone," presumably kidney stone surgery. It contains a pledge of confidentiality committing the Hippocratic physician from disclosing "those thing that ought not be spread abroad." While this implies that some things perhaps ought to be "spread abroad," it at least shows ancient roots for the notion of confidentiality in medical ethics. Extremely complex questions arise regarding the authorship, dating, meaning, and philosophical context of the Oath. In the opening essay, historian Ludwig Edelstein provides a plausible account of the origins of the Oath.

The Oath has gone through many revisions and updatings. Medieval Christians were aware of it. In fact some scholars have suggested that the Hippocratic perspective in Greek medical ethics emerged as dominant because of its compatability with Judeo-Christian thought. On the other hand, there is very little evidence of early Christians accepting the Oath. There are extremely few references to Hippocrates in early Christian literature, and they tend to separate Christian medical ethics from Hippocratic. A medieval attempt to write a Christian version of the Oath contains many significant changes.

Regardless of its origin and compatibility with Judeo-Christianity, the Oath has been viewed by Western physicians as the source document of the essence of ethics for physicians. The World Medical Association in 1948 adopted the Declaration of Geneva, which is clearly a recasting of the Hippocratic Oath in modern language. The core Hippocratic principle is rendered, "The health of my patient will be my first consideration."

By the middle of the twentieth century the Hippocratic ethic was beginning to be called into question in a number of ways. It focused almost exclusively on the welfare of individual patients. The physician in the Oath was seen as dealing with individual, isolated patients. In reality medicine was becoming a much more complex, social, institutional entity with hospitals, group practices, health-care teams, complex insurance mechanisms, and critical resource-allocation problems. The isolated individual doctor-patient relationship was becoming a thing of the past. Furthermore, patients and lay people generally were more educated. They were beginning to insist on a more active role in decisionmaking and shaping of the moral norms for the physician-patient relationship. The very idea that ethics was simply a matter of producing benefits and avoiding harms was challenged by those in ethical traditions deemed more "deontological," that is, more oriented to duties and rights that are not determined solely by the consequences of actions. Edmund Pellegrino is one of the first to sense the trends that call into question the ancient ethic of the Hippocratic tradition. His essay in this chapter traces these problems.

The American Medical Association (AMA), still very much within the Hippocratic tradition, began to reassess its ethical commitments during this period. In 1957 a major revision of its principles of medical ethics was adopted. It changed the form of the ethical code from a long, detailed series of injunctions to a brief set of principles. It made explicit the physician's obligation and commitment to the community. Still, service to the patient and promotion of patient-well-being were central to this verison of the AMA's principles.

By 1980, tension had grown even greater. Broader cultural influences made the 1957 principles sound dated, especially the use of masculine pronouns. More fundamental changes in ethical theory were brewing. For the first time in the history of organized Western medicine there was discussion of "rights," rather than simply "benefits and harms." Compassion and respect for human dignity were identified as the virtues of the physician rather than the more traditional virtues of purity and holiness, as expressed in the Hippocratic Oath, or more paternalistic early AMA codes.

The scholar who has contributed most to the modern understanding of the Hippocratic tradition is the medical historian Ludwig Edelstein. His essay, "The Hippocratic Oath," which was first published in 1943, helped generations of physicians,
historians, and medical ethicists understand that the Hippocratic Oath is not a
document that can be understood apart from its historical context. Edelstein applies
the skills of the classicist to show that the Hippocratic Oath is quite different from
many other Hippocratic writings. Also, it is written somewhat later than some of the
other, more scientific treatises attributed to the historical figure Hippocrates; quite
possibly, it dates from the fourth century BC. Edelstein argues that the Oath is best
understood as a code reflecting the views of a minority group of physicians, probably of Pythagorean persuasion. Although other scholars have called into question
some of the details of Edelstein's interpretation, the main points are widely accepted
today. A much shortened version of Edelstein's essay is reprinted here without the
extensive references that include detailed comparisons of ancient and modern texts.

The Hippocratic Oath: Text, Translation, and Interpretation

LUDWIG EDELSTEIN

OATH

I swear by Apollo Physician and Hygieia and Panaceia and all the gods and god-
desses, making them my witnesses, that I will fulfill according to my ability and
judgment this oath and this covenant:

To hold him who has taught me this art as equal to my parents and to live my
life in partnership with him, and if he is in need of money to give him a share of
mine, and to regard his offspring as equal to my brothers in male lineage and to
teach them this art—if they desire to learn it—without fee and covenant; to give a
share of precepts and oral instruction and all the other learning to my sons and to
the sons of him who has instructed me and to pupils who have signed the covenant
and have taken an oath according to the medical law, but to no one else.

I will apply dietetic measures for the benefit of the sick according to my ability and
judgment; I will keep them from harm and injustice.

I will neither give a deadly drug to anybody if asked for it, nor will I make a
suggestion to this effect. Similarly I will not give to a woman an abortive
remedy. In purity and holiness I will guard my life and my art.
I will not use the knife, not even on sufferers from stone, but will withdraw in favor
of such men as are engaged in this work.
Whatever houses I may visit, I will come for the benefit of the sick, remaining free of
all intentional injustice, of all mischief and in particular of sexual relations
with both female and male persons, be they free or slaves.

What I may see or hear in the course of the treatment or even outside of the
treatment in regard to the life of men, which on no account one must spread
abroad, I will keep to myself holding such things shameful to be spoken about.

If I fulfill this oath and do not violate it, may it be granted to me to enjoy life and
art, being honored with fame among all men for all time to come; if I transgress it
and swear falsely, may the opposite of all this be my lot.

INTERPRETATION

The Hippocratic Oath clearly falls into two parts. The first specifies the duties of the
pupil toward his teacher and his teacher's family and the pupil's obligations in
transmitting medical knowledge. The second gives a number of rules to be observed
in the treatment of diseases, a short summary of medical ethics as it were. Most
scholars consider these two sections to be only superficially connected or at least
determined by different moral standards. Be this as it may, the two parts certainly
diverge in their subject matter, and, for the purpose of analyzing their content, it is
advantageous first to discuss them separately and then to ask how they are related to
each other. Again for the sake of convenience, I shall deal with the so-called ethical
code first, the main question being whether the historical setting in which these
rules of conduct were conceived can be ferreted out.

Unfortunately, most of the statements contained in the document are worded in
rather general terms; they are vague in their commending of justice, of purity and
holiness, concepts which in themselves do not imply any distinct meaning but may
be understood in various ways. Yet there are two stipulations that have a more
definite character and seem to point to the basic beliefs underlying the whole
program which is here evolved: the rules concerning the application of poison and
of abortive remedies. Their interpretation should therefore provide a clue for a
historical identification of the views embodied in the Oath of Hippocrates.

I. The Ethical Code

A. *Rules Concerning Poison and Abortion.* "I will neither give a deadly
drug to anybody if asked for it, nor will I make a suggestion to this effect. Similarly I
will not give to a woman an abortive remedy. In purity and holiness I will guard my

life and my art."–such is the vow made. It concerns the physician not so much in his capacity as the healer of diseases but rather in that of the pharmacist who is in possession of the drugs which he prescribes. Poison is a drug and so is the pessary. The physician agrees not to deliver either one to his patient. The term used on both instances is the same; just as he will not *give* the pessary to a woman who comes to seek his help, he will not *give* poison to anyone who is under his care.

Why regulations concerning cases of abortion are introduced into the document is immediately understandable. Under ancient conditions the physician was often presented with the problem as to whether he should give an abortive remedy. But what about the physician's supplying poison? Did he so frequently have occasion to give poison that it seemed worthwhile to ordain what he should do in such instances? What exactly is the situation referred to in the Oath?

All modern interpreters assume that the interdiction of the supplying of poisons means that the physician is charged not to assist his patient in a suicide which he might contemplate. Some interpreters claim that here the physician is also, or even primarily, asked to refrain from any criminal attempt on his patient's life. Cases of poisoning, they say, were very frequent in antiquity; the law, though of course it threatened punishment for murder, was of little avail because the lack of proper scientific methods made it impossible to ascertain whether poison had been administered or not. As a means of strengthening civil jurisdiction, therefore, a clause was introduced into the ancient medical code which today would be entirely out of place. There is no evidence, however, that the Oath refers to anybody except patient and physician. The words in question, then can mean only that the doctor promises not to supply his patient with poison if asked by him to do so nor to suggest that he take it. It is the prevention of suicide, not of murder that is here implied.

But was suicide an instance to be reckoned with in medical practice? Could the doctor ever advise such an act to his patient? In antiquity this was indeed the case. If the sick felt that their pains had become intolerable, if no help could be expected, they often put an end to their own lives. This fact is repeatedly attested and not only in general terms; even the diseases are specified which in the opinion of the ancients gave justification for a voluntary death. Moreover, the taking of poison was the most usual means of committing suicide, and the patient was likely to demand the poison from his physician who was in possession of deadly drugs and knew those which brought about an easy and painless end. On the other hand, such a resolution naturally was not taken without due deliberation, except perhaps in a few cases of great distress or mental strain. The sick wished to be sure that further treatment would be of no avail, and to render this verdict was the physician's task. The patient, therefore, consulted with him, or urged his friends to speak to the doctor. If the latter, in such a consultation, confirmed the seriousness or hopelessness of the case, he suggested directly or indirectly that the patient commit suicide.

Of course, I do not mean to claim that everybody whose illness had become desperate thought of ending his own life. Even if human aid was no longer effectual, recourse to the gods was still possible, and men did seek succor in the sanctuaries;

even if the pain was excruciating and relief was to be had neither from human nor from divine physicians, men could, and did go on living in spite of all their suffering. Yet the fact remains that throughout antiquity many people preferred voluntary death to endless agony. This form of "euthanasia" was an everyday reality. Consequently it is quite understandable that the Oath deals with the attitude which the physician should take in regard to the possible suicide of his patient. From a practical point of view it was no less important to tell the ancient doctor what to do when faced with such a situation than it was to advise him about cases of abortion.

The relevance of the "pharmacological rules" for a medical oath having been established, one may now ask why the Oath forbids the physician to assist in suicide or in abortion. Apparently these prohibitions did not echo the general feeling of the public. Suicide was not censured in antiquity. Abortion was practiced in Greek times no less than in the Roman era, and it was resorted to without scruple. Small wonder! In a world in which it was held justifiable to expose children immediately after birth, it would hardly seem objectionable to destroy the embryo. Why then should the physician not give a helping hand to those of his patients who wanted to end their own lives or to those who did not wish to have offspring?

For a moment one might harbor the idea that the interdiction of poison and of abortive remedies was simply the outgrowth of medical ethics. After all, medicine is the art of healing, of preserving life. Should the physician assist in bringing about death? I do not propose to discuss this issue in general terms. It suffices here to state that in antiquity many physicians actually gave their patients the poison for which they were asked. Apparently *qua* physicians they felt no compunction about doing so. Although in later centuries some refused to participate in an attempt on men's lives, because, as they said, it was unfitting for their sect "to be responsible for anyone's death or destruction," it is not reported that they ever employed the same reasoning in cases of self-murder. As for abortions, many physicians prescribed and gave abortive remedies. Medical writings of all periods mention the means for the destruction of the embryo and the occasions where they are to be employed. In later centuries some physicians rejected abortion under all circumstances; they supported their decision with a reference to the prohibition in the Hippocratic Oath and added that it was the duty of the doctor to preserve the products of nature. Soranus, the greatest of the ancient gynecologists, had little patience with these colleagues of his. In agreement with many other physicians he contended that it was necessary to think of the life of the mother first, and he resorted to abortion whenever it seemed necessary, much as he deprecated it if performed for no other reason than the wish to preserve beauty or to hide the consequences of adultery. In short, the strict attitude upheld by the Oath was not uncontested even from the medical point of view. In antiquity it was not generally considered a violation of medical ethics to do what the Oath forbade. An ancient doctor who accepted the rules laid down by "Hippocrates" was by no means in agreement with the opinion of all his fellow physicians; on the contrary, he adhered to a dogma which was much stricter than that embraced by many, if not by most of his colleagues. Simple reflection on the duties of the physician, on the task of medicine alone, under these circumstances, can hardly have led to the formulation and adoption of the "pharmacological stipulations."

In my opinion, the Oath itself points to other, more fundamental considerations that must have been instrumental in outlining the prohibitions under discussion. For the physician, when forswearing the use of poison and of abortive remedies, adds: "In purity and in holiness I will guard my life and my art." It might be possible to construe purity as a quality insisted upon by the craftsman who is conscious of the obligations of his art. The demand for holiness, however, can hardly be understood as resulting from practical thinking or technical responsibility. Holiness belongs to another realm of values and is indicative of standards of a different, a more elevated character.

Yet certainly not such purity and holiness are meant as might accrue to men from obedience to civil law or common religion. Ancient jurisdiction did not discriminate against suicide; it did not attach any disgrace to it, provided that there was sufficient reason for such an act. And self-murder as a relief from illness was regarded as justifiable, so much so that in some states it was an institution duty legalized by the authorities. Nor did Greek or Roman law protect the unborn child. If, in certain cities, abortion was prosecuted, it was because the father's right to his offspring had been violated by the mother's action. Ancient religion did not proscribe suicide. It did not know of any eternal punishment for those who voluntarily ended their lives. Likewise it remained indifferent to foeticide. Its tenets did not include the dogma of an immortal soul for which men must render account to their creator. Law and religion then left the physician free to do whatever seemed best to him.

From all these considerations it follows that a specific philosophical conviction must have dictated the rules laid down in the Oath. Is it possible to determine this particular philosophy? To take the problem of suicide first: Platonists, Cynics and Stoics can be eliminated at once. They held suicide permissible for the diseased. Some of these philosophers even extolled such an act as the greatest triumph of men over fate. Aristotle, on the other hand, claimed that it was cowardly to give in to bodily pain, and Epicurus admonished men not to be subdued by illness. But does that mean that the Oath is determined by Aristotelian or Epicurean ideas? I shall not insist that it is hard to imagine a physician resisting the adjurations of his patients if he has nothing but Aristotle's or Epicurus' exhortations to courage to quote to them and to himself. It is more important to stress the fact that the Aristotelian and Epicurean opposition to suicide did not involve moral censure. If men decided to take their lives, they were within their rights as sovereign masters of themselves. The Aristotelian and Epicurean schools condoned suicide. Later on the Aristotelians even gave up their leader's teaching, and under the onslaught of the Stoic attack withdrew their disapproval of self-murder. At any rate, Aristotelianism and Epicureanism do not explain a rejection of suicide which apparently is based on a moral creed and a belief in the divine.

Pythagoreanism, then, remains the only philosophical dogma that can possibly account for the attitude advocated in the Hippocratic Oath. For indeed among all

Greek thinkers the Pythagoreans alone outlawed suicide and did so without qualification. The Platonic Socrates can adduce no other witness than the Pythagorean Philolaus for the view that men, whatever their fate, are not allowed to take their own lives. And even in later centuries the Pythagorean school is the only one represented as absolutely opposed to suicide. Moreover, for the Pythagorean, suicide was a sin against God who had allocated to man his position in life as a post to be held and to be defended. Punishment threatened those who did not obey the divine command to live; it was considered neither lawful nor holy to seek release, "to bestow this blessing upon oneself." Any physician who accepts such a dogma naturally must abstain from assisting in suicide or even from suggesting it. Otherwise he would be guilty of a crime, he no less than his patient, and in this moral and religious conviction the doctor can well find the courage to remain deaf to his patient's insistence, to his sufferings, and even to the clamor of the world which disagrees almost unanimously with the stand taken by him. It seems safe to state this much: the fact that in the Hippocratic Oath the physician is enjoined to refrain from aiding or advising suicide points to an influence of Pythagorean doctrines.

In my opinion the same can be asserted of the rule forbidding abortion and rejecting it without qualification. Most of the Greek philosophers even commended abortion.

It was different with the Pythagoreans. They held that the embryo was an animate being from the moment of conception. That they did so is expressly attested by a writer of the third century AD. The same can be concluded from the Pythagorean system of physiology as it was outlined in the Hellenistic period by Alexander Polyhistor: the germ is a clot of brain containing hot vapors within it, and soul and sensation are supposed to originate from this vapor. Similar views were previously accepted by Philolaus in the fourth century BC. Consequently, for the Pythagoreans, abortion, whenever practiced, meant destruction of a living being. Granted that the righteousness of abortion depends on whether the embryo is animate or not, the Pythagoreans could not but reject abortion unconditionally.

Furthermore, abortion was irreconcilable with their ethical beliefs no less than with their scientific views. In their ascetic rigorism, in their strictness concerning sexual matters and regarding matrimony in particular, they went further than any other sect. They banned extra-marital relations. Even in matrimony coitus was held justifiable only for the purpose of producing offspring. Besides, children to them were more than future members of a community or citizens of a state. It was considered man's duty to beget children so as to leave behind in his own place another worshiper of the gods. With such convictions how could the Pythagoreans ever allow abortive remedies to be applied? How could they fail to condemn practices of this kind, so common among their compatriots?

It stands to reason, then, that the Hippocratic Oath, in its abortion-clause no less than in its prohibition of suicide, echoes Pythagorean doctrines. In no other stratum of Greek opinion were such views held or proposed in the same spirit of uncompromising austerity. When the physician, after having forsworn ever to give poison or abortive remedies, adds: "In purity and holiness I will guard my life and my art," it must be the purity and holiness of the "Pythagorean way of life" to which he dedicates himself.

B.   *The General Rules of the Ethical Code.*   The question now arises whether what is true of certain of the ethical clauses of the Hippocratic Oath is true of all of them, in other words, whether the whole medical code is in agreement with Pythagorean philosophy. By this latter term I mean Pythagoreanism as it was understood in the fourth century BC. It is to this form of the dogma that the rules discussed so far were related, and it seems fair to assume that the rest of the stipulations, if at all influenced by Pythagorean thinking, correspond to the same concept of Pythagoreanism. At any rate, wherever I shall speak of Pythagorean doctrines without qualification, it is neither the teachings of the "historical" Pythagoras, nor those of the later so-called Neo-Pythagoreans which I have in mind, but rather those theories and beliefs which writers of the fourth century BC, men like Plato, Aristotle and their pupils, attributed to Pythagoras and his followers.

1.   *The Tripartite Division of Medicine.* To start, then, with the analysis of that section of the ethical code which deals with the treatment of diseases proper: here mention is made of diet, drugs and cutting. In a more technical language, medicine is viewed as comprising dietetics, pharmacology and surgery. Consequently those matters are discussed which seem most important for the attitude of the physician within these three departments of his art. Now a division of medicine into the branches is not unusual and in itself is not indicative of any particular medical or philosophical school. But, according to Aristoxenus, the Pythagoreans were among those who accepted this particular classification of medicine; moreover, the sequence of the various parts of the healing art in the Pythagorean doctrine is the same as it is in the Hippocratic Oath, dietetics coming first, pharmacology next, surgery last.

a.   DIETETIC MEANS. In detail, the physician is asked to use dietetic means to the advantage of his patients as his judgment and capacity permit; moreover he is enjoined to keep them from mischief and injustice. That the doctor's dietetic prescriptions should be given to help the patient is an obvious truth. It is the goal of all good craftsmanship to seek the best for the object with which the craftsman is concerned. Every ancient physician would have subscribed to such a formulation. It suffices to say that the Pythagorean physicians did not feel differently, for this school acknowledged the useful and the advantageous as second among the aims of human endeavor.

But what exactly is meant by the promise to keep the patient from mischief and injustice? Can this really imply, as some scholars have suggested, that the physician shall enforce his treatment even against the resistance or indifference of his patient's family? It is true, interference of others may occur and the physician may have to contend with it, but this happens rarely, too seldom indeed to have been considered in the medical code. Moreover, while mischief may be done to the sick by his friends, why should this danger be any greater in regard to the dietetic treatment of diseases for which case alone mention is made of it, than it would be in regard to everything else the physician may prescribe or do? No, it can scarcely be protection from the wrong done by others that the physician vows to give to his patients. But since it can neither be protection from the wrong which he himself may do, one must conclude that he promises to guard his patients against the evil which they may suffer through themselves. That men by nature are liable to inflict upon themselves injustice and mischief, and that this tendency becomes apparent in all matters concerned with their regimen, this is indeed an axiom of Pythagorean dietetics.

The Pythagoreans defined all bodily appetites as propensities of the soul, as a craving for the presence or absence of certain things. Most of these appetites they considered as acquired or created by men themselves, and therefore they thought human desires were to be watched closely and to be scrutinized severely. As a natural process they acknowledged only that the body should take in an appropriate amount of food and should be cleansed again appropriately after it had been filled. To overload oneself with superfluous food and drink was regarded as an acquired inclination of the soul.

But unfortunately all bodily passions have the tendency to increase indefinitely. Of themselves they become "idle, irreverent, harmful and licentious," as one can readily see in those who are in the position to live according to their wishes. In order to live right from early youth on, one must learn to hold in contempt those things that are "idle and superfluous." It is necessary, therefore, to select the nourishment of the body with great caution, to determine its quality and quantity most carefully, a supreme wisdom entrusted to the physicians.

This is the Pythagorean doctrine concerning the regimen of the healthy. It is clear, I think, that in such a theory bodily and psychic factors are blended in a peculiar way. At the same time there is a moral element involved: unhealthy desire is uncontrolled desire; a decision is to be made between those appetites which ought to be satisfied and those which ought to be disregarded. Moreover, the Pythagorean teaching, in a strange manner, insists on negative instances. Not that alone which one does is important; that which one does not do, or is not allowed to do, carries just as much consequence. Right living is brought about not only, not even primarily, through positive actions, but rather through avoidance of those steps that are dangerous, through the repression of insatiable desires which if left to themselves would cause damage.

The same consideration for body and soul, the same combination of precepts and prohibitions seems to be characteristic of the Pythagorean treatment of diseases. Most illnesses, in the opinion of these philosophers, are due to opulent living; too much food is consumed which cannot be digested properly, and thus extravagance destroys the body, just as it destroys wealth. If health, the retention of the form, changes into disease, the destruction of the form, the body needs purification through medicine, just as the sick soul needs purification through music. The physician in such a case must give assistance by changing the patient's regimen. He must use dietetical means, as the Hippocratic Oath says. In choosing them he will be intent on his patient's benefit according to the best of his judgment and ability. Whatever he prescribes, as a true follower of Pythagoras he will remember one fundamental truth: everything that is given to the body creates a certain disposition of the soul. Men in general, though they are aware of the fact that some things, such as wine, may suddenly bring about a striking change in a person's behavior, do not apprehend that every kind of food or drink causes a certain mental habit, slight as the variations may be. But the physician knows that his art primarily consists in this knowledge. Consequently, he must see to it that the soul of the sick, through a wrong diet, does not fall into "idle, irreverent, harmful and licentious passions." Since he acts according to this principle when assisting the healthy, he must certainly do likewise when treating the sick. Or in the words of the Hippocratic Oath: the physician must protect his patient from the mischief and injustice which he may inflict upon himself if his diet is not properly chosen. He must be a physician of the soul no less than of the body; he must not overlook the moral implications of his actions, nor even the negative indices to be watched; for the regimen followed by a person concerns both his bodily and his psychic constitution.

The rules concerning dietetics, then, agree with Pythagoreanism, in fact they acquire meaning only if seen in the light of Pythagorean teaching. That the pharmacological precepts, the stipulations concerning poison and abortion, are Pythagorean in origin has already been demonstrated. It remains to be shown that the laws laid down for surgery, too, are most easily understandable on the theory that they are founded in Pythagorean doctrine.

b. SURGERY. The physician vows: "I will not use the knife either on sufferers from stone, but I will give place to such as are craftsmen therein"; this at least is the most common rendering of the words in question. Supposing that it be correct, what should be the reason for the prohibition here pronounced? The treatment of stone-diseases by operation, in Greek medicine, seems to have been an old-established procedure; at any rate, since the rise of Alexandrian medicine, such an operation was performed throughout the centuries. Why then is it forbidden in the Oath?

The words must mean what in the opinion of all early interpreters they seemed to mean: lithotomy is here excluded because the performance of operations is held to be incompatible with the physician's craft, and by the one example given the Oath intends to exclude surgery in general from the field of the physician. It is possible that originally more operations were named as forbidden, that these references are missing only in the preserved text. But such a hypothesis cannot be verified. It is more probable, however, that the statement as it stands is intact but in itself carries broader implications. For instead of translating "I will not use the knife either on sufferers from stone," it is equally well possible to translate "I will not use the knife, not even on sufferers from stone." This would signify that the physician directly renounces operative surgery altogether. He will not resort to it even in the case of that disease which more than any other, according to the testimony of the ancients, drove men to suicide. The prohibition could not be formulated in more emphatic and solemn words.

Whatever rendering is chosen, the statement under discussion enjoins a separation of medicine and surgery. Driven back to this interpretation which no doubt is drastically at variance with reality, one feels almost inclined to say with Littre that such an explanation must be rejected, and that consequently the motive for the interdiction of lithotomy in the Oath remains obscure. It is likewise true, however, that one medical sect valued surgery less highly than dietetics and pharmacology, I mean the Pythagorean physicians. As Aristoxenus says, they believed "most of all" in dietetics; they applied poultices more liberally than did their predecessors, but "thought less" of the efficacy of drugs; "they believed least of all in using the knife and in cauterizing." In other words, according to Aristoxenus, the Pythagoreans attributed different values to the various branches of medicine, and in their classification operative surgery together with cauterization was ranked lowest. If one remembers that in Aristoxenus' opinion the Pythagoreans explained most diseases as the result of unreasonable living, one is at first inclined to conclude that they were the more appropriate means of treatment. Still this can hardly be the whole truth. For Plato in the *Timaeus,* when outlining the Pythagorean treatment of diseases, does not mention cutting or cauterizing at all, though he agrees with Aristoxenus in placing the importance of pharmacology after that of dietetics. Evidently, then there must have been Pythagoreans who refused to apply any surgical means of treatment which were otherwise so universally used in Greek medicine. This inference from the Platonic *Timaeus* seems quite certain though no express statement to this effect is preserved.

It is most likely that Aristoxenus' report is one of his typical attempts to reconcile the rigorous Pythagorean attitude with the demands of common sense and the exigencies of daily life: such compromises he introduces in many instances where other sources attest the uncompromising attitude of the Pythagoreans. Seen from this angle, the stipulation of the Oath appears as another compromise, more lenient and at the same time more rigid than that reported by Aristoxenus: the use of cauterization obviously is allowed, operative surgery is completely eliminated. On the other hand, the Pythagorean physician will allow others to help his patient in his extremity. The stipulation against operating is valid only for him who has dedicated himself to a holy life. The Pythagoreans recognized that men in general could not observe any elaborate rules of purity; in this fact they say no argument against that which they considered right for themselves. To give place to another craftsman, especially in such instances where the patient might fall prey to a sinful temptation, certainly was a duty demanded by philanthropy, by commiseration with those who suffered.

But why should the Pythagorean have avoided the use of the knife? The answer can only be conjecture: he who believed that bloody sacrifices should not be offered to the gods and saw in them a defilement of divine purity could well believe that he himself would be defiled in his purity and holiness by using the knife in bloody operations. However that may be, it is only in connection with Pythagorean medicine that the injunction of the Hippocratic Oath, according to which operative surgery was forbidden to the physician, acquires any meaning and plausibility at all. The rules given in regard to surgery no less than those concerning dietetics and pharmacology are Pythagorean in character.

    2.   *Two General Provisions.* Those stipulations of the Oath which deal with

the medical treatment proper are finally followed by two more general provisions bearing on medical ethics in the strict sense of the word. The behavior of the physician toward his patient and the patient's family is regulated; reticence is imposed upon him in regard to whatever he may see or hear. Is it really true that in non-medical literature no parallels can be found to these postulates? In my opinion these ethical rules, too, in their specific wording are understandable only in connection with Pythagorean doctrine.

a.   REFRAINING FROM INJUSTICE AND MISCHIEF. As for the first vow, he who swears the Oath promises to come, into whatever house he enters, to help the sick, refraining from injustice and mischief, especially from all sexual incontinence. That the physician should act for the sole purpose of assisting his patient, is a demand that seems self-evident. It certainly is as compatible with any ethical standard to which a doctor may subscribe, as it is with Pythagorean ethics. It may seem equally natural that the physician is bidden to refrain from all injustice and mischief. Yet, the appropriateness of the statement does not imply that it is not in need of further explanation, be it in regard to its meaning or its motivation.

Those who believe that only medical parallels can be adduced for the stipulations of the Oath point to seemingly similar utterances in one of the so-called Hippocratic writings, the book "On the Physician." Here it is stated that in his relations with the sick the doctor ought to be just, for the patients have no small dealings with their physician. They put themselves into his hands, and the physician comes in contact with women and maidens and with very precious possessions indeed; so toward all these self-control should be used. I do not wish to raise the issue, whether justice is here commended for utilitarian rather than moral reasons. Nor do I emphasize the fact that only if it had a moral bent could this assertion be likened to the Oath. In refutation of the argument of modern interpreters it is enough to say that the parallel referred to is by far less comprehensive and less rigorous than the statement which it is supposed to explain. The Oath, unlike the Hippocratic treatise "On the Physician," does not speak only of the avoidance of injustice, it also excludes mischief. Moreover, the oath enjoins continence in regard to women and men alike; it stresses that the same continence must be observed toward free-born people and slaves, features that are entirely missing in the other passage. A more satisfactory interpretation of the words in question, therefore, must be sought.

Now a plea for justice and continence may of course be derived from many ancient philosophical systems. As for justice, the Platonists and the Aristotelians praised its dignity no less than did the Pythagoreans. But so much it is safe to claim: that the physician is required to abstain from all intentional injustice and mischief—such a formulation savors of the famous Pythagorean sayings by which injustice and mischief are proscribed, even if committed against animals and plants. And indeed, to blend the concept of justice with that of forbearance is characteristic of the Pythagoreans. They abhorred violence; only if provoked by injustice would they resort to force. In this recoiling from aggression the asceticism of Pythagorean ethics culminated. Moreover, the consequences drawn in the Oath from the ethical standards there imposed are in strict keeping with those principles which the Pythagoreans enforced upon their followers. Their views on sexual matters were severer than those of all other ancient philosophers. They alone judged sexual relations in terms of justice, meaning thereby not that which is forbidden or allowed by law: for the husband to be unfaithful to his wife was considered to be unjust toward her. The Pythagoreans upheld the equality of men and women. They alone condemned sodomy. Besides, in the performance of moral duties, they did not discriminate between social ranks. In that respect free-born people and slaves, for the Pythagoreans, were on equal footing. Everything, then, that the Oath stipulates in regard to sexual continence agrees with the tenets of Pythagorean ethics, in fact with the ideals of these philosophers alone.

Finally, as a Pythagorean postulate the clause takes on a peculiar significance for the physician. It is justice first of all that is required from him. This virtue, to the average people, meant to live in accordance with the laws of the state. To Plato, wherever he does not speak of justice in his own peculiar usage as the perfect working of the human soul in all its functions, justice was mainly a civic virtue. Aristotle tried to establish justice as a political virtue, and as one that applies to contracts and dealings in the law-courts. All these aspects are also inherent in the Pythagorean concept of justice, and they certainly are of some concern for the physician. While in his direct dealing with men, in his personal contact with them and their households, it may be of less importance whether generally speaking he is a law-abiding citizen, it makes a great difference indeed, whether he is an honest man or not. It is in this sense that even the author of the Hippocratic book "On the Physician" counsels the doctor not to infringe upon the possessions of others with whom he is doing business. But such justice, essential as it may be for good morals, is not all that the Pythagorean ideal of justice implies. To the adherents of this dogma, justice was the social virtue par excellence. As Aristoxenus reports, they believed that "in any relation with others" some kind of justice is involved. "In all intercourse" it is possible to take "a well-timed and ill-timed attitude." In order to do what is proper, one must differentiate according to circumstances. Speech and actions necessarily vary depending on the particular situation and the persons concerned. From the right decision result timeliness, appropriateness, and fitness of behavior, and it is justice that reveals itself in good manners. Interpreted in the light of Pythagorean teaching, then, the recommendation of justice epitomized all duties of the physician toward his patient in the contacts of daily life, all he should do or say in the course of his practice; it gives the rules of medical deportment in a nutshell.

b.   THE PROMISE OF SILENCE. Last but not least: The promise of silence. The physician accepts the obligation to keep to himself all that he sees or hears during the treatment; he also swears not to divulge whatever comes to his knowledge outside of his medical activity in the life of men. The latter phrase in particular has always seemed strange. It is so far-reaching in scope that it can hardly be explained by professional considerations alone. To be sure, other medical writings also advise the physician to be reticent. The motive in doing so is the concern for the physician's renommée which might suffer if he is a prattler. But the Oath demands silence in regard to that "which on no account one must spread abroad." It insists on secrecy not as precaution but as a duty. In the same way silence about things which are not to be communicated to others was considered a moral obligation by the Pythagoreans. They did not tell everything to everybody. They did not indiscriminately impart their knowledge to others. They expected the scientist to be reticent and ready to listen. Certainly if the doctor who promises not to talk about anything that he may see or hear is to be placed in any philosophical school, it must be the Pythagorean.

To sum up the results of the analysis of the ethical code: the provisions concerning the application of poison and of abortive remedies, in their inflexibility, intimated that the second part of the Oath is influenced by Pythagorean ideas. The interpretation of the other medical and ethical stipulations showed that they, too, are tinged by Pythagorean theories. All statements can be understood only, or at any rate they can be understood best, as adaptations of Pythagorean teaching to the specific task of the physician. Even from a formal point of view, these rules are reminiscent of Pythagoreanism: just as in the Oath the doctor is told what to do and what not to do. Far from being the expression of the common Greek attitude toward medicine or of the natural duties of the physician, the ethical code rather reflects opinions which were peculiarly those of a small and isolated group.

II.   The Covenant

The ethical code by the acceptance of which the physician gives a higher sanction to his practical endeavor is preceded by a solemn agreement concerning medical education. The pupil promises to regard his teacher as equal to his parents, to share his life with him, to support him with money if he should be in need of it. Next he vows to hold his teacher's children as equals to his brothers and to teach them the art without fee and covenant if they should wish to learn it. Finally he takes upon himself the obligation to impart precepts, oral instruction and all the other learning to his own sons, to those of his teacher and to pupils who have signed the covenant and have taken an oath according to the medical law, to all these, but to no one else.

Whatever the precise purport of the single terms and phrases used in this covenant, so much is immediately clear in regard to its general meaning and is commonly admitted: the teacher here is made the adopted father of the pupil, the teacher's family becomes the pupil's adopted family. In other words, the covenant establishes between teacher and pupil the closest and most sacred relationship that can be imagined between men, and it does so for no other apparent reason than that the pupil is being instructed in the art.

In explaining this stipulation modern interpreters usually allege that in Greece, in early centuries, medicine like all the other arts was passed on from father to son in closed family guilds. When at a certain time these organizations began to receive outsiders in to their midst, they are said to have demanded from them full participation in the responsibilities of the "real" children. Consequently those who wished to be admitted to all the privileges and rights of the family had to become its members through adoption. The Hippocratic covenant, then, it is claimed, is an engagement which was signed by newcomers joining one of the medical artisan families, and it was probably the family of the Asclepiads in which this formula held good.

The evidence for such a theory, in my opinion, is insufficient. Galen is the only ancient author who asserts that the Asclepiads, after having been for generations the sole possessors of medicine, later shared their knowledge with people not belonging to their clan. And even he says that these outsiders were men whom the family esteemed "on account of their virtue"; he does not contend that they were made members of the family or forced to accept any obligations. It is hardly by chance, therefore, that Galen himself does not refer to the Hippocratic Oath as bearing out the truth of his story. In any case, his words cannot be adduced as corroborative proof for the assumptions of modern scholars. Nor does it increase the strength of the modern argument if Galen's testimony is combined with that of Plato, according to whom "physicians taught their sons medicine and . . . Hippocrates taught out-side pupils for a fee." Though Plato says this, it still does not follow that the outsiders became the adopted children of their masters. On the contrary, who will believe that the young Athenian aristocrat Hippocrates of whom Plato speaks would have considered paying a fee to the great Hippocrates for instruction, had that meant that he should enter the family of the Coan physician!

There is one particular historical setting, however, one particular province of Greek pedagogics where a counterpart of the Hippocratic covenant can be found: the Pythagoreans of the fourth century apparently were wont to honor those by whom they had been instructed as their fathers by adoption. So Epaminondas is said to have done; and in Epaminondas' time it was told of Pythagoras himself that he had revered his teacher as a son reveres his father. If the Hippocratic covenant is viewed against the background of such testimony, the specific form in which the pupil is here bound to his teacher is no longer an unexplainable and isolated phenomenon. Compared with Pythagorean concepts of teaching and learning as they were evolved in the fourth century BC, the vow of the medical student assumes definite historical meaning.

This result seems to imply that the covenant as a whole must be influenced by Pythagorean philosophy. The agreement between the Hippocratic treatise and the Pythagorean reports concerns so unusual a circumstance that they are most unlikely to be independent of each other. Nor is it probable that the Pythagoreans derived their pattern of instruction from a medical manifesto that in the range of medical education and indeed of general education is without parallel. Nevertheless one should hesitate to claim Pythagorean origin for the covenant by reason of one feature only, even if it be the main feature of this document. But as matters stand, all the other demands enjoined upon the pupil may likewise by explained only in connection with Pythagorean views and customs, or at least they are compatible with them.

To take those duties first which the pupil acknowledged in regard to his mentor: he is asked to share his life with his teacher and to support him with money if need be. That the Pythagorean pupil shared his money with his teacher if necessary, one may readily believe. To support his father was the son's duty, even according to common law. This obligation was the more binding for the Pythagorean, who was taught to honor his parents above all others. But the Pythagorean also came to his teacher's assistance in all the vicissitudes of life, wherever and whenever he was needed: he tended him in illness; he procured burial for him. All this is admiringly reported of Pythagoras himself. The Pythagorean pupil was indeed supposed to share his life with his master, as the son does with his father. He did much more than advance money to him in case of an emergency.

Next, the Hippocratic covenant admonishes the pupil to regard his teacher's offspring as his brothers, and without fee and covenant to teach them his art if they wish to learn it. That the teacher's children should be the pupil's brothers naturally follows from the fact that the disciple acknowledges his master as his father. Thus the teacher's sons and his pupils become one flesh and blood. But the preference shown for the interest of the members of the family, the unselfishness commended in the relationship to them, the confidence put in their reliability without any insistence on formal guarantees—all these features are characteristic of Pythagorean ethics. The Pythagoreans were admonished to turn to their brothers first, and to make friends with them before all others outside the family. Moreover, all Pythagoreans considered themselves brothers and were believed, like brothers, to have divided their earthly goods among themselves. Their unquestioned belief in their brothers' trustworthiness did not falter even in the face of death. Under these circumstances, how could the Pythagorean do other than teach his adopted brothers without fee the knowledge which he had acquired? What assurances could he expect or ask of them before he instructed them in the art that he had learned from their father?

Finally, the fact that in the Hippocratic covenant teaching is divided into precepts, oral instruction and the other learning, is best understood as a Pythagorean classification. The precepts of Pythagoras, handed down from one generation to the other, were greatly renowned throughout the centuries. "Oral instruction" and "learning" were the two categories under which Aristoxenus listed all that was "taught and said" in Pythagorean circles, and all that the members of the school tried "to learn and remember." That knowledge, according to the covenant, is to be imparted to a closed circle of selected people alone, most assuredly is in agreement with those principles on which the transmission of Pythagorean doctrine was based. The Pythagoreans differed from all other philosophical sects in that they did not divulge their teaching to everybody. They carefully examined those who wished to join them. It is attested even that they exacted an oath from the pupil who was to be admitted, just as the Hippocratic treatise speaks of outsiders who sign the covenant and take an oath before they are allowed to participate in the course of studies.

To sum up: not only the main feature of the covenant, the father-son relationship between teacher and pupil, but also all the detailed stipulations concerning the duties of the pupil can be paralleled by doctrines peculiar to the followers of Pythagoras. If related to Pythagoreanism, the specific formulas used in the covenant acquire meaning and definiteness. What otherwise appears exaggerated, or strange, or even fictitious, thus becomes the adequate expression of a real situation. Since the rules proposed show no affinity with any other Greek educational theory or practice, it seems permissible to claim that the Hippocratic covenant is inspired by Pythagorean doctrine.

III. The Unity of the Document

Covenant and ethical code, the two parts of which the so-called Hippocratic Oath consists, in the preserved text form a unity. Without any marked transition the first section is followed by the second. Is there any reason for believing that the two have not always belonged together?

It seems certain that the obligations laid down in the covenant and in the ethical code are assumed by the physician simultaneously, that is, at the moment of his entering the medical profession as a practitioner in his own right. The promise to help the teacher and the stipulation concerning the teaching to be given to others point to the fact that he who takes the Oath has become an independent craftsman. In the same way the rules regarding the practitioner's behavior are best understandable if imposed upon the doctor who is now starting out on his career. For as long as the pupil is still under the supervision of his teacher, his actions of necessity are regulated by his master's orders. In short, covenant and ethical code are signed together, not by the beginner but rather by the student who has completed his course.

Moreover the two parts are a spiritual unity. For it is not true, contrary to what is sometimes claimed, that the covenant exhibits a realistic business attitude, whereas the ethical code is determined by a lofty and exalted standard of conduct. The agreement concerning teaching and the rules of professional behavior both reflect the same idealistic outlook on human affairs, they are steeped in Pythagorean doctrine. The same can be said of the preamble and the peroration by which the document is introduced and concluded as one coherent formula.

At this point, I think, I can say without hesitation that the so-called Oath of Hippocrates is a document uniformly conceived and thoroughly saturated with Pythagorean philosophy. In spirit and in letter, in form and content, it is a Pythagorean manifesto. The main features of the Oath are understandable only in connection with Pythagoreanism; all its details are in complete agreement with this system of thought. If only one or another characteristic had been uncovered, one might consider the coincidence fortuitous. Since the concord is complete, and since there is no counterinstance of any other influence, all indications point to the conclusion that the Oath is a Pythagorean document.

IV. Date and Purpose of the Oath

The origin of the Hippocratic Oath having been established, it should now be possible to determine the time when the Oath was written and the purpose for which it was intended. What answers regarding these questions are to be deduced from the analysis of the document?

As for the date, it seems one must conclude that the Oath was not composed

before the fourth century BC. All the doctrines followed in the treatise are characteristic of Pythagoreanism as it was envisaged in the fourth century BC. It is most
probable even that the Oath was outlined only in the second half or toward the end
of the fourth century, for the greater part of the parallels adduced are taken from the
works of pupils of Aristotle.

Two of the main provisions of the Oath are connected with theories that are
attributed either directly or indirectly to Philolaus, a contemporary of Plato. This
makes the turn of the fifth to the fourth century the *terminus post quem* for the
composition of the Oath. Moreover, even if one or another ethical precept ascribed
to the Pythagoreans by Aristoxenus and accepted in the Hippocratic Oath was held
also by older Pythagoreans, the whole program of instruction envisaged in the Oath
in conformity with the Pythagorean model is characteristic of fourth century
Pythagoreanism; for it presupposes the destruction of the Pythagorean society in the
last decades of the fifth century. As Aristoxenus related, it was after the uprising in
Italy that Lysis went to Thebes where he taught Epaminondas and was revered by
him as his adopted father. In a letter ascribed to him, Lysis protests against those
who after the dissolution of the society made the Pythagorean dogma available to
everybody. Pythagoras himself, Lysis asserts, had charged his daughter never to give
his writings to those "outside of the house." Whether this letter is genuine or not, it
must have been for some such reasons that Lysis bound Epaminondas to himself as
his adopted son. This afforded the only solution which made it possible to initiate
outsiders into the Pythagorean doctrine, and yet to keep it a secret, a "family secret,"
as is also the intention of the Oath. But such a relationship between teacher and
pupil could be instituted only after the disappearance of the great fraternity that had
existed before. Only at that moment did the transmission of the Pythagorean doctrine become the concern of the individual Pythagorean; in earlier times it had been
promoted by the society itself. The Hippocratic Oath, which calls the teacher the
adopted father of the pupil, can hardly have been composed, therefore, before the
fourth century BC.

Nor is it likely that the document is of later origin. In the fourth century BC
Pythagoreanism reached the peak of its importance. Its influence gradually began to
wane from the beginning of the Hellenistic period. When in the first century BC the
Pythagorean system was revived and again became a potent factor in philosophical
speculation, it took on traits very different from those which are characteristic of the
earlier dogma and the prescripts of the Oath. Moreover, in Alexandria medical
ethics was integrated into the teaching of the medical sects. Closely connected as
these newly established schools were with philosophy, Pythagoreanism played no
part in their teaching. A direct influence of Pythagorean philosophy on medicine,
however, is not probable.

Yet in the fourth century BC the Hippocratic Oath in every respect was a timely
manifesto. It stands to reason, then, that it was in the fourth century BC that Pythagorean
philosophy led to the formulation of the Hippocratic Oath. Does this imply that the
document must have been outlined by a philosopher rather than by a physician? Not at
all. The Hippocratic Oath is a program of medical ethics, and there is no reason to

question that it was composed by a doctor. But ancient physicians often belonged to philosophical schools or studied with philosophers. The Pythagorean teaching aroused considerable interest among the physicians of the fourth century. It is quite possible that a physician, strongly impressed by what he had learned from the Pythagoreans either through personal contact or through books, conceived this medical code in conformity with Pythagorean ideals.

V. Conclusion

The so-called Hippocratic Oath has always been regarded as a message of timeless validity. From the interpretation given it follows that the document originated in a group representing a small segment of Greek opinion. That the Oath at first was not accepted by all ancient physicians is certain. Medical writings, from the time of Hippocrates down to that of Galen, give evidence of the violation of almost every one of its injunctions. This is true not only in regard to the general rules concerning helpfulness, continence and secrecy. Such deviations one would naturally expect. But for centuries ancient physicians, in opposition to the demands made in the Oath, put poison in the hands of those among their patients who intended to commit suicide; they administered abortive remedies; they practiced surgery.

At the end of antiquity a decided change took place. Medical practice began to conform to that state of affairs which the Oath had envisaged. Surgery was separated from general practice. Resistance against suicide, against abortion, became common. Now the Oath began to be popular. It circulated in various forms adapted to the varying circumstances and purposes of the centuries. Generally considered the work of the great Hippocrates, its study became part of the medical curriculum. The commentators supposed that the master had written the Oath as the first of all his books and made it incumbent on the beginner to read this treatise first.

Small wonder! A new religion arose that changed the very foundations of ancient civilization. Yet, Pythagoreanism seemed to bridge the gulf between heathendom and the new belief. Christianity found itself in agreement with the principles of Pythagorean ethics, its concepts of holiness and purity, justice and forbearance. The Pythagorean god who forbade suicide to men, his creatures, was also the God of the Jews and the Christians. As early as in the "Teaching of the Twelve Apostles" the command was given: "Thou shalt not use philtres; thou shalt not procure abortion; nor commit infanticide." Even the Church Fathers abounded in praise of the high-mindedness of Hippocrates and his regulations for the practice of medicine.

As time went on, the Hippocratic Oath became the nucleus of all medical ethics. In all countries, in all epochs in which monotheism, in its purely religious or in its more secularized form, was the accepted creed, the Hippocratic Oath was applauded as the embodiment of truth. Not only Jews and Christians, but the Arabs, the mediaeval doctors, men of the Renaissance, scientists of the Enlightenment, and scholars of the nineteenth century embraced the ideals of the Oath. I am not qualified to outline the successive stages of this historical process. But I venture to suggest that he who undertakes to study this development will find it better understandable if he realizes that the Hippocratic Oath is a Pythagorean manifesto and not the expression of an absolute standard of medical conduct.

The Hippocratic Oath is only the first of a long line of codes and oaths adopted by Western physicians. The Declaration of Geneva, which is written to be a modern version of the Hippocratic Oath by the World Medical Association, shows a quite conscious connection to the Oath. The Declaration of Geneva is explicit in its commitment that the first duty of the physician is the health of the patient. Certain changes are reflected in the modernization in addition to the removal of the obvious references to the Greek deities. The commitment to keeping the knowledge of medicine secret has been dropped; confidentiality seems more bluntly protected without exception; the prohibition on giving abortive pessaries was (after considerable dispute) softened to a commitment to respect life from the moment of conception; and the prohibition on surgery for stones has been dropped. Still the Declaration is very much in the Hippocratic tradition.

Declaration of Geneva

WORLD MEDICAL ASSOCIATION

At the time of being admitted as a Member of the Medical Profession:

I SOLEMNLY PLEDGE myself to consecrate my life to the service of humanity.
I WILL GIVE to my teachers the respect and gratitude which is their due;
I WILL PRACTICE my profession with conscience and dignity;
THE HEALTH OF MY PATIENT will be my first consideration;
I WILL RESPECT the secrets which are confided in me;
I WILL MAINTAIN by all the means in my power, the honor and the noble traditions of the medical profession;
MY COLLEAGUES will be my brothers;
I WILL NOT PERMIT considerations of religion, nationality, race, party politics or social standing to intervene between my duty and my patient;
I WILL MAINTAIN the utmost respect for human life, from the time of conception; even under threat, I will not use my medical knowledge, contrary to the laws of humanity;
I MAKE THESE PROMISES solemnly, freely and upon my honor.

(Adopted by the General Assembly of THE WORLD MEDICAL ASSOCIATION at Geneva, Switzerland, September, 1948)

By the 1970s the problems with the Hippocratic tradition manifest in the Hippocratic Oath and the Declaration of Geneva began to emerge. Edmund Pellegrino, a physician and medical humanist who is the Director of the Kennedy Institute of Ethics at Georgetown University, exposes these problems in his essay "Toward an Expanded Medical Ethics: The Hippocratic Ethic Revisited." He shows that the exclusive focus on the individual is only one of the potential problems with the Hippocratic tradition as received. He argues that in the modern world the patient increasingly is capable of and desires to participate in decisions. He warns the physician against assuming that his or her own judgments about what is beneficial will be shared by patients. He warns that the modern situation requires a more conscious theory of values and awareness of the possibility of conflicting values. Finally, he observes that medicine today is much more institutionalized than it was in the time of Greek medicine. This means that new, more social ethical problems such as cost containment and competition for resources must be addressed, problems not in the consciousness of the Greek Hippocratic physician.

Toward an Expanded Medical Ethics: The Hippocratic Ethic Revisited

EDMUND D. PELLEGRINO

MORE IS NEEDED

Custom without truth is but the seniority of error.
Saint Cyprian, *Epistles LXXIV*

The good physician is by the nature of his vocation called to practice his art within a framework of high moral sensitivity. For two millennia this sensitivity was provided by the Oath and the other ethical writings of the Hippocratic corpus. No code has been more influential in heightening the moral reflexes of ordinary men. Every subsequent medical code is essentially a footnote to the Hippocratic precepts, which even to this day remain the paradigm of how the good physician should behave.

The Hippocratic ethic is marked by a unique combination of humanistic concern and practical wisdom admirably suited to the physician's tasks in society. In a simpler world, that ethic long sufficed to guide the physician in his service to patient and community. Today, the intersections of medicine with contemporary science, technology, social organization, and changed human values have revealed significant missing dimensions in the ancient ethic. The reverence we rightly accord the Hippocratic precepts must not obscure the need for a critical examination of their missing dimensions—those most pertinent for contemporary physicians and society. The need for expanding traditional medical ethics is already well-established. It was first underscored by the shocking revelations of the Nuremberg trials. A spate of new codes has appeared which attempt to deal more responsibly with the promise and the dangers of human experimentation; the inquiry is well under way.[1-3]

More recently, further ethical inquiries have been initiated to reflect the change in moral climate and medical attitudes toward abortion, population control, euthanasia, transplanting organs, and manipulating human behavior and genetic constitution.[1-5]

In actual fact, some of the major proscriptions of the Hippocratic Oath are already being consciously compromised: confidentiality can be violated under certain conditions of law and public safety; abortion is being legalized; dangerous drugs are used everywhere; and a conscious but controlled invasion of the patient's rights in human experimentation is now permitted.

This essay will examine some important dimensions of medical ethics not included in the Hippocratic ethic and, in some ways, even obscured by its too rigorous application. To be considered here are the ethics of participation, the questions raised by institutionalizing medical care, the need for an axiology of medical ethics, the changing ethics of competence, and the tensions between individual and social ethics.

An analysis of these questions will reveal the urgent need for expanding medical ethical concerns far beyond those traditionally observed. A deeper ethic of social and corporate responsibility is needed to guide the profession to levels of moral sensitivity more congruent with the expanded duties of the physician in contemporary culture.

THE HIPPOCRATIC ETHIC

The normative principles which constitute what may loosely be termed the Hippocratic ethic are contained in the Oath and the deontological books: *Law, Decorum, Precepts,* and *The Physician.* These treatises are of varied origin and combine behavioral imperatives derived from a variety of sources—the schools at Cos and Cnidus, intermingled with Pythagorean, Epicurean, and Stoic influences.[6-7]

The Oath[8] speaks of the relationships of the student and his teacher, advises the physician never to harm the patient, enjoins confidentiality, and proscribes abortion, euthanasia, and the use of the knife. It forbids sexual commerce with the women in the household of the homesick. The doctor is a member of a select brotherhood dedicated to the care of the sick, and his major reward is a good reputation.

Law discusses the qualities of mind and the diligence required of the prospective physician from early life.[9] *The Physician* emphasizes the need for dignified comportment, a healthy body, a grave and kind mien, and a regular life.[9(pp. 311–313)] In *Decorum,* we are shown the unique practical wisdom rooted in experience which is essential to good medicine and absent in the quack; proper comportment in the sick room dictates a reserved, authoritative, composed air; much practical advice is given on the arts and techniques of clinical medicine.[9(pp. 279–301)] *Precepts* again warns against theorizing without fact, inveighs against quackery, urges consideration in setting fees, and encourages consultation in difficult cases.[8(pp. 313–333)]

Similar admonitions can be found scattered throughout the Hippocratic corpus, but it is these few brief ethical treatises which have formed the character of the physician for so many centuries. From them, we can extract what can loosely be called the Hippocratic ethic—a mixture of high ideals, common sense, and practical wisdom. A few principles of genuine ethics are often repeated and intermingled with etiquette and homespun advice of all sorts. The good physician emerges as an authoritative and competent practitioner, devoted to his patient's well-being. He is a benevolent and sole arbiter who knows what is best for the patient and makes all decisions for him.

There is in the Hippocratic corpus little explicit reference to the responsibilities of medicine as a corporate entity with responsibility for its members and duties to the greater human community. The ethic of the profession as a whole is assured largely by the moral behavior of its individual members. There is no explicit delineation of the corporate responsibility of physicians for one another's ethical behavior. On the whole, the need for maintaining competence is indirectly stated. There are, in short, few explicit recommendations about what we would today call "social ethics."

These characteristics of the Hippocratic ethic have been carried forward to our day. They are extended in the code of Thomas Percival, which formed the basis of the first code of ethics adopted by the American Medical Association in 1847.[10] They were sufficient for the less complex societies of the ancient and modern worlds but not for the contemporary twentieth-century experience. The Hippocratic norms can no longer be regarded as unchanging absolutes but as partial statements of ideals, in need of constant reevaluation, amplification, and evolution.

Without in any way denigrating the essential worth of the Hippocratic ethic, it is increasingly apparent that the ideas conveyed about the physician are simplistic and incomplete for today's needs. In some ways, it is even antipathetic to the social and political spirit of our times. For example, the notion of the physician as a benevolent and paternalistic figure who decides all for the patient is inconsistent with today's educated public. It is surely incongruous in a democratic society in which the rights of self-determination are being assured by law. In a day when the remote effects of individual medical acts are so consequential, we cannot be satisfied with an ethic which is so inexplicit about social responsibilities. Nowhere in the Hippocratic Oath is the physician recognized as a member of a corporate entity which can accomplish good ends for man that are more than the sum of individual good acts. The necessity for a stringent ethic of competence and a new ethic of shared responsibility which flows from team and institutional medical care are understandably not addressed.

It is useful to examine some of these missing ethical dimensions as examples of the kind of organic development long overdue in professional medical ethical codes.

THE ETHICS OF PARTICIPATION

The central and most admirable feature of the Oath is the respect it inculcates for the patient. In the Oath, the doctor is pledged always to help the patient and keep him from harm. This duty is then exemplified by specific prohibitions against abortion, use of deadly drugs, surgery, breaches of confidence, and indulgence in sexual relations with members of the sick person's household. Elsewhere, in *The Physician, Decorum,* and *Precepts,* the physician is further enjoined to be humble, careful in observation, calm and sober in thought and speech. These admonitions have the same validity today that they had centuries ago and are still much in need of cultivation.

But in one of these same works, *Decorum,* we find an excellent example of how drastically the relationship between physician and patient has changed since Hippocrates' time. The doctor is advised to "Perform all things calmly and adroitly, concealing most things from the patient while you are attending him." A little further on, the physician is told to treat the patient with solicitude, "revealing nothing of the patient's present and future condition."[9(pp. 297, 299)] This advice is at variance with social and political trends and with the desires of most educated patients. It is still too often the modus operandi of physicians dreaming of a simpler world in which authority and paternalistic benevolence were the order of the day.

Indeed, a major criticism of physicians today centers on this very question of disclosure of essential information. Many educated patients feel frustrated in their desire to participate in decisions which affect them as intimately as medical decisions invariably do. The matter really turns on establishing new bases for the patient's trust. The knowledgeable patient can trust the physician only if he feels the latter is competent and uses that competence with integrity and for ends which have value for the patient. Today's educated patient wants to understand what the physician is doing, why he is doing it, what the alternatives may be, and what choices are open. In a democratic society, people expect the widest protection of their rights to self-determination. Hence, the contemporary patient has a right to know the decisions involved in managing his case.

When treatment is specific, with few choices open, the prognosis good, and side effects minimal, disclosing the essential information is an easy matter. Unfortunately, medicine frequently deals with indefinite diagnoses and nonspecific treatments of unspecific value. Several alternatives are usually open; prognosis may not be altered by treatment; side effects are often considerable and discomfort significant. The patient certainly has the right to know these data before therapeutic interventions are initiated. The Nuremberg Code and others were designed to protect the subject in the course of human experimentation by insisting on the right of informed and free consent. The same right should be guaranteed in the course of ordinary medical treatment as well.

So fundamental is this right of self-determination in a democratic society that to limit it, even in ordinary medical transactions, is to propagate an injustice. This is not to ignore the usual objections to disclosure: the fear of inducing anxiety in the patient, the inability of the sick patient to participate in the decision, the technical nature of medical knowledge, and the possibility of litigation. These objections deserve serious consideration but will, on close analysis, not justify concealment except under special circumstances. Obviously, the fear of indiscriminate disclosure cannot obfuscate the invasion of a right, even when concealment is in the interest of the patient.

Surely, the physician is expected by the patient and society to use disclosure prudently. For the very ill, the very anxious, the poorly educated, the too young, or the very old, he will permit himself varying degrees of disclosure. The modes of doing so must be adapted to the patient's educational level, psychologic responses, and physiologic state. It must be emphatically stated that the purpose of disclosure of alternatives, costs, and benefits in medical diagnosis and treatment is not to relieve the physician of the onus of decision or displace it on the patient. Rather, it permits the physician to function as the technical expert and adviser, inviting the patient's participation and understanding as aids in the acceptance of the decision and its consequences. This is the only basis for a mature, just, and understandable physician-patient relationship.

DEONTOLOGIC VERSUS AXIOLOGIC ETHICS

The most important human reason for enabling the patient to participate in the decisions which affect him is to allow consideration of his personal values. Here, the Hippocratic tradition is explicitly lacking since its spirit is almost wholly deontological, that is, obligations are stated as absolutes without reference to any theory of values. Underlying value systems are not stated or discussed. The need for examining the intersection of values inherent in every medical transaction is unrecognized. The values of the physician or of medicine are assumed to prevail as absolutes, and an operational attitude of "noblesse oblige" is encouraged.

A deontologic ethic was not inappropriate for Greek medicine, which did not have to face so many complex and antithetical courses of action. But a relevant ethic for our times must be more axiologic than deontologic, that is, based in a more conscious theory of values. The values upon which any action is based are of enormous personal and social consequence. An analysis of conflicting values underlies the choice of a noxious treatment for a chronic illness, the question of prolonging life in an incurable disease, or setting priorities for using limited medical resources. Instead of absolute values, we deal more frequently with an intersection of several sets and subsets of values: those of the patient, the physician, sciences, and society. Which shall prevail when these values are in conflict? How do we decide?

The patient's values must be respected whenever possible and whenever they do not create injustice for others. The patient is free to delegate the decision to his physicians, but he must do this consciously and freely. To the extent that he is educated, responsible, and thoughtful, modern man will increasingly want the opportunity to examine relative values in each transaction. When the patient is unconscious or otherwise unable to participate, the physician or the family acts as his surrogate, charged as closely as possible to preserve his values.

The Hippocratic principle of *primum non nocere,* therefore, must be expanded to encompass the patient's value system if it is to have genuine meaning. To impose the doctor's value system is an intrusion on the patient; it may be harmful, unethical, and result in an error in diagnosis and treatment.

Disclosure is, therefore, a necessary condition if we really respect each patient as a unique being whose values, as a part of his person, are no more to be violated than his body. The deontologic thrust of traditional medical ethics is too restrictive in a time when the reexamination of all values is universal. It even defeats the very purposes of the traditional ethic, which are to preserve the integrity of the patient as a person.

INDIVIDUAL VERSUS SOCIAL ETHICS

Another notably unexplored area in the Hippocratic ethic is the social responsibility of the physician. Its emphasis on the welfare of the individual patient is exemplary, and this is firmly explicated in the Oath and elsewhere. Indeed, in *Precepts,* this respect for the individual patient is placed at the very heart of medicine: "Where there is love of one's fellow man, there is love of the Art."[8](p. 319)

As Ford has shown, today too the physician's sense of responsibility is directed overwhelmingly toward his own patient.[11] This is one of the most admirable features of medicine, and it must always remain the central ethical imperative in medical transactions. But it must now be set in a context entirely alien to that in which ancient medicine was practiced. In earlier eras the remote effects of medical acts were of little concern, and the rights of the individual patient could be the exclusive and absolute base of the physician's actions. Today, the growing interdependence of all humans and the effectiveness of medical techniques have drastically altered the simplistic arrangements of traditional ethics. The aggregate effects of individual medical acts have already changed the ecology of man. Every death prevented or life prolonged alters the number, kind, and distribution of human beings. The resultant competition for living space, food, and conveniences already imperils our hope for a life of satisfaction for all mankind.

Even more vexing questions in social ethics are posed when we attempt to allocate our resources among the many new possibilities for good inherent in medical progress and technology. Do we pool our limited resources and manpower to apply curative medicine to all now deprived of it or continue to multiply the complexity of services for the privileged? Do we apply mass prophylaxis against streptococcal diseases, or repair damaged valves with expensive heart surgery after they are damaged? Is it preferable to change cultural patterns in favor of a more reasonable diet for Americans or develop better surgical techniques for unplugging fat-occluded coronary arteries? Every health planner and concerned public official has his own set of similar questions. It is clear that we cannot have all these things simultaneously.

This dimension of ethics becomes even more immediate when we inquire into the responsibility of medicine for meeting the urgent sociomedical needs of large segments of our population. Can we absolve ourselves from responsibility for deficiencies in distribution, quality, and accessibility of even ordinary medical care for the poor, the uneducated and the disenfranchised? Do we direct our health care system to the care of the young in ghettos and underdeveloped countries or to the affluent aged? Which course will make for a better world? These are vexing questions of the utmost social concern. Physicians have an ethical responsibility to raise these questions and, in answering them, to work with the community in ordering its priorities or make optimal use of available medical skills.

It is not enough to hope that the good of the community will grow fortuitously out of the summation of good acts of each physician for his own patients. Societies are necessary to insure enrichment of the life of each of their members. But they are more than the aggregate of persons within them. As T. S. Eliot puts it, "What life have you if you have not life together? There is no life that is not in community."[12]

Society supports the doctor in the expectation that he will direct himself to socially relevant health problems, not just those he finds interesting or remunerative. The commitment to social egalitarianism demands a greater sensitivity to social ethics than is to be found in traditional codes. Section ten of the American Medical Association Principles of Medical Ethics (1946) explicitly recognizes the profession's responsibility to society. But a more explicit analysis of the relationships of individual and social ethics should be undertaken. Medicine, which touches on the most human problems of both the individual and society, cannot serve man without attending to both his personal and communal needs.

The Hippocratic ethic and its later modifications were not required to confront such paradoxes. Today's conscientious physician is very much in need of an expanded ethic to cope with his double responsibility to the individual and to the community.

THE ETHICS OF INSTITUTIONALIZED MEDICINE

The institutionalization of all aspects of medical care is an established fact. With increasing frequency, the personal contract inherent in patient care is made with institutions, groups of physicians, or teams of health professionals. The patient now often expects the institution or group to select his physician or consultant and to assume responsibility for the quality and quantity of care provided.

Within the institution itself, the health care team is essential to the practice of comprehensive medicine. Physicians and nonphysicians now cooperate in providing the spectrum of special services made possible by modern technology. The responsibility for even the most intimate care of the patient is shared. Some of the most important clinical decisions are made by team members who may have no personal contact at all with the patient. The team itself is not a stable entity of unchanging composition. Its membership changes in response to the patient's needs, and so may its leadership. Preserving the traditional rights of the patient, formerly vested in a single identifiable physician, is now sometimes spread anonymously over a group. Competence, confidentiality, integrity, and personal concern are far more difficult to assure with a group of diverse professionals enjoying variable degrees of personal contact with the patient.

No current code of ethics fully defines how the traditional rights of the medical transaction are to be protected when responsibility is diffused within a team and an institution. Clearly, no health profession can elaborate such a code of team ethics by itself. We need a new medical ethic which permits the cooperative definition of normative guides to protect the person of the patient served by a group, none of whose members may have sole responsibility for care. Laymen, too, must participate, since boards of trustees set the overall policies which affect patient care. Few trustees truly recognize that they are the ethical and legal surrogates of society for the patients who come to their institutions seeking help.

Thus, the most delicate of the physician's responsibilities, protecting the patient's welfare, must now be fulfilled in a new and complicated context. Instead of the familiar one-to-one unique relationship, the physician finds himself coordinator of a team, sharing with others some of the most sensitive areas of patient care. The physician is still bound to see that group assessment and management are rational, safe, and personalized. He must especially guard against the dehumanization so easily and inadvertently perpetrated by a group in the name of efficiency.

The doctor must acquire new attitudes. Since ancient times, he has been the sole dominant and authoritarian figure in the care of his patient. He has been supported in this position by traditional ethics. In the clinical emergency, his dominant role is still unchallenged, since he is well trained to make quick decisions in ambiguous situations. What he is not prepared for are the negotiations, analysis, and ultimate compromise fundamental to group efforts and essential in non-emergency situations. A whole new set of clinical perspectives must be introduced, perspectives difficult for the classically trained physician to accept, but necessary if the patient is to benefit from contemporary technology and organization of health care.

THE ETHICS OF COMPETENCE

A central aim of the Oath and other ethical treatises is to protect the patient and the profession from quackery and incompetence. In the main, competence is assumed as basic fulfillment of the Hippocratic ideal of *primum non nocere*.

The Hippocratic works preach the wholly admirable common-sense ethos of the good artisan: careful work, maturation of skills, simplicity of approach, and knowledge of limitations. This was sound advice at a time when new discoveries were so often the product of speculation untainted by observation or experience.

The speculative astringency of the Hippocratic ethic was a potent and necessary safeguard against the quackery of fanciful and dangerous "new" cures.

With the scientific era in medicine, the efficacy of new techniques and information in changing the natural history of disease was dramatically demonstrated. Today, the patient has a right to access to the vast stores of new knowledge useful to medicine. Failure of the physician to make this reservoir available and accessible is a moral failure. The ethos of the artisan, while still a necessary safeguard, is now far from being a sufficient one.

Maintaining competence today is a prime ethical challenge. Only the highest standard of initial and continuing professional proficiency is acceptable in a technological world. This imperative is now so essential a feature of the patient-physician transaction that the ancient mandate, "Do no harm," must be supplemented: "Do all things essential to optimal solution of the patient's problem." Anything less makes the doctor's professional declaration a sham and a scandal.

Competence now has a far wider definition than in ancient times. Not only must the physician encompass expertly the knowledge pertinent to his own field, but he must be the instrument for bringing all other knowledge to bear on his patient's needs. He now functions as one element in a vast matrix of consultants, technicians, apparatus, and institutions, all of which may contribute to his patient's well-being. He cannot provide all these things himself. To attempt to do so is to pursue the romantic and vanishing illusion of the physician as Renaissance man.

The enormous difficulties of its achievement notwithstanding, competence has become the first ethical precept for the modern physician after integrity. It is also the prime human precept and the one most peculiar to the physician's function in society. Even the current justifiable demands of patients and medical students for greater compassion must not obfuscate the centrality of competence in the physician's existence. The simple intention to help others is commendable but, by itself, not only insufficient but positively dangerous. What is more inhumane or more a violation of trust than incompetence? The consequence of a lack of compassion may be remediable, while a lack of competence may cost the patient his chance for recovery of life, function, and happiness. Clearly, medicine cannot attain the ethical eminence to which it is called without both compassion and competence.

Within this framework, a more rigorous ethic of competence must be elaborated. Continuing education, periodic recertification, and renewal of clinical privileges have become moral mandates, not just hopeful hortatory devices dependent upon individual physician responses. The Hippocratic ethic of the good artisan is now just the point of departure for the wide options technology holds out for individual and social health.

TOWARD A CORPORATE ETHIC AND AN ETHICAL SYNCYTIUM

The whole of the Hippocratic corpus, including the ethical treatises, is the work of many authors writing in different historical periods. Thus, the ethical precepts cannot be considered the formal position of a profession in today's sense. There is no evidence of recognition of true corporate responsibility for larger social issues or of sanctions to deter miscreant members.

The Greek physician seems to have regarded himself as the member of an informal aristocratic brotherhood, in which each individual was expected to act ethically and to do so for love of the profession and respect of the patient. His reward was *doxa*, a good reputation, which in turn assured a successful practice. There is notably no sense of the larger responsibilities as a profession for the behavior of each member. Nowhere stated are the potentialities and responsibilities of a group of high-minded individuals to effect reforms and achieve purposes transcending the interests of individual members. In short, the Greek medical profession relied on the sum total of individual ethical behaviors to assure the ethical behavior of the group.

This is still the dominant view of many physicians in the Western world who limit their ethical perspectives to their relationships with their own patients. Medical societies do censure unethical members with varying alacrity for the grosser forms of misconduct or breaches of professional etiquette. But there is as yet insufficient assumption of a corporate and shared responsibility for the actions of each member of the group. The power of physicians as a polity to effect reforms in quality of care, its organization, and its relevance to needs of society is as yet unrealized.

Yet many of the dimensions of medical ethics touched upon in this essay can only be secured by the conscious assumption of a corporate responsibility on the part of all physicians for the final pertinence of their individual acts to promote better life for all. There is the need to develop, as it were, a functioning ethical syncytium in which the actions of each physician would touch upon those of all physicians and in which it is clear that the ethical failings of each member would diminish the stature of every other physician to some degree. This syncytial framework is at variance with the traditional notion that each physician acts as an individual and is primarily responsible only to himself and his patient.

This shift of emphasis is dictated by the metamorphosis of all professions in our complex, highly organized, highly integrated, and egalitarian social order. For most of its history medicine has existed as a select and loosely organized brotherhood. For the past hundred years in our country, it has been more formally organized in the American Medical Association and countless other professional organizations dedicated to a high order of individual ethics. A new stage in the evolution of medicine as a profession is about to begin as a consequence of three clear trends.

First, all professions are increasingly being regarded as services, even as public utilities, dedicated to fulfilling specific social needs not entirely defined by the profession. Professions themselves will acquire dignity and standing in the future, not so much from the tasks they perform, but from the intimacy of the connection between those tasks and the social life of which the profession is a part. Second, the professions are being democratized, and it will be ever more difficult for any group to hold a privileged position. The automatic primacy of medicine is being challenged by the other health professions, whose functions are of increasing importance in patient care. This functionalization of the professions tends to emphasize what is done for a patient and not who does it. Moreover, many tasks formerly performed only by the physicians are being done by other professionals and non-professionals. Last, the socialization of all mankind affects the professions as well. Hence, the collectivity will increasingly be expected to take responsibility for how well or poorly the profession carries out the purposes for which it is supported by society.

These changes will threaten medicine only if physicians hold to a simplistic ethic in which the agony of choices among individual and social values is dismissed as spurious or imaginary. The physician is the most highly educated of health professionals. He should be first to take on the burdens of continuing self-reformation in terms of a new ethos—one in which the problematics of priorities and values are openly faced as common responsibilities of the entire profession. We must recognize the continuing validity of traditional ethics for the personal dimensions of patient care and their inadequacy for the newer social dimensions of health in contemporary life. It is the failure to appreciate this distinction that stimulates so much criticism of the profession at the same time that individual physicians are highly respected.

One of the gravest and most easily visible social inequities today is the mal-distribution of medical services among portions of our population. This is another sphere in which the profession as a whole must assume responsibility for what individual physicians cannot do alone. The civil rights movement and the revolt of the black minority populations have punctuated the problem. Individual physicians have always tried to redress this evil, some in heroic ways. Now, however, the problem is a major ethical responsibility for the whole profession: we cannot dismiss the issue. We must engender a feeling of ethical diminution of the entire profession whenever there are segments of the population without adequate and accesible medical care. This extends to the provision of primary care for all, insistence on a system of coverage for all communities every hour of the day, proper distribution of the various medical specialties and facilities, and a system of fees no longer based on the usual imponderables, but on more standardized norms.

There are, perforce, reasonable limits to the social ills to which the individual physician and the profession can be expected to attend qua physician. Some have suggested that medicine concern itself with the Vietnam war, the root causes of poverty, environmental pollution, drugs, housing, and racial injustice. It would be difficult to argue that all of these social ills are primary ethical responsibilities of individual physicians or even of the profession. To do so would hopelessly diffuse medical energies and manpower from their proper object—the promotion of health and the cure of illness. The profession can fight poverty, injustice, and war through medicine.

A distinction, therefore, must clearly be made between the physician's primary ethical responsibilities, which derive from the nature of his profession, and those which do not. Each physician must strike for himself an optimal balance between professional and civic responsibilities.

SUMMARY

We have attempted a brief analysis of some of the limitations and omissions in traditional medical ethics as embodied in the Hippocratic corpus and its later exemplifications. These limitations are largely in the realm of social and corporate ethics, realms of increasing significance in an egalitarian, highly structured, and exquisitely interlocked social order.

The individual physician needs more explicit guidelines than traditional codes afford to meet today's new problems. The Hippocratic ethic is one of the most admirable codes in the history of man. But even its ethical sensibilities and high moral tone are insufficient for the complexities of today's problems.

An evolving, constantly refurbished system of medical ethics is requisite in the twentieth century. An axiologic, rather than a deontologic, bias is more in harmony with the questions raised in a world society whose values are in continual flux and reexamination. There is ample opportunity for a critical reappraisal of the Hippocratic ethic and for the elaboration of a fuller and more comprehensive medical ethic suited to our profession as it nears the twenty-first century. This fuller ethic will build upon the noble precepts set forth so long ago in the Hippocratic corpus. It will explicate, complement, and develop those precepts, but it must not be delimited in its evolution by an unwarranted reluctance to question even so ancient and honorable a code as that of the Hippocratic writings.

NOTES

1. *American Academy of Arts and Sciences.* "Proceedings" 98:No. 2, 1969.
2. Pellegrino, E. D. "The Necessity, Promise, and Dangers of Human Experimentation." *Experiments With Man—World Council Studies, No. 6,* New York: Geneva and Friendship Press, 1969.
3. *Annals of the New York Academy of Arts and Sciences.* "New Dimensions in Legal and Ethical Concepts for Human Research." 169:293–593, 1970.
4. Torrey, E. F. *Ethical Issues in Medicine.* Boston: Little, Brown, 1968.
5. Pellegrino, E. D. "Physicians, Patients, and Society: Some New Tensions in Medical Ethics." In *Human Aspects of Biomedical Innovation,* edited by Everett Mendelsohn, Judith P. Swazey, and Irene Taviss. Cambridge, Mass.: Harvard University Press, 1971, pp. 77–97, 291–220.
6. Sigerest, H. E. *The History of Medicine,* vol. 11. New York: Oxford University Press, 1961, pp. 260, 298.
7. Heidel, W. A. *Hippocratic Medicine: Its Spirit and Method.* New York: Columbia University Press, 1941, p. 149.
8. Jones, W. H. S. *Hippocrates,* vol. I. Cambridge, Mass.: Harvard University Press, 1923, pp. 299–301, 313–333.
9. Jones, W. H. S. *Hippocrates,* vol. II. Cambridge, Mass.: Harvard University Press, 1923, pp. 263–265, 279–301, 311–313.
10. Leake, C., ed. *Percival's Medical Ethics.* Baltimore: William & Wilkins, 1927, p. 291.
11. Ford, et al. *The Doctor's Perspective.* New York: Year Book, 1967.
12. Eliot, T. S. "The Rock." *The Complete Poems and Plays, 1909–1950.* New York: Harcourt & Brace, 1952, p. 101.

The American Medical Association, at its first meetings in Philadelphia in 1847 adopted a long statement on ethics adopted in large part from a document written by Thomas Percival in 1797 as part of the adjudication of a dispute among physicians, surgeons, and apothecaries. Several revisions of the AMA's statements on ethics were adopted over the years. In 1957 the AMA adopted a new set of principles expressed in a shorter, more abstract form. Some of the concerns raised by Edmund Pellegrino are reflected in it. One of the themes that begins to emerge in the early codes of Percival and the AMA is the tension between the duty of the physician to the patient and the social duty the physician may owe to the society. This theme, totally absent from the original Hippocratic Oath, is already present in Percival's writing and becomes a more critical issue in the versions of the AMA's codes written in the twentieth century. This is particularly apparent in the tenth principle of the 1957 version of the AMA Principles.

Principles of Medical Ethics (1957)

AMERICAN MEDICAL ASSOCIATION

PREAMBLE

These principles are intended to aid physicians individually and collectively in maintaining a high level of ethical conduct. They are not laws but standards by which a physician may determine the propriety of his conduct in his relationship with patients, with colleagues, with members of allied professions, and with the public.

Section 1:
The principle objective of the medical profession is to render service to humanity with full respect for the dignity of man. Physicians should merit the confidence of patients entrusted to their care, rendering to each a full measure of service and devotion.

Section 2:
Physicians should strive continually to improve medical knowledge and skill, and should make available to their patients and colleagues the benefits of their professional attainments.

Section 3:
A physician should practice a method of healing founded on a scientific basis; and he should not voluntarily associate professionally with anyone who violates this principle.

Section 4:

The medical profession should safeguard the public and itself against physicians deficient in moral character or professional competence. Physicians should observe all laws, uphold the dignity and honor of the profession and accept its self-imposed disciplines. They should expose, without hesitation, illegal or unethical conduct of fellow members of the profession.

Section 5:

A physician may choose whom he will serve. In an emergency, however, he should render service to the best of his ability. Having undertaken the care of a patient, he may not neglect him; and unless he has been discharged he may discontinue his services only after giving adequate notice. He should not solicit patients.

Section 6:

A physician should not dispose of his services under terms or conditions which tend to interfere with or impair the free and complete exercise of his medical judgment and skill or tend to cause a deterioration of the quality of medical care.

Section 7:

In the practice of medicine a physician should limit the source of his professional income to medical services actually rendered by him, or under his supervision, to his patients. His fee should be commensurate with the services rendered and the patient's ability to pay. He should neither pay nor receive a commission for referral of patients. Drugs, remedies or appliances may be dispensed or supplied by the physician provided it is in the best interest of the patient.

Section 8:

A physician should seek consultation upon request; in doubtful or difficult cases; or whenever it appears that the quality of medical service may be enhanced thereby.

Section 9:

A physician may not reveal confidences entrusted to him in the course of medical attendance, or the deficiencies he may observe in the character of patients, unless he is required to do so by law or unless it becomes necessary in order to protect the welfare of the individual or of the community.

Section 10:

The honored ideals of the medical profession imply that the responsibilities of the physician extend not only to the individual, but also to society where these responsibilities deserve his interest and participation in activities which have the purpose of improving both the health and the well-being of the individual and the community.

In 1980 the AMA adopted a completely new set of medical ethical principles. It shows how these concerns with the problems of the original Hippocratic perspective have manifested themselves and gradually emerged to dominate the medical ethics of organized medicine at least in the United States. The committee of the AMA responsible for the writing of the new Principles was chaired by James Todd, who is now AMA Assistant Executive Vice President. The committee reported that medical ethics must be seen increasingly as something to which all members of the society must contribute. It called into question the earlier paternalism of the Hippocratic tradition and emphasized the responsibility of the profession to the society as well as to the individual patient. The new Principles for the first time in any code written by physicians, adopt the language of rights rather than staying exclusively with the more traditional language of benefits and harms. The idea that rights are relevant to morality as well as benefits and harms is alien to professional codes of medical ethics in the Hippocratic tradition. The new Principles show the beginnings of the influence of other ethical theories, especially the ethics of modern Western liberalism.

Principles of Medical Ethics (1980)

American Medical Association

PREAMBLE

The medical profession has long subscribed to a body of ethical statements developed primarily for the benefit of the patient. As a member of this profession, a physician must recognize responsibility not only to patients, but also to society, to other health professionals, and to self. The following Principles adopted by the American Medical Association are not laws, but standards of conduct which define the essentials of honorable behavior for the physician.

   I.   A physician shall be dedicated to providing competent medical service with compassion and respect for human dignity.
   II. A physician shall deal honestly with patients and colleagues, and strive to expose those physicians deficient in character or competence, or who engage in fraud or deception.
   III. A physician shall respect the law and also recognize a responsibility to seek changes in those requirements which are contrary to the best interests of the patient.

IV.   A physician shall respect the rights of patients, of colleagues, and of other health professionals, and shall safeguard patient confidences within the constraints of the law.

V.   A physician shall continue to study, apply and advance scientific knowledge, make relevant information available to patients, colleagues, and the public, obtain consultation, and use the talents of other health professionals when indicated.

VI.   A physician shall, in the provision of appropriate patient care, except in emergencies, be free to choose whom to serve, with whom to associate, and the environment in which to provide medical services.

VII.   A physician shall recognize a responsibility to participate in activities contributing to an improved community.

The Dominant Western Competitors

INTRODUCTION

When the Hippocratic tradition was challenged for its individualism and its lack of commitment to the autonomy of the patient as a decisionmaker, we began to discover other traditions in Western thought, some of which had well developed medical ethical traditions of their own. These include the major religious traditions as well as modern secular liberal political philosophy.

Judaism and Catholicism have long held richly nuanced medical ethical systems. They have manifest themselves in hospitals and medical schools within these traditions, but also in the thinking of health-care professionals and lay persons from within these traditions. As the Hippocratic tradition has become more problematic, we have found it necessary to reexamine the positions and the moral premises of these religious traditions. This is true not only for institutions and individuals who stand within them, but also for health-care providers and public-policy makers who must deal with patients who express judgments about medical care based on these traditions. We are seeing increasingly that they offer coherent, well-considered alternative views about the way health care ought to be provided.

Protestantism, being inherently more pluralistic and more diverse, has not developed as fully articulated a medical ethic as Judaism and Catholicism. Its medical ethical positions, like its theology, are much more diverse. Nevertheless, there are positions that Protestants tend to share. They sometimes stand in contrast to the dominant professional medical ethical positions within the Hippocratic tradition. For example, Protestants tend to emphasize the importance of the lay person as one who is capable of "reading the text," of looking at information and making decisions for himself or herself. Other positions of mainstream Protestantism provide the foundations for a medical ethical system that in turn provides an alternative to the Hippocratic tradition.

Secular thought also has the potential of providing an alternative to Hippocratic medical ethics. The most important secular philosophical system is that of liberal political philosophy. It manifests itself in such crucial political documents as the Declaration of Independence and the Bill of Rights of the Constitution. It provides the philosophical underpinnings of the hundreds of court decisions that have essentially overturned the core ethical positions of the Hippocratic tradition. It stands behind the moral notions of the rights of patients to consent to treatment, to have information about themselves held in privacy regardless of professional judgments about the benefit of such privacy, and the right to refuse treatment. The readings in this chapter provide examples of some of the major religious and secular alternatives to the Hippocratic tradition in the Anglo-American West.

One of the most ancient and richly developed alternatives to the Hippocratic tradition is the medical ethic of Judaism. Judaism derives its medical ethical positions from its classical sources—the Old Testament (especially the Torah) and the Talmudic sources and their commentaries. Not only are the sources different from Hippocratic professional medical ethics, the authoritative interpreters are different. Whereas professional medical groups have tended to turn to the profession itself to interpret moral imperatives, Judaism turns to rabbinical authorities and Jewish councils. As we see in the following essay, the moral norms are also quite different. In particular there is a rigorous commitment to the sacredness of life and the duty to preserve it, a duty that is much more emphatic than in Hippocratic, Christian, or secular traditions. What follows is a shortened form of an essay that originally addressed ethical decisionmaking in the care of defective newborns. The portion reprinted traces the key moral commitments of Jewish ethics applied to medicine.

The Obligation to Heal in the Judaic Tradition

J. David Bleich

In recent years medical science and technology have made tremendous strides. Some diseases have been virtually eradicated; for others effective remedies have been virtually eradicated; for others effective remedies have been found. Concomitantly, ways and means have been developed which enable physicians to sustain life even when known cures do not exist. Maladies and deformities often appear in associated syndromes. While heretofore untreatable conditions now respond to medical ministration, such response is often less than total. Particularly in the case of defective newborns, methods now exist which make it possible to correct certain problems only to leave the patient in a deformed or debilitated state. In such cases questions with regard to the value of the life which is preserved become very real.

The physician's practical dilemma can be stated in simple terms: to treat or not to treat. In deciding whether or not to initiate or maintain such treatment the physician is called upon to make not only medical, but also moral, determinations. There are at least two distinguishable components which present themselves in all such quandaries. The first is a value judgment. Is it desirable that the patient be treated? Should value judgments be made with regard to the quality of life to be preserved? The second question pertains to the physician's personal responsibilities.

Under what circumstances and to what extent is the physician morally obligated to persist in rendering aggressive professional care?

The value with which human life is regarded in the Jewish tradition is maximized far beyond the value placed upon human life in the Christian tradition or in Anglo-Saxon common law. In Jewish law and moral teaching, the value of human life is supreme and takes precedence over virtually all other considerations. This attitude is most eloquently summed up in a Talmudic passage regarding the creation of Adam:

> Therefore only a single human being was created in the world, to teach that if any person has caused a single soul of Israel to perish, Scripture regards him as if he had caused an entire world to perish; and if any human being saves a single soul of Israel, Scripture regards him as if he had saved an entire world.[1]

Human life is not a good to be preserved as a condition of other values but as an absolute basic and precious good in its own stead. The obligation to preserve life is commensurately all-encompassing.

Life with suffering is regarded as being, in many cases, preferable to cessation of life and with it elimination of suffering. The Talmud, *Sotah* 22a, and Maimonides, *Hilkhot Sotah* 3:20, indicate that the adulterous woman who was made to drink "the bitter waters" (Num. 6:11–31) did not always die immediately. If she possessed other merit, even though guilty of the offense with which she was charged, the waters, rather than causing her to perish immediately, produced a debilitating and degenerative state which led to a protracted termination of life. The added longevity, although accompanied by pain and suffering, is viewed as a privilege bestowed in recognition of meritorious actions. Life accompanied by pain is thus viewed as preferable to death.

Man does not possess absolute title to his life or to his body. He is but the steward of the life which he has been privileged to receive. Man is charged with preserving, dignifying and hallowing that life. He is obliged to seek food and sustenance in order to safeguard the life he has been granted; when falling victim to an illness and disease, he is obliged to seek a cure in order to sustain life. Never is he called upon to determine whether life is worth living—this is a question over which God remains the sole arbiter.

The value placed upon human life is reflected in Halakhah, the corpus of Jewish law, which provides for the suspension of all religious precepts (with the exception of the prohibition against commission of the three cardinal sins: idolatry, murder and certain sexual offenses) when necessary in order to save life.[2] Even the mere possibility of saving human life mandates violation of such laws "however remote the likelihood of saving human life may be."[3] The quality of life which is thus preserved is never a factor to be taken into consideration. Neither is the length of the survivor's life expectancy a controlling factor. Judaism regards not only human life in general as being of infinite and inestimable value, but regards every moment of life as being of infinite value.[4] Obligations with regard to treatment and cure are one and the same whether the person's life is likely to be prolonged for a matter of years or merely for a few seconds. Thus, even on the Sabbath, efforts to free a victim buried under a collapsed building must be maintained even if the victim is found in circumstances such that he cannot survive longer than a brief period of time.[5] Sectarians such as the Sadducees who lived during the period of the Second Commonwealth and the Karaites of the Geonic period who challenged these provisions of Jewish law and, by implication, the value system upon which they are predicated, were branded heretics.[6]

Defective newborns are known and discussed in rabbinic literature. *Sefer Chasidim*, n. 186, a thirteenth-century compendium authored by R. Judah the Pious, describes the case of a child born with severest of physical deformities and mental deficiencies—a monster-like creature which obviously had no human potential whatsoever. A question was raised as the whether or not the monster-birth might be destroyed. The answer was an emphatic negative. The answer is not at all surprising. Noteworthy is the question. The desire to destroy this creature was predicated upon the fact that the monster-like child was born with ferocious-looking teeth and an elongated tail. In light of these characteristics and in view of the general demeanor of the monster-birth, it was felt by some that this creature constituted a life-threatening menace to the community. In circumstances of lesser gravity it would not have occurred to anyone to raise the question. An early nineteenth-century responsum authored by R. Eliezer Fleckeles, *Teshuvah mei-Ahavah*, I, n. 53, makes much the same point in connection with a somewhat less dramatic situation. A child born of a human mother, despite the possession of animal-like organs and features, is a human being whose life must be protected and preserved.[7] Such a creature may not be killed, nor may it, despite its deformity, be permitted to die as a result of benign neglect.

The obligation to save the life of an endangered person is derived by the Talmud from the verse, "Neither shalt thou stand idly by the blood of thy neighbor" (Lev. 19:16).[8] The Talmud and the various codes of Jewish law offer specific examples of situations in which moral obligation exists with regard to rendering aid. These include the rescue of a person drowning in a river, assistance to one being mauled by wild beasts and aid to a person under attack by bandits.

Application of this principle to medical intervention for the purposes of preserving life is not without theological and philosophical difficulties. It is to be anticipated that a theology which ascribes providential concern to the Deity will view sickness as part of the divine scheme. A personal God does not allow his creatures, over whom He exercises providential guardianship, to become ill unless the affliction is divinely ordained as a means of punishment, for purposes of expiation of sin or for some other beneficial purpose entirely comprehensible to the Deity, if not to man. Thus, while the ancient Greeks regarded illness as a curse and the sick as inferior persons because, to them, malady represented the disruption of the harmony of the body which is synonymous with health, in Christianity suffering was deemed to be a manifestation of divine grace because it effected purification of the afflicted and served as an ennobling process. Since illness resulted in a state of enhanced spiritual perfection, the sick man was viewed as marked by divine favor.

Human intervention in causing or speeding the therapeutic process is, then, in a sense, interference with the deliberate design of providence. The patient in seeking medical attention betrays a lack of faith in failing to put his trust in God. This attitude is reflected in the teaching of a number of early and medieval Christian theologians who counseled against seeking medical attention.[9] The Karaites rejected all forms of human healing and relied entirely upon prayer. Consistent with their fundamentalist orientation, they based their position upon a quite liberal reading of Exodus, chapter 16, verse 26. A literal translation of the Hebrew text of the passage reads as follows. "I will put none of the diseases upon thee which I have put upon the Egyptians, for I am the Lord the physician."[10] Hence, the Karaites taught that God alone should be sought as physician.[11]

This view was rejected by rabbinic Judaism, but not without due recognition of the cogency of the theological argument upon which it is based. Rabbinic teaching recognized that intervention for the purposes of thwarting the natural course of the disease could be sanctioned only on the basis of specific divine dispensation. Such license is found, on the basis of Talmudic exegesis, in the scriptural passage dealing with compensation for personal injury:

> And if other men quarrel with one another and one smiteth the other with a stone or with the fist and he die not, but has to keep in bed . . . he must pay the loss entailed by absence from work and cause him to be thoroughly healed (Exod. 21:19–20).

Ostensibly, this passage refers simply to financial liability incurred as the result of an act of assault. However, since specific reference is made to liability for medical expenses, it follows that liability for such expenses implies biblical license to incur those expenses in the course of seeking the ministrations of a practitioner of the healing arts. Thus, the Talmud, Baba Kama 85a, comments "From here [it is derived] that the physician is granted permission to cure." Specific authorization is required, comments Rashi, in order to teach us that ". . . we are not to say, 'How is it that God smites and man heals?'" In much the same vein, Tosafot and R. Samuel ben Aderet state that without such sanction, "He who heals might appear as if he invalidated a divine decree."[12]

Nontherapeutic lifesaving intervention is Talmudically mandated on independent grounds. The Talmud, Sanhedrin 73a, posits an obligation to rescue a neighbor from danger such as drowning or being mauled by an animal. This obligation is predicated upon spiritual exhortation with regard to the restoration of lost property, "And thou shalt return it to him" (Deut. 22:2). On the basis of a pleanism in the Hebrew text, the Talmud declares that this verse includes an obligation to restore a fellowman's body as well as his property. Hence, there is created an obligation to come to the aid of one's fellowman in a life-threatening situation. Noteworthy is the fact that Maimonides,[13] going beyond the examples supplied by the Talmud, posits this source as the basis of the obligation to render medical care. Maimonides declares that the biblical commandment "And thou shalt return it to him" establishes an obligation requiring the physician to render professional services in the life-threatening situations. Every individual, insofar as he is able, is obligated to restore the health of a fellowman no less than he is obligated to restore his property. Maimonides views this as a binding religious obligation.

Noteworthy is not only Maimonides' expression of this concept to cover medical matters but also his failure to allude at all to the verse "And he shall surely heal." It would appear that Maimonides is of the opinion that without the granting of specific permission, one would not be permitted to tamper with physiological processes; obligations derived from Deuteronomy, chapter 22, verse 2 would be limited to prevention of accident or assault by man or beast. Dispensation to intervene in the natural order is derived from Exodus, chapter 21, verse 20; but once such license is given, medical therapy is not simply elective but acquires the status of a positive obligation.[14] As indicated by Sanhedrin 73a, this obligation mandates not only the rendering of personal assistance as is the case with regard to the restoration of lost property, but, by virtue of the negative commandment, "You shall not stand idly by the blood of your neighbor" (Lev. 19:16), the obligation is expanded to encompass expenditure of financial resources for the sake of preserving the life of one's fellowman. This seems to have been the interpretation given to Maimonides' comments by Rabbi Joseph Karo who, in his code of Jewish law, combined both concepts in stating:

> The Torah gave permission to the physician to heal; moreover, this is a religious precept and it is included in the category of saving life; and if the physician withholds this services it is considered as shedding blood.[15]

Nachmanides also finds that the obligation of the physician to heal is inherent in the commandment, "And thou shalt love thy neighbor as thyself" (Lev. 19:18).[16] As an instantiation of the general obligation to manifest love and concern for one's neighbor, the obligation to heal encompasses not only situations posing a threat to life or limb or demanding restoration of impaired health but also situations of lesser gravity warranting medical attention for relief of pain and promotion of well-being.[17]

Despite the unequivocal and authoritative rulings of both Maimonides and Rabbi Joseph Karo, there do exist within the rabbinic tradition dissonant views which look somewhat askance at the practice of the healing arts. Abraham Ibn Ezra[18] finds a contradiction between the injunction "And he shall cause to be thoroughly healed" and the account given in II Chronicles, chapter 16, verse 12. Scripture reports that Asa, King of Judah, became severely ill and in his sickness "he sought not to the Lord, but to the physicians." According to Ibn Ezra, Scripture grants license for therapeutic intervention only for treatment of external wounds. Wounds inflicted by man, either by design or by accident, may legitimately be treated by any means known to mankind. That which has been inflicted by man may be cured by man. However, internal wounds or physiological disorders, according to this view, are not encompassed in the injunction "and he shall cause to be thoroughly healed." Such afflictions are presumed to be manifestations of divine rebuke or punishment and only God, Who afflicts, may heal.

Needless to say, Ibn Ezra's position was rejected by normative Judaism as is most eloquently demonstrated by the ruling recorded in *Shulchan Arukh, Orach Chayyim* 328:3. Jewish law not only sanctions but requires suspension of Sabbath restrictions for treatment of a person afflicted by a life-threatening malady. Orach Chayyim 328:3 rules blanketly that all "internal wounds" are to be presumed to be life-threatening for purposes of Halakhah. Quite obviously, Jewish law as coded mandates treatment of even internal disorders by means of all therapeutic techniques. R. Zemach Duran, while acknowledging Ibn Ezra's outstanding competence as a biblical exegete, had little regard for the latter's legal acumen and dismisses him as "not having been proficient in the laws."[19]

Of greater relevance in the formulation of Jewish thought are the comments of Nachmanides in his *Commentary of the Bible,* Leviticus, chapter 26, verse 11.

It is, however, entirely possible that Nachmanides' comments are intended only as a description of conditions prevailing in a spiritual utopia. In developing his theory of providence, Maimonides explains that the quality of providential guardianship extended to man is directly correlative with man's spiritual attainment. To the extent that man is lacking in perfection his condition is regulated by the laws of nature.[20] Thus a pious person privileged to be the recipient of a high degree of providential guardianship would not require medication, but might expect to be healed by God directly. Other individuals, not beneficiaries of this degree of providence, are perforce required to seek a cure by natural means. In doing so they incur no censure whatsoever. Indeed, Nachmanides prefaces his comments with a reference to such times when the people of "Israel are perfect" and specifically states that failure to seek medical attention was normative only "for the righteous" and even for them solely "during the time of prophecy." Lesser individuals living in spiritually imperfect epochs are duty-bound to seek the cures made available by medical science. Understood in this manner, there is no contradiction between Nachmanides and the Talmudic references cited, or, for that manner, between Nachmanides and Maimonides.[21] In terms of normative Jewish law, there is no question that there exists a positive obligation to seek medical care.[22]

However, in the absence of specific spiritual license to practice and to seek the benefits of the healing arts, the Jewish faith community would be a community of faith healers.[23] Thus, despite the serious nature of the halakhic imperative with regard to the preservation of human life, it is not surprising that this imperative is somewhat circumscribed insofar as therapeutic preservation of life is concerned. The limited situation in which treatment may be withheld must be carefully delineated.

There is no basis in Jewish teaching for a distinction between ordinary versus extraordinary forms of therapy per se, and, in fact, no rabbinic authority draws such a distinction which is of great relevance. A patient may be compelled to submit to medically indicated therapy. However, declares R. Jacob Emden, *Mor u-Ketziah, Orach Chayyim* 328, a distinction must be made between therapeutic procedures of proven efficacy and those of unproven therapeutic value. Acceptance of a therapeutic procedure of known efficacy, known as *refuah bedukah,* is a moral and halakhic imperative. The patient may not terminate or shorten his life either actively or passively. Since God grants dispensation to seek medical cure, use of medicaments or acceptance of surgical intervention in such situations is mandatory. Man may no more abstain from the use of drugs to cure illness than he may abstain from food and drink. However, if the proposed therapy is of unproven value the patient may legitmately refuse treatment. This is true not only when the treatment itself is potentially hazardous, but even if there is no reason to suspect that the proposed treatment may be harmful in any way. In such instances treatment is discretionary; the patient may licitly decline treatment and rely exclusively upon divine providence. R. Emden declares that one who consistently abstains from such modes of therapy "and does not rely upon a human healer and his cure but leaves the matter in the hands of the trustworthy . . . Healer" is praiseworthy. R. Emden, an eighteenth century authority, himself believed that all medical procedures designed to cure internal afflictions were of the latter category. While R. Emden's position must undoubtedly be modified in the light of present-day medical knowledge, the underlying principle is entirely applicable. The patient is morally bound only with regard to the use of medicaments and procedures of demonstrated efficacy. Applying this principle, the patient may legitimately decline a drug or procedure whose curative powers are questionable. This is not to say that a moral obligation to seek a cure exists only if the physician is in a position to guarantee with certainty that a recovery will ensue. The examples given of demonstrable efficacy, viz., amputation of a limb or applications of salves and bandages, certainly are not of absolute curative power. Despite the most attentive medical ministrations, some patients do not recover. However, the procedures enumerated are of known value in treating certain afflictions and hence must be pursued. Nevertheless, drugs or surgical procedures whose causal efficacy is not known with certitude may be rejected by the patient. Experimental procedures, including those which are non-hazardous in nature, certainly fall within this category.

Although there is clear dispensation to intervene in physiological processes for purposes of effecting a cure, it does not follow that a physician may subject a patient to, or that a patient may voluntarily accept, a mode of therapy which involves an element of risk. The question of the moral propriety of hazardous procedures arises in three different contexts.

1. Situations in which the existing condition is such that if the patient is left untreated he will certainly succumb as a result of his illness.
2. Situations in which the prognosis is uncertain. In such cases, the patient, if not treated, or if treated by non-hazardous procedures, may or may not survive, whereas if treated, the hazards of the illness are replaced by the hazards of the treatment.
3. Situations in which the malady is not a life-threatening one, but treatment which is hazardous in nature is indicated as a means of relieving agony, discomfort or disfigurement.

It is a principle of Jewish law that the obligation to cure and to preserve life is not limited to situations in which it may be anticipated that subsequent to therapy the patient will have a normal life expectancy. As noted, the *Talmud, Yoma* 85a, clearly indicates that a victim trapped under the debris of a fallen wall is to be rescued even if as a result of such efforts his life will be prolonged only a matter of moments. Not only is every human life of infinite value, but every moment of human life is of infinite value. Accordingly, ritual restrictions such as Sabbath laws are suspended even for the most minimal prolongation of life.

However, when minimal duration of life (*chayyei sha'ah*) is weighed against the possibility of cure accompanied by normal life expectancy, Jewish teaching accepts the principle that reasonable risks may be incurred in order to effect a recovery. This is the case even if the proposed therapy is of such a nature that the drug or procedure may prove to be ineffective and the patient's life shortened thereby. Based upon Talmudic discussion, R. Meir Posner, *Bet Meir, Yoreh De'ah* 339:1 and R. Jacob Reisher, *Shevut Ya'akov*, III, n. 84,[24] specifically permit use of a hazardous drug which might cause death to result "within an hour or two" on behalf of a patient who would otherwise have lived for "a day or two days." Despite the brevity of the period of time which the patient might have been expected to live without therapy, *Shevut Ya'akov* mandated consultation with "proficient medical specialists in the city" and ruled that therapy was to be instituted only if the physicians recommended it by at least a majority of two to one. He further required that the approval of the local rabbinic authority be obtained before such recommendations are acted upon.

An apparent contradiction to this position is found in *Sefer Chasidim*, n. 467. This source describes a folk remedy consisting of "grasses" or herbs administered by "women" in treatment of certain maladies which either cured or killed the person so threatened within a period of days. *Sefer Chasidim* admonishes that they "will certainly be punished for they have killed a person before his time." R. Shlomo Mordechai Shwadron, *Orchot Chayyim, Orach Chayyim* 318:10, resolves this contradiction by stating that the instance discussed by *Sefer Chasidim* involved a situation in which there was clearly a possibility for cure without hazardous intervention. According to this analysis *Sefer Chasidim* set forth the commonsense approach that hazardous procedures dare not be instituted unless conventional, non-hazardous approaches have been exhausted.

In none of these sources does one find a discussion or a consideration of the statistical probability of prolonging life versus the mortality rate or the odds of shortening life. Yet certainly, in weighing the advisability of instituting hazardous therapy, the relative possibility of achieving a cure is a factor to be considered. *Bet David* II, n. 340, permits intervention even if there exists but one chance in a thousand that the proposed drug will be efficacious whereas there are nine hundred and ninety-nine chances that it will hasten the death of the patient. A differing view is presented by R. Joseph Hochgelerenter, *Mishnat Chakhamin,* who refuses to sanction hazardous therapy unless there is at least a fifty percent chance of survival.[25] He further requires, as did Shevut Ya'akov, that dispensation be obtained from ecclesiastical authorities on each occasion that such therapy is administered. Rabbi Moses Feinstein, a foremost contemporary authority, however, rules that, where in the absence of intervention death is imminent, a hazardous procedure may be instituted as long as there is a "slim" (*safek rachok*) chance of a cure, even though the chances of survival are "much less than even" and it is in fact almost certain that the patient will die.[26]

A much earlier authority, R. Moses Sofer, refused to sanction a hazardous procedure in which the chances of effecting a cure were "remote"[27] but offers no mathematical criteria with regard to the nature of mortality risks which may be properly assumed.

Tiferet Yisrael raises a quite different question in discussing the permissibility of prophylactic innoculations which are themselves hazardous. In the situation described, the patient, at the time of treatment, is at no risk whatsoever. The fear is that he will contact a potentially fatal disease, apparently smallpox. The innoculation, however, does carry with it a certain degree of immediate risk. *Tiferet Yisrael* justifies acceptance of the risk which he estimates as being "one in a thousand" because the statistical danger of future contagious infection is greater.[28]

At least one contemporary author differentiates between various cases on the basis of the nature of the risk involved, rather than on the basis of anticipated rates of survival. Rabbi Moshe Dov Welner[29] argues that hazardous procedures may be undertaken despite inherent risks only if therapeutic nature of the procedure has been demonstrated. For example, a situation might present itself which calls for administration of a drug with known curative potential but which is also toxic in nature. The efficacy of the drug is known but its toxicity may, under certain conditions, kill the patient. The drug may be administered in anticipation of a cure despite the known statistical risk, argues Rabbi Welner, could not be sanctioned in administering an experimental drug whose curative powers are unknown or have heretofore not been demonstrated.

A related problem is the attitude toward hazardous therapy for alleviation of pain or other symptoms rather than for the cure of a potentially fatal illness. R. Jacob Emden adopts a somewhat ambivalent position with respect to the question.[30] This authority refers specifically to the surgical removal of gall stones, a procedure designed to correct a condition which he viewed as presenting no hazard to life or health but recognized as being excruciatingly painful. He remarks that, in the absence of danger to life, those who submit to surgery "do not act correctly" and that the procedure is not "entirely permissible." R. Emden carefully stops short of branding the procedure sinful.

The permissibility of placing one's life in danger when not afflicted by a life-threatening malady does, however, require justification. The great value placed upon preservation of life augurs against placing oneself in a risk situation. In general, Jewish law teaches that man may not expose himself to danger. An entire section of the Code of Laws (*Yoreh De'ah* II, 116,) is devoted to an enumeration of actions and situations which must be avoided because they present an element of risk. One hypothesis which may be advanced in sanctioning risks undertaken in a medical context is that the verse "and he shall cause to be thoroughly healed" grants blanket dispensation for any sound medical practice. That such dispensation is included within the framework of this mandate may be demonstrated in the following manner: It is beyond dispute that an aggressor is liable for medical expenses even if the wound inflicted is not potentially lethal. It follows that the physician is permitted, and indeed obligated, to treat patients who suffer from afflictions which are not life-threatening. This is certainly the case when the treatment itself poses no danger. The sole question is with regard to justification of hazardous treatment on non-life-threatening afflictions.

Justification for this position may be found in statements of Nachmanides[31] and Rabbenu Nissim Gerondi.[32] These authorities both comment that all modes of therapy are potentially dangerous. In the words of Rabbenu Nissim, "All modes of therapy are a danger for the patient for it is possible that if the physician errs with regard to a specific drug, it will kill the patient." Nachmanides states even more explicitly, "With regard to cures there is naught but danger; what heals one kills another." Nevertheless, healing—even of non-life-threatening afflictions—is sanctioned by Scripture. Apparently then, since even therapy is fraught with danger, the hazards of treatment are specifically sanctioned when incurred in conjunction with a therapeutic protocol. Accordingly, the practice of the healing arts, despite the hazards involved, cannot be branded as sinful even if designed simply for the alleviation of pain.

Utilizations of medical procedures which are ordinary and usual but which carry with them an element of risk may perhaps be justified on other grounds as well. The Talmud in a variety of instance[33] indicates that a person may engage in commonplace activities even though he places himself in a position of danger on doing so. In justifying such conduct the Talmud declares, "Since many have trodden thereon 'the Lord preserveth the simple'" (Ps. 116:6). The principle enunciated in this dictum is that man is justified in placing his trust in God provided that the risk involved is of a type which is commonly accepted as a reasonable one by society at large. It may readily be argued that any accepted therapeutic procedure may be classified in this manner.[34]

The physician may withhold otherwise mandatory treatment only when the patient has reached the state of gesisah, i.e. the patient has become moribund and death is imminent. Jewish laws with regard to care of the dying are spelled out with care and precision. One must not pry his jaws, anoint him, wash him, plug his orifices, remove the pillow from underneath him or place on the ground.[35] It is also forbidden to close his eyes "for whoever closes the eyes with the onset of death is a shedder of blood."[36] Each of these acts is forbidden because the slightest movement of the patient may hasten death. As the Talmud puts it, "The matter may be compared to a flickering flame: as soon as one touches it, the light is extinguished."[37] Accordingly, any movement or manipulation of the dying person is forbidden.

Although euthanasia in any form is forbidden and the hastening of death even by a matter of moment is regarded as tantamount to murder, there is one situation in which treatment may be withheld from the moribund patient in order to provide an unimpeded death. While the death of a goses may not be speeded, there is no obligation to perform any action which will lengthen the life of the patient in this state. The distinction between an active and a passive act applies to a goses and to a goses only. When a patient is, as it were, actually in the clutches of the angel of death and the death process has actually begun, there is no obligation to heal. Therefore, Rema permits the removal of "anything which constitutes a hindrance to the departure of the soul, such as a clattering noise or salt upon his tongue . . . since such acts involve no active hastening of death but only the removal of the impediment."[38] Some authorities not only sanction withholding of treatment but prohibit any action which may prolong the agony of a goses.[39]

It cannot be overemphasized that even acts of omission are permitted only when the patient is in a state of gesisah. At any earlier stage withholding of treatment is tantamount to euthanasia. What are the criteria indicative of the onset of this state? Rema defines this state as being that of the patient who brings up a secretion in his throat on account of the narrowing of his chest."[40] Of course, if the condition is reversible there is an obligation to heal. When the condition of gesisah is irreversible there is no obligation to continue treatment and according to some authorities, even a prohibition against prolonging the life of the moribund patient.

It appears that this state is not determined by a patient's ability to survive solely by natural means for this period unaided by drugs or medication. The implication is that goses is one who cannot, under any circumstances, be maintained alive for a period of seventy-two hours. Testimony with regard to the existence of a state of gesisah as conclusive evidence of impending death implies that the state is not only irreversible but also prolongable even by artificial means. Otherwise there would exist a legal suspicion that life may have been prolonged artificially by means of extraordinary medical treatment. The obvious conclusion to be drawn is that if it medically feasible to prolong life the patient is indeed not a goses and, therefore, in such instances there is a concomitant obligation to preserve the life of the patient as long as possible.

It follows that a specific physiological condition may or may not correspond to a state of gesisah depending upon the state of medical knowledge of the day. When medicine is of no avail and the patient will expire within seventy-two hours, he is deemed to be in the process of "dying." When, however, medication can prolong life such medicine, in effect, delays the onset of the death process. Accordingly, the patient who receives medical treatment enabling him to survive for a period of three days or more is not yet in the process of "dying." It follows, therefore, that those responsible for his care are not relieved of their duty to minister to his needs and to postpone the onset of death by means of medical treatment.

The aggressiveness with which Judaism teaches that life must be preserved is not at all incompatible with the awareness that the human condition is such that there are circumstances in which man would prefer death to life. The Talmud reports[41] that Rabbi Judah the Prince, redactor of the *Mishnah*, was afflicted by what appears to have been an incurable intestinal disorder and as a result suffered from an apparently debilitating form of dysentery. R. Judah had a female servant who is depicted in rabbinic writings as being a woman of exemplary piety and moral character. This woman is reported to have prayed for the death of R. Judah. On the basis of this narrative, a thirteenth century commentator, Rabbenu Nissim Gerondi[42] states that it is permissible and even praiseworthy to pray for the death of a patient who is gravely ill and in extreme pain. He chides those who are remiss in discharging the obligation of visiting the sick, remarking of such an individual ". . . not only does he not aid [the patient] in living but even when [the patient] would [derive] benefit from death, even that small benefit [prayer for his demise] he does not bestow upon him."

The gift of life, bestowed by God, can be reclaimed only by Him. Man dare not push the divine hand, so to speak, through an overt action but may, through prayer, presume to tell God what to do.

There is one responsum in particular which deals with the question of prayer for termination of suffering through death, but which has important implications for decision making in general. R. Chaim Palaggi, *Chikekei Lev*, I, *Yoreh De'ah*, n. 50, accepts the view of Rabbenu Nissim but expresses an important laveat. According to this authority only totally disinterested parties may lead to a premature termination of life. Husband, children, family, and those charged with the care of the patient, according to R. Palaggi, may not pray for death. The considerations underlying this reservation are twofold in nature. (1) Those who are emotionally involved, if they are permitted even such nonphysical methods of intervention as prayer, may be prompted to perform an overt act which would have the effect of shortening life and thus be tantamount to euthanasia; (2) Precisely because of their closeness to the situation they are psychologically incapable of reaching a detached, dispassionate and objective opinion in which considerations of patient benefit are the sole controlling motives. The human psyche is such that the intrusion of emotional involvement and subjective interest preclude a totally objective and disinterested decision.

Decisions that are available therapeutic methods shall not be employed because they are hazardous or of insufficiently demonstrated efficacy or a decision that the patient is already in a state of gesisah are also subject to unconscious bias because of the inability of the family and physician totally to transcend their personal and emotional involvement with the patient. It is entirely in keeping with these considerations that Jewish scholars have insisted that the pertinent facts be placed before a rabbinic decision for adjudication on a case by case basis.

The thrust of the material which has been presented argues in favor of aggressive treatment of defective newborns regardless of the extent of their impairment or the quality of life which may be conserved by such treatment. It is unlikely that its impact upon these physicians who, to a greater or lesser extent, practice selective nontreatment on a routine basis will be sufficiently strong to effect a dramatic volteface. Nevertheless, this modest effort will have achieved a modicum of success if those engaged in the practice of medicine become sensitized to the issues which have been raised and achieve an awareness of the existence of a rich theological and ethical tradition which cannot acquiesce, much less sanction, the current practice of many physicians.

When analyzing treatment versus nontreatment, informed consent, if it is to be fully informed, should entail an awareness on the part of the person granting consent not only of the medical hazards involved but also of the moral dilemmas present in such a decision. The patient or next of kin should be fully informed with regard to conflicting medical opinion and counsel; He should be equally aware of moral traditions which conflict with a course of action advocated by the medical practitioners. The physician seeking consent is bound in conscience to be absolutely certain that the patient of next of kin is fully informed, both medically and morally.

The rabbinic tradition was fully cognizant of these factors in its insistence upon multiple medical consultation and in its demand that the medical data be placed before a competent rabbinic authority prior to initiation of hazardous therapy or withholding of life-supporting measures. The rabbi served as an ethicist, a qualified expert capable of dispassionate examination of the data and of reaching a determination based upon the ethical principle of his moral tradition.

The rabbi-ethicist presents a role model which might be emulated by society with great moral profit. A qualified and professionally trained ethicist could be an invaluable addition to the hospital staff. In a pluralistic society the ethicist would most emphatically not serve as a decision maker. He would, however, be singularly qualified to analyze and interpret the medical information upon which decision making is based so the patient and his family would be in a position to make an informed medical decision. He would be available to analyze and discuss any moral issues which might be confronted in making such decisions. The ethicist's position would be that of analyst and discussant—not that of advisor. The information transmitted by a trained ethicist in an objective and impartial manner would enable the patient and his family to turn to their own moral and spiritual counselors, if they should desire to do so, for advice consonant with their own religious traditions. The inclusion of an ethicist as a member of the health care team would assure that the decision reached is both a medically and morally informed decision.

NOTES

1. Sanhedrin 37a.
2. Yoreh De'ah 157:1.
3. Orach Chayyim 329:3.
4. See R. Yechiel Michal Tucatzinsky, *The Death Penalty According to the Torah in the Past and the Present*, Ha-Torah ve-ha-Medinah 2 IV, 34 (1952) and V–VI 331–334 (1953–1954).
5. Orach Chayyim 329:4.
6. See Hamburger, Real-Encyclopaedie fur Bibel und Talmud, Supplement II 37 (1901); Zimmels, Magicians, Theologians and Doctors 172 n. 72 (1952).
7. It is of interest to compare this view with that of Martin Luther who refused to baptize deformed children and who declared that they ought to be drowned because they have no soul. See McKenzie, *The Infancy of Medicine: An Enquiry into the Influence of Folklore Upon the Evolution of Scientific Medicine* 313 (1927).

8. Sanhedrin 73a.

9. See Allbutt, Greek Medicine in Rome 402 (1921).

10. See Abraham Ibn Ezra, Commentary on the Bible, ad locum.

11. See A. Harkavy, Likutei Kadmoniyot II, 148 (1903); Harry Friedenwald, The Jews and Medicine 9 (1944).

12. See commentaries of Tosafot and Rashba, ad locum.

13. Commentary on the Mishnah, Nedarim 4:4; cf. Maimonides, Mishneh Torah, Hilkhot Nedarim 6:8.

14. Cf. R. Barukh Ha-Levi Epstein, Torah Temimah, Exodus 21:19 and Deuteronomy 22:2. This explanation of Maimonides' apparent contradiction of the Talmudic text as well as the comments of Torah Temimah contradict Jakobivits' statement to the effect that Maimonides' system does not require biblical sanction for the practice of medicine. See Immanuel Jackobovits, *Jewish Medical Ethics* 260 n. 8 (1959). See infra note 83.

15. Yoreh De'ah 336:1. See Eliezer Waldenberg, *Ramat Rachel* no. 21 and id. *Tritz Eliezer* X, n. 25, chap. 7.

16. Nachmanides, Torah Ha-Adam, Kitvei Ramban II, 43 (B. Cheval ed. 5724).

17. Waldenberg, Ramat Rachel n. 21.

18. Ibn Ezra, *supra note* 67, Exodus 21:19.

19. R. Zemach Duran, Teshuvot Tashbatz I, n. 51. Nevertheless Ibn Ezra's interpretation of Exodus 21:19 is followed by the fourteenth-century biblical exegete, Rabbenu Bachya, in his commentary on that passage and R. Johnathan Eybeschutz, Kereiti U-Peleiti, Tiferet Yisra'El, Yoreh De'Ah 188:5.

20. Maimonides, Guide of the Perplexed III, chaps. 17–18.

21. This appears to be the manner in which Nachmanides was interpreted by R. David Ben Shmuel Ha-Levi, Taz, Yoreh De'Ah 336:1; see also R. Eliyahu Dessler, Mikhtav Mei-Eliyahu III, 170–175 (5725) and Waldenberg, supra note 74, n. 20, 3.

22. See Bachya Ibn Pakuda, Chovat Ha-Levavot, Sha'Ar Ha-Bitachon chap. 4; R. Simon Ben Zemach Duran, Teshuvot Tashbatz III, n. 82; R. Joel Serkes, Bayit Chadash, Yoreh De'Ah 336: R. Abraham Gumbiner, Magen Avraham, Orach Chayyim 328:6; R. Moses Sofer, Teshuvot Chatam Sofer, Orach Chayyim n. 176; Besamim Rosh n. 386; R. Ya'akov Ettlinger, Binyan Zion n. 111; R. Nissim Abraham Ashkenazi, Ma'Aseh Avraham, Yoreh De'Ah n. 55; R. Nathan Nate Landau, Kenaf Renanah, Orach Chayyim n. 60; R. Ovadiah Yosef, Yabi'a Omer, IV, Choshen Mishpat n. 6, 4; R. Moses Ben Abraham Mat, Matteh Mosheh IV, chap. 3; R. Samson Morpug, Shemesh Tzdakah, Yoreh De'Ah n. 29; R. Chaim Yosef David Azulai, Birkei Yosef, Yoreh De'Ah 336:2; R. Yehudah Eyash, Shivtei Yehudah n. 336; Waldenberg supra note 74 n. 20; id. tzitz Eli'ezer IX, n. 17, chap. 6, 17; X, n. 25, chap. 19; XI, n. 41, chap. 20; R. Ya'Akov Prager, Sheilat Ya-Akov n. 5.

23. See R. Abraham Danzig, Chokhmat Adam 141:25.

24. See also Ettlinger, supra note 82; Waldenberg, supra note 82, IV, n. 13; R. Israel Lipshitz, Tiferet Yisrael, YOMA, 8:41; R. Shlomo Eger, Gilyon Maharsha, Yoreh De'Ah 155:1.

25. This is also the position of Waldenberg, supra note 82, X, n. 25, chap. 5, 5. Cf. R. Chaim Ozer Grodzinski, Teshuvot Achi'Ezer, Yoreh De'Ah n. 16, 8.

26. Igrot Moshe, Yoreh De'Ah II, n. 58.

27. Teshuvot Chatam Sofer, Yoreh De'Ah n. 76.

28. Bo'Az, Yoma 8:3.

29. Ha-Torah Ve-Ha-Medinah VII–VIII, 314 (1956–1957).

30. R. Jacob Embden, Mor U-Ketziah, Orach Chayyim 338.

31. Nachmanides, supra note 73.

32. Rabbenu Nissim Gerondi, Commentary to Sanhedrin 84b.

33. Shabbat 128b; Avodah Zarah 30b; Niddah 31a; & Yevamot 72a.

34. Cf. R. Ya'Akov Breish, Chelkat Ya'Akov III, n. 11.

35. Yoreh De'Ah 339:1.

36. Id.
37. Shabbat 151b: & Semachot 1:4.
38. Yoreh De'Ah 339:1.
39. Teshuvot Bet Ya'Akov n. 59; Moshe, supra note 86, II, n. 174; cf. also R. Moses Isserles, Darkei Mosheh, Yoreh De'Ah 339; however, Shevut Ya'Akov I, n. 13, Bi'Ur Halakhah, Orach Chayyim 329:2; and Waldenberg, supra note 74, n. 28, see no prohibition against prolonging the life of a goses; the latter two authorities view prolongation by means of accepted medical treatment as obligatory.
40. Even Ha'Ezer 121:7 and Choshen Mishpat 221:2.
41. Ketubot 104a.
42. Rabbenu Nissim Gerondi, Commentary to Nedarim 40a.

Roman Catholic moral theology also has a long history of interest in medical ethics. Like Judaism its medical ethic is derived from its systematic theological commitments. As such, it may not always be compatible with the Hippocratic tradition. Moreover, its source of authority is more appropriately the church authority rather than medical authority. There are centuries of writings articulating positions within Catholicism on classical moral dilemmas including not only abortion and contraception, but also the care of the terminally ill and all other categories of medical problems. In the selection that follows, a code of ethics adopted by the United States Catholic Conference demonstrates many of the classical Catholic positions including the doctrine of double effect, the distinction between ordinary and extraordinary means, and the criterion of proportionality.

Ethical and Religious Directives for Catholic Health Facilities

PREAMBLE

Catholic health facilities witness to the saving presence of Christ and His church in a variety of ways: by testifying to transcendent spiritual beliefs concerning life, suffering, and death; by humble service to humanity and especially to the poor; by medical competence and leadership; and by fidelity to the Church's teachings while ministering to the good of the whole person.

The total good of the patient, which includes his higher spiritual as well as his bodily welfare, is the primary concern of those entrusted with the management of a Catholic health facility. So important is this, in fact, that if an institution could not fulfill its basic mission in this regard, it would have no justification for continuing its existence as a Catholic health facility. Trustees and administrators of Catholic health facilities should understand that this responsibility affects their relationship with every patient, regardless of religion, and is seriously binding in conscience.

A Catholic-sponsored health facility, its board of trustees, and administration face today a serious difficulty as, with community support, the Catholic health facility exists side by side with other medical facilities not committed to the same moral code, or stands alone as the one facility serving the community. However the health facility identified as Catholic exists today and serves the community in a large part because of the past dedication and sacrifice of countless individuals whose lives have been inspired by the Gospel and the teachings of the Catholic Church.

And just as it bears responsibility to the past, so does the Catholic health facility carry special responsibility for the present and future. Any facility identified as Catholic assumes with this identification the responsibility to reflect in its policies and practices the moral teachings of the Church, under the guidance of the local bishop. Within the community the Catholic health facility is needed as a courageous witness to the highest ethical and moral principles in its pursuit of excellence.

The Catholic-sponsored health facility and its board of trustees, acting through its chief executive officer, further, carry an overriding responsibility in conscience to prohibit those procedures which are morally and spiritually harmful. The basic norms delineating this moral responsibility are listed in these Ethical and Religious Directives for Catholic Health Facilities. It should be understood that patients and those who accept board membership, staff appointment or privileges, or employment in a Catholic health facility will respect and agree to abide by its policies and these Directives. Any attempt to use a Catholic health facility for procedures contrary to these norms would indeed compromise the board and administration in its responsibility to seek and protect the total good of its patients, under the guidance of the Church.

The Directives prohibit those procedures which, according to present knowledge, are recognized as clearly wrong. The basic moral absolutes which underlie these Directives are not subject to change, although particular applications might be modified as scientific investigation and theological development open up new problems or cast new light on old ones.

In addition to consultations among theologians, physicians, and other medical and scientific personnel in local areas, The Committees on Health Affairs of the United States Catholic Conference, with the widest consultation possible, should regularly receive suggestions and recommendations from the field, and should periodically discuss any possible need for an updated revision of these Directives.

The moral evaluation of new scientific developments and legitimately debated questions must be finally submitted to the teaching authority of the Church in the person of the local bishop, who has the ultimate responsibility for teaching Catholic doctrine.

SECTION I: ETHICAL AND RELIGIOUS DIRECTIVES

1. General

Directive

1. The procedures listed in these Directives as permissible require the consent at least implied or reasonably presumed, of the patient or his guardians. This condition is to be understood in all cases.

2. No person may be obliged to take part in a medical or surgical procedure which he judges in conscience to be immoral; nor may a health facility or any of its staff be obliged to provide a medical or surgical procedure which violates their conscience or these directives.

3. Every patient, regardless of the extent of his physical or psychic disability, has a right to be treated with a respect consonant with his dignity as a person.

4. Man has the right and the duty to protect the integrity of his body together with all of its bodily functions.

5. Any procedure potentially harmful to the patient is morally justified only insofar as it is designed to produce a proportionate good.

6. Ordinarily the proportionate good that justifies a medical or surgical procedure should be the total good of the patient himself.

7. Adequate consultation is recommended, not only where there is doubt concerning the morality of some procedure, but also with regard to all procedures involving serious consequences, even though such procedures are listed here as permissible. The health facility has the right to insist on such consultations.

8. Everyone has the right and the duty to prepare for the solemn moment of death. Unless it is clear, therefore, that a dying patient is already well-prepared for death as regards both spiritual and temporal affairs, it is the physician's duty to inform him of his critical condition or to have some other responsible person impart this information.

9. The obligation of professional secrecy must be carefully fulfilled not only as regards the information on the patient's charts and records but also as regards confidential matters learned in the exercise of professional duties. Moreover, the charts and records must be duly safeguarded against inspection by those who have no right to see them.

10. The indirectly intended termination of any patient's life, even at his own request, is always morally wrong.

11. From the moment of conception, life must be guarded with the greatest care. Any deliberate medical procedure, the purpose of which is to deprive a fetus or an embryo of its life, is immoral.

12. Abortion, that is, the directly intended termination of pregnancy before viability, is never permitted nor is the directly intended destruction of a viable fetus. Every procedure whose sole immediate effect is the termination of pregnancy before viability is an abortion, which, in its moral context, includes the interval between conception and the implantation of the embryo.

13. Operations, treatments, and medications, which do not directly intend termination of pregnancy but which have as their purpose the cure of a proportionately serious pathological condition of the mother, are permitted when they cannot be safely postponed until the fetus is viable, even though they may or will result in the death of the fetus. If the fetus is not certainly dead, it should be baptized.

14. Regarding the treatment of hemorrhage during pregnancy and before the fetus is viable: Procedures that are designed to empty the uterus of a living fetus still effectively attached to the mother are not permitted; procedures designed to stop hemorrhage (as distinguished from those designed precisely to expel the living and attached fetus) are permitted insofar as necessary, even if fetal death is inevitably a side effect.

15. Cesarean section for the removal of a viable fetus is permitted, even with risk to the life of the mother, when necessary for successful delivery. It is likewise permitted, even with risk to the child, when necessary for the safety of the mother.

16. In extrauterine pregnancy the dangerously affected part of the mother (e.g., cervix, ovary, or fallopian tube) may be removed, even though fetal death is foreseen, provided that:
    (a) the affected part is presumed already to be so damaged and dangerously affected as to warrant its removal, and that
    (b) the operation is not just a separation of the embryo or fetus from its site within the part (which would be a direct abortion from a uterine appendage), and that
    (c) The operation cannot be postponed without notably increasing the danger to the mother.

17. Hysterectomy, in the presence of pregnancy and even before viability, is permitted when directed to the removal of a dangerous pathological condition of the uterus of such serious nature that the operation cannot be safely postponed until the fetus is viable.

2. Procedures Involving Reproductive Organs and Functions

18. Sterilization, whether permanent or temporary for men or for women, may not be used as a means of contraception.

19. Similarly excluded is every action which, either in anticipation of the conjugal act, or in its accomplishment, or in the development of its natural consequences, proposes, whether as an end or as a means, to render procreation impossible.

20. Procedures that induce sterility, whether permanent or temporary, are permitted when: (a) they are immediately directed to the cure, diminution, or prevention of a serious pathological condition and are not directly contraceptive

(that is, contraception is not the purpose); and (b) a simple treatment is not reasonably available. Hence, for example, oophorectomy or irradiation of the ovaries may be allowed in treating carcinoma of the breast and metastatis therefrom; and orchidectomy is permitted in the treatment of carcinoma of the prostate.

21. Because the ultimate personal expression of conjugal love in the marital act is viewed as the only fitting context for the human sharing of the divine act of creation, donor insemination and insemination that is totally artificial are morally objectionable. However, help may be given to a normally performed conjugal act to attain its purpose. The use of the sex faculty outside the legitimate use by married partners is never permitted even for medical or other laudable purpose, e.g., masturbation as a means of obtaining seminal specimens.

22. Hysterectomy is permitted when it is sincerely judged to be a necessary means of removing some serious uterine pathological condition. In these cases, the pathological condition of each patient must be considered individually and care must be taken that a hysterectomy is not performed merely as a contraceptive measure, or as a routine procedure after any definite number of Cesarean section.

23. For a proportionate reason, labor may be induced after the fetus is viable.

24. In all cases in which the presence of pregnancy would render some procedure illicit (e.g., curettage), the physician must make use of such pregnancy tests and consultation as may be needed in order to be reasonably certain that the patient is not pregnant. It is to be noted that curettage of the endometrium after rape to prevent implantation of a possible embyro is morally equivalent to abortion.

25. Radiation therapy of the mother's reproductive organs is permitted during pregnancy only when necessary to suppress a dangerous pathological condition.

3. Other Procedures

26. Therapeutic procedures which are likely to be dangerous are morally justifiable for proportionate reasons.

27. Experimentation on patients without due consent is morally objectionable, and even the moral right of the patient to consent is limited by his duties of stewardship.

28. Euthanasia ("mercy killing") in all its forms is forbidden. The failure to supply the ordinary means of preserving life is equivalent to euthanasia. However, neither the physician nor the patient is obliged to use extraordinary means.

29. It is not euthanasia to give a dying person sedatives or analgesics for the alleviation of pain, when such a measure is judged necessary, even though they may deprive the patient of the use of reason, or shorten his life.

30. The transplantation of organs from living donors is morally permissible when the anticipated benefit to the recipient is proportionate to the harm done to the donor, provided that the loss of such organ(s) does not deprive the donor of life itself nor of the functional integrity of his body.

31. Post-mortem examinations must not begin until death is morally certain. Vital organs, that is, organs necessary to sustain life, may not be removed until death has taken place. The determination of the time of death must be made in accordance with responsible and commonly accepted scientific criteria. In accordance with current medical practice, to prevent any conflict of interest, the dying patient's doctor or doctors should ordinarily be distinct from the transplant team.

32. Ghost surgery, which implies the calculated deception of the patient as to the identity of the operating surgeon, is morally objectionable.

33. Unnecessary procedures, whether diagnostic or therapeutic, are morally objectionable. A procedure is unnecessary when no proportionate reason justifies. A procedure is unnecessary when no proportionate reason justifies it. A fortiori, any procedure that is contra-indicated by sound medical standards is unnecessary.

SECTION II: THE RELIGIOUS CARE OF PATIENTS

34. The administration should be certain that patients in a health facility receive appropriate spiritual care.

35. Except in cases of emergency (i.e., danger of death), all requests for baptism made by adults or for infants should be referred to the chaplain of the health facility.

36. If a priest is not available, anyone having the use of reason and proper intention can baptize. The ordinary method of conferring emergency baptism is as follows: the person baptizing pours water on the head in such a way that it will flow on the skin, and, while the water is being poured, must pronounce these words audibly: I baptize you in the name of the Father, and of the Son, and of the Holy Spirit. The same person who pours the water must pronounce the words.

37. When emergency baptism is conferred, the chaplain should be notified.

38. It is the mind of the Church that the sick should have the widest possible liberty to receive the sacraments frequently. The generous cooperation of the entire staff and personnel is requested for this purpose.

39. While providing the sick abundant opportunity to receive Holy Communion, there should be no interference with the freedom of the faithful to communicate or not to communicate.

40. In wards and semi-private rooms, every effort should be made to provide sufficient privacy for confession.

41. Special care and concern should be shown that those who are seriously ill or are dangerously ill due to sickness or old age receive the Sacrament of Anoint-

ing. A prudent or probable judgment about the seriousness of the sickness is sufficient. If necessary a doctor may be consulted, although there should be no reason for scruples.

A sick person should be anointed before surgery whenever a dangerous illness is the reason for the surgery. Old people may be anointed if they are in weak condition although no dangerous illness is present. Sick children may be anointed if they have sufficient use of reason to be comforted by this sacrament.

The sacrament may be repeated if the sick person recovers after anointing or, during the same illness, the danger becomes more serious.

Normally the sacrament is celebrated when the sick person is fully conscious. It may be conferred upon the sick who have lost consciousness or the use of reason, if, as Christian believers, they would have asked for it if they were in control of their faculties.

41a.   All baptized Christians who can receive communion are bound to receive viaticum. Those in danger of death from any cause are obliged to receive communion. The administration of this sacrament is not to be delayed for the faithful are to be nourished by it while still in full possession of their faculties.

41b.   For special cases, when sudden illness or some other cause has unexpectedly placed one of the faithful in danger of death, the continuous rite should be used by which the sick person may be given the sacraments of penance, anointing, and eucharist as viaticum in one service.

42.   Personnel of a Catholic health facility should make every effort to satisfy the spiritual needs and desires of non-Catholics. Therefore, in hospitals and similar institutions conducted by Catholics, the authorities in charge should, with the consent of the patient, promptly advise ministers of other communions of the presence of their communicants and afford them every facility for visiting the sick and giving them spiritual and sacramental ministrations.

43.   If there is a reasonable cause present for not burying a fetus or member of the human body, these may be cremated in a manner consonant with the dignity of the deceased human body.

REFERENCES

Final paragraph of the Preamble: Vatican II *Constitution on the Church,* #27.
Directive
3.   *Pacem in Terris,* n. 11.
11.   Vatican II: *The Church in the Modern World,* n. 51.
18.   *Humanae Vitae,* n. 14.
19.   *Humanae Vitae,* n. 14.
20.   *Humanae Vitae,* n. 15.
28.   Vatican II: *The Church in the Modern World,* n. 27.
42.   Directory for the Application of the Decisions of the Second Ecumenical Council of the Vatican Concerning Ecumenical Matters, n. 63.
43.   *Canon Law Digest,* Vol. 6, p. 669.

Protestants reflect very great diversity in their ethical and religious positions. As such it is difficult to identify any one representative Protestant medical ethic. Part of the core commitment of Protestantism is a respect for the lay person's capacity to develop and articulate his or her own moral and religious positions. On any given issue there can be a wide range of often conflicting views.

While positions vary tremendously, there is a common orientation and method shared by many working explicitly within the Protestant context. The following essay by Paul Ramsey, a former professor of religion at Princeton and Protestant scholar, is taken from the preface to his pioneering book, *The Patient as Person*. It traces key Protestant themes—covenant fidelity, faithfulness defined by covenant, the role of all, including lay persons, in decisions, and the uniqueness of the religious perspective.

The Patient as Person

Paul Ramsey

The problems of medical ethics that are especially urgent in the present day . . . are by no means technical problems on which only the expert (in this case, the physician) can have an opinion. They are rather the problems of human beings in situations in which medical care is needed. Birth and death, illness and injury are not simply events the doctor attends. They are moments in every human life. The doctor makes decisions as an expert but also as a man among men; and his patient is a human being coming to his birth or to his death, or being rescued from illness or injury in between.

Therefore, the doctor who attends *the case* has reason to be attentive to the patient as person. Resonating throughout his professional actions, and crucial in some of them, will be a view of man, an understanding of the meaning of the life at whose first or second exodus he is present, a care for the life he attends in its afflictions. In this respect the doctor is quite like the rest of us, who must yet depend wholly on him to diagnose the options, perhaps the narrow range of options, and to conduct us through the one that is taken.

To take up for scrutiny some of the problems of medical ethics is, therefore, to bring under examination at once a number of crucial human moral problems. These are not narrowly defined issues of medical ethics alone. Thus this volume has—if I may say so—the widest possible audience. It is addressed to patients as persons, to physicians of patients who are persons—in short, to everyone who has had or will have to do with disease or death. The question, What ought the doctor to do? is only a particular form of the question, What should be done?

This, then, is a book *about ethics,* written by a Christian ethicist. I hold that medical ethics is consonant with the ethics of a wider human community. The former is (however special) only a particular case of the latter. The moral requirements governing the relations of physician to patients and researcher to subjects are only a special case of the moral requirements governing any relations between man and man. Canons of loyalty to patients or to joint adventurers in medical research are simply particular manifestations of canons of loyalty of person to person generally. Therefore, in the following chapters I undertake to explore a number of medical covenants among men. These are the covenant between physician and patient, the covenant between researcher and "subject" in experiments with human beings, the covenant between men and a child in need of care, the covenant between the living and the dying, the covenant between the well and the ill or with those in need of some extraordinary therapy.

We are born within covenants of life with life. By nature, choice, or need we live with our fellowmen in roles or relations. Therefore we must ask, What is the meaning of the *faithfulness* of one human being to another in every one of these relations? This is the ethical question.

At crucial points in the analysis of medical ethics, I shall not be embarrassed to use as an interpretative principle the Biblical norm of *fidelity to covenant,* with the meaning it gives to *righteousness* between man and man. This is not a very prominent feature in the pages that follow since it is also necessary for an ethicist to go as far as possible into the technical and other particular aspects of the problems he ventures to take up. Also, in the midst of any of these urgent human problems, an ethicist finds that he has been joined—whether in agreement or with some disagreement—by men of various persuasions, often quite different ones. There is in actuality a community of moral discourse concerning the claims of persons. This is the main appeal in the pages that follow.

Still we should be clear about the moral and religious premises here at the outset. I hold with Karl Barth that covenant-fidelity is the inner meaning and purpose of our creation as human beings, while the whole of creation is the external basis and condition of the possibility of covenant. This means that the conscious acceptance of covenant responsibilities is the inner meaning of even the "natural" or systemic relations or roles we enter by choice, while this fabric provides the external framework for human fulfillment in explicit covenants among men. The practice of medicine is one such covenant. *Justice, fairness, righteousness, faithfulness, canons of loyalty, the sanctity of life, hesed, agape or charity* are some of the names given to the moral quality of attitude and of action owed to all men by any man who steps into a covenant with another man—by any man who, so far as he is a religious man, explicitly acknowledges that we are a covenant people on a common pilgrimage.

The chief aim of the chapters to follow is, then, simply to explore the meaning of *care,* to find the actions and abstentions that come from adherence to *covenant,* to ask the meaning of the *sanctity* of life, to articulate the requirements of steadfast *faithfulness* to a fellow man. We shall ask, What are the moral claims upon us in crucial medical situations and human relations in which some decision must be made about how to show respect for, protect, preserve, and honor the life of fellow man?

Just as man is a *sacredness in the social and political order,* so he is a *sacredness in the natural, biological order.* He is a sacredness in bodily life. He is a person who within the ambience of the flesh claims our care. He is an embodied soul or ensouled body. He is therefore a sacredness in illness and in his dying. He is a sacredness in the fruits of the generative processes. (From some point he is this if he has any sanctity, since it is undeniably the case that men are never more than, from generation to generation, the products of human generation.) The sanctity of human life prevents ultimate trespass upon him even for the sake of treating his bodily life, or for the sake of others who are also only a sacredness in their bodily lives. Only a being who is a sacredness in the social order can withstand complete dominion by "society" for the sake of engineering civilizational goals—withstand, in the sense that the engineering of civilizational goals cannot be accomplished without denying the sacredness of the human being. So also in the use of medical or scientific techniques.

It is of first importance that this be understood, since we live in an age in which *hesed* (steadfast love) has become *maybe* and the "sanctity" of human life has been reduced to the ever more reducible motion of the "dignity" of human life. The latter is a sliver of a shield in comparison with the awesome respect required of men in all their dealings with men if man has a touch of sanctity in this his fetal, mortal, bodily, living and dying life.

Today someone is likely to say: "Another 'semanticism' which is somewhat of an argument-stopper has to do with the sacredness of inviolability of the individual."[1] If such a principle is asserted in gatherings of physicians, it is likely to be met with another argument-stopper: It is immoral not to do research (or this experiment must be done despite its necessary deception of human beings). This is then a standoff of contrary moral judgments or intuitions or commitments.

The next step may be for someone to say that medical advancement is hampered because our "society" makes an absolute of the inviolability of the individual. This raises the spectre of a medical and scientific community freed from the shackles of that cultural norm, and proceeding upon the basis of an ethos all its own. Alternatively, the next move may for someone to say: Our major task is to reconcile the welfare of the individual with the welfare of mankind; both must be served. This, indeed, is the principal task of medical ethics. However, there is no "unseen hand" guaranteeing that, for example, *good* experimental designs will always be morally *justifiable.* It is better not to begin with the laissez-faire assumption that the rights of men and the needs of future progress are always reconcilable. Indeed, the contrary assumption may be more salutary.

Several statements of this viewpoint may well stand as mottos over all that follows in this volume. "In the end we may have to accept the fact that some limits do exist to the search for knowledge."[2] "The end does not always justify the means, and the good things a man does can be made complete only by the things he refuses to do."[3] "There may be valuable scientific knowledge which it is morally impossible to obtain. There may be truths which would be of great and lasting benefit to mankind if they could be discovered, but which cannot be discovered without systematic and sustained violation of legitimate moral imperatives. It may be necessary to choose between knowledge and morality, in opposition to our long-standing prejudice that the two must go together."[4] "To justify whatever practice we think is technically demanded by showing that we are doing it for a good end . . . is both the best defense and the last refuge of a scoundrel."[5] "A[n experimental] study is ethical or not in its inception; it does not become ethical or not because it turned up valuable data."[6] These are salutary warnings precisely because by them we are driven to make the most searching inquiry concerning more basic ethical principles governing medical practice.

Because physicians deal with life and death, health and maiming, they cannot avoid being conscious or deliberate in their ethics to some degree. However, it is important to call attention to the fact that medical ethics cannot remain at the level of surface intuitions or in an impasse of conversation-stoppers. At this point there can be no other resort than to ethical theory—as that elder statesman of medical ethics, Dr. Chauncey D. Leake, Professor of Pharmacology at the University of California Medical Center, San Francisco, so often reminds us. At this point physicians must in greater measure become moral philosophers, asking themselves some quite profound questions about the nature of proper moral reasoning, and how moral dilemmas are rightly to be resolved. If they do not, the existing medical ethics will be eroded more and more by what it is alleged *must* be done and technically *can* be done.

In the medical literature there are many articles on ethics which are greatly to be admired. Yet I know that these are not part of the daily fare of medical students, or of members of the profession when they gather together as professionals or even for purposes of conviviality. I do not believe that either the codes of medical ethics or the physicians who have undertaken to comment on them and to give fresh analysis of the physician's moral decisions will suffice to withstand the omnivorous appetite of scientific research or of a therapeutic technology that has a momentum and a life of its own.

The Nuremberg Code, The Declaration of Helsinki, various "guidelines" of the American Medical Association, and other "codes" governing medical practice constitute a sort of "catechism" in the ethics of the medical profession. These codes exhibit a professional ethics which ministers and theologians and members of other professions can only profoundly respect and admire. Still, a catechism never sufficed. Unless these principles are constantly pondered and enlivened in their application they become dead letters. There is also need that these principles be deepened and sensitized and opened to further humane revision in face of all the ordinary and the newly emerging situations which a doctor confronts—as do we all—in the present day. In this task none of the sources of moral insight, no understanding of the humanity of man or for answering questions of life and death, can rightfully be neglected.

There is, in any case, no way to avoid the moral pluralism of our society. There is no avoiding the fact that today no one can do medical ethics until someone first does so. Due to the uncertainties in Roman Catholic moral theology since Vatican II, even the traditional medical ethics courses in schools under Catholic auspices are undergoing vast changes, abandonment, or severe crisis. The medical profession now finds itself without one of the ancient landmarks—or without one opponent. Research and therapies and actionable schemes for the self-creation of our species mount exponentially, while Nuremberg recedes.

The last state of the patient (medical ethics) may be worse than the first. Still there is evidence that this can be a moment of great opportunity. An increasing number of moralists—Catholic, Protestant, Jewish and unlabeled men—are manifesting interest, devoting their trained powers of ethical reasoning to questions of medical practice and technology. This same galloping technology gives all mankind reason to ask how much longer we can go on assuming that what can be done or should be, without uncovering the ethical principles we mean to abide by. These questions are now completely in the public forum, no longer the province of scientific experts alone.

The day is past when one could write a manual on medical ethics. Such books by Roman Catholic moralists are not to be criticized for being deductive. They were not; rather they were commendable attempts to deal with concrete cases. These manuals were written with the conviction that moral reasoning can encompass hard cases, that ethical deliberation need not remain highfalutin but can "subsume" concrete situations under the illuminating power of human moral reason. However, the manuals can be criticized for seeding finally to "resolve" innumerable cases and to give the once and for all "solution" to them. This attempt left the impression that a rule book could be written for medical practice. In a sense, this impression was the consequence of a chief virtue of the authors, i.e., that they were resolved to think through a problem, if possible, *to the end* and precisely with relevance and applicability in concrete cases. Past medical moralists can still be profitably read by anyone who wishes to face the challenge of how he would go about prolonging ethical reflection into action.

Medical ethics today must, indeed, be "casuistry"; it must deal as competently and exhaustively as possible with the concrete features of actual moral decisions of life and death and medical care. But we can no longer be so confident that "resolution" or "solution" will be forthcoming.

To take up the questions of medical ethics for probing, to try to enter into the heart of these problems with reasonable and compassionate moral reflection, is to engage in the greatest of joint ventures: the moral becoming of man. This is to see in the prism of medical cases the claims of any man to be honored and respected. So might we enter thoughtfully and actively into the moral history of mankind's fidelity to covenants. In this everyone is engaged.

NOTES

1. Wolf Wolfensberger, "Ethical Issues in Research with Human Subjects." *Science* 155:48, January 6, 1967.
2. Paul A. Freund, *Is the Law Ready for Human Experimentation?* Trial 2 (October–November 1966):49; "Ethical Problems in Human Experimentation." *New England Journal of Medicine* 273 (No. 10):692, 10 September 1965.
3. Dunlop (1965), quoted in Douglass Hubble, "Medical Science, Society and Human Values." *British Medical Journal* 5485:476, 19 February 1966.
4. James P. Scanlan, "The Morality of Deception in Experiments." *Bucknell Review* 13 (No. 1):26, March 1965.
5. John E. Smith, "Panel Discussion: Moral Issues in Clinical Research." *Yale Journal of Biology and Medicine* 36:463, June 1964.
6. Henry K. Beecher, *Research and the Individual: Human Studies*. Boston: Little, Brown, 1970, p. 25.

The differences on certain issues between Catholic and Protestant medical ethics are well known. The methods and concepts used in the two traditions are less thoroughly analyzed. In the following essay Lisa Sowle Cahill, a scholar familiar with both traditions, compares the work of Paul Ramsey with that of Richard McCormick, one of the leading Catholic scholars working in medical ethics today. She shows how Ramsey insists on working within explicitly Christian sources like the Bible while McCormick, taking a more traditional Catholic position, makes use of rational ethics as well as Christian sources. McCormick's Catholic ethics is teleological; the focus is on the end, the highest good. Ramsey, by contrast, is more deontological; he focuses on moral obligation and obedience to covenant, rather than good ends. Cahill traces other contrasts in their ethics including the relative priority of the individual and the common good and the role of moral rules. She concludes that they are "within shouting distance."

Within Shouting Distance: Paul Ramsey and Richard McCormick on Method

LISA SOWLE CAHILL

Those reflecting on medical ethics from the perspective of religious commitment and its theological elucidation are confronted with the peculiar problem of reconciling the language of a community of faith and obligation with a perceived responsibility to and for the larger human community and with a concomitant need for public discourse. In their medical-ethical arguments, two prominent Christian ethicists, Paul Ramsey and Richard McCormick, develop working paradigms for successful public conversation. Ramsey is not only a representative of themes which often characterize Protestant ethics, but also has contributed a quantity of recent and detailed analyses of the crises of values in research and health care. McCormick affirms the major historical and systematic influences within Roman Catholicism. Moreover, he develops, from within natural law moral theology itself, revisions not only of past moral judgments but of formal principles and metaphysical foundations of the former. Ramsey's vision remains distinctively Christian, even when this weakens his case for a universal ethical appeal; McCormick forcefully correlates religious and secular values, but does not so clearly demonstrate the functional significance for ethics of his theology, precisely as Christian. The purpose of the present analysis is to determine to what extent the ethics of each author is informed by his theological commitments, and how the differences between the two illustrate underlying theological disputes.

THE SOURCES AND SCOPE OF CHRISTIAN ETHICS

Ramsey is committed to develop for Christian decision making the biblical norm of agape, or self-sacrificial neighbor love. He disclaims interest in discovering secular translations of it, but does expect a "convergence" of religion and humanism at the level of concrete judgments. Thus Ramsey makes the peculiar claim that, while his reasoning has a unique and nonreducible source, his conclusions may well convince those who reject his presuppositions (Ramsey 1970b, p. xi; 1977b, p. 59; 1978a, p. xiii). So does Ramsey modify his "confessional" Christian position as he engages in the task of effective proclamation in a pluralistic setting.

McCormick, on the other hand, defines his position within a theological ethics which systematically has anticipated a coincidence between natural or rational ethics and Christian ethics. The premise of the "law of nature" is, as he states it, an objective moral order discernible both prediscursively and reflectively (McCormick 1978a, pp. 250–253). Human consciousness grasps in actual experience "the goods or values man can seek, the values that define his human opportunity, his flourishing" (1978b, p. 217). The revelation in Jesus Christ discloses the coherence of these values in God, friendship with whom is the destiny to which persons are invited. This revelation does not, however, generate distinct moral norms which supersede those discernible by reason (McCormick 1977, p. 69; 1978c, p. 100; 1979, pp. 98–99). Rational discourse about obligation in medical practice, as in other personal and social relationships, is in principle an adequate basis of ethics for both Christian and secular humanist.

If a move toward at least a practical universalism is needed to avoid the "separatism" of theological ethics in relation to public ethics, Ramsey must find an alternative to McCormick's reasonable order of values which will compromise his own presuppositions and concerns. He therefore buttresses his expectation of confluence between religious and humanistic ethics by several innovative qualifications of his original particularistic position. On this issue, Ramsey's perspective develops chronologically and in relation to specific problems which have absorbed his attention.

In his first major and only foundational work, *Basic Christian Ethics*, Ramsey envisions Christian ethics as witness to Christ in its practical dimensions. The righteousness and faithfulness of God establish the covenant to which the human response is "obedient love" (1951, pp. xi, 13). Ramsey's more topical writings manifest three modifications of, albeit not departures from, his original insistence that the Christian moral ought is not evident to reason (1951, p. 14; see also 1967a, pp. 108–109; 1977b, p. 59). These are: (1) the derivation of moral norms from natural "covenants" distinct from but congruent with revealed ones; (2) the affirmation of Christian values in Western culture; and (3) the suggestion that God's redemptive covenant itself is all-inclusive.

In *Deeds and Rules in Christian Ethics*, Ramsey explains his own ethics as "mixed agapism" relying on reason as well as revelation, not because these are independent sources, but because God's covenant is established with all persons in Christ (Ramsey 1967, pp. 29, 122). Therefore "traces of agapistic attitudes and actions" characterize "our common humanity" (1967, p. 43). Appeals to a universal covenant abound, but are introduced briefly and rhetorically, rather than systematically.[1]

Recent writings also presuppose a comprehensive moral community, suggested in conjunction with Ramsey's appropriation of "performative language analysis" (see esp. Evans 1963; cf. Ramsey 1968a, pp. 121–125; 1977b, pp. 60–66; see also a section of an unpublished manuscript entitled "Religious Faith a Performative Morality," available from author) to interpret God's covenantal initiative and humankind's obedient response. Ramsey's premise of a covenant revealed to a particular community but effectively established for "all" persons backs up an inclusive understanding of obligation without abandoning his biblical base. A similar inclusiveness can be defended by the "natural law" affirmation of God as the end toward which all persons implicitly are oriented in their actualization of ordered finite values.

DEONTOLOGY "VERSUS" TELEOLOGY

Ramsey's and McCormick's latest controversies have focused at the formal level on an issue which has long been fundamental for both, that is, a paradigm to interpret human moral agency and derive concrete norms. In terms also appropriate to the parallel Anglo-American philosophical debate, the choice lies between a teleological model and a deontological one (see Broad 1944, esp. pp. 206–207). This controversy is relevant to theological ethics, insofar as deontology historically has been associated with scriptural confessionalism, and teleology with the Aristotelian-

Thomistic ethics of natural virtue. The discussion rapidly proceeds to whether and when teleologists can be characterized as utilitarians, the latter having become a distinctly pejorative epithet in Christian ethics. In teleology, as concerned with some *goal*, it is precisely consequences which determine normative moral evaluation, although not necessarily measurable consequences for specific historical communities, as is assumed by those who would paint all teleologists with a utilitarian brush. Deontologists frequently insist that considerations of justice, equality, or fairness are essential in the fulfillment of moral *duty*. Thus those actions which treat persons as means to desirable social states ought to be prohibited absolutely. However, not every *telos* excludes some persons from participation for the benefit of others, or justifies any conceivable act given the right configuration of social-benefits-producing circumstances. For example, Aristotle's "happiness" or Aquinas's "friendship with God" are not quantifiable, nor limited in their possible range of distribution, and not reserved for some at the expense of others.

Ramsey has been committed consistently to a deontological model of ethics, as alone expressing the character of Christian moral obligation as obedient response in covenant. Consideration of consequences remains secondary to the determination of the unconditional demands of agape or covenant fidelity (Ramsey 1951, pp. 107, 115–116, 124, 130; 1961c, p. 3, 8; 1967, pp. 108, 109; 1970a, pp. 29–31; 1970b, pp. 2, 25, 58, 256; 1971, pp. 700–706; 1975, pp. xv–xvi, 13; 1979, pp. 8–10). The "ethics of agent agape" and of "agent care" in *Ethics at the Edges of Life* reaffirms obligation as the starting point for medical ethics, not any calculation of the good or harmful consequences of affording treatment to any individual, especially on the basis of social usefulness or merit (Ramsey 1978a, p. 218).

McCormick, by contrast, models moral agency teleologically, God is loved and pursued through the free realization of values which participate in the absolute good, God (*summum bonum*). Moral choice is the preference of some values over others and may be evaluated by an intelligent perception of their objective hierarchical relations (*ordo bonorum*). Those acts are good acts which realize the highest available good in a given situation. McCormick has been accused of utilitarianism (e.g., Carney 1978), because it appears occasionally that his criterion for concrete value preference is an empirical and relatively immediate social good rather that the comprehensive transcendent good, God. (I shall return to the merits of this accusation and to the general characterization of McCormick as a teleologist in a later portion of this essay.)

The debate over teleology "versus" deontology will be pursued here through the issues remaining, namely, the function of moral rules, the relative priority of the individual and the common good, and the ethics of causing death in a medical setting. These are specifics about which Ramsey and McCormick claim that certain conclusions are coherent with, or even entailed by, the teleological and deontological perspectives. My own perception is that the usefulness of the distinction is largely limited to descriptions of the basic character of moral agency (e.g., as responsive obedience to divine mandates or as purposive striving toward union with God).

INDIVIDUAL AND SOCIETY

McCormick's teleology of common moral experience and Ramsey's theological deontology become differentiated more precisely when focused on a problem endemic to social ethics: the relative priority of individual and community. Disagreements between these colleagues have been pronounced regarding proxy consent to nontherapeutic research on children and fetuses.[2] Themes coalesce there which are also represented in other analyses by both. Ramsey essentially asserts that both natural and Christian covenant-fidelity yield "informed consent" an inviolable requirement of medical practice. The sacredness of the individual must not be compromised for the sake of benefits to others. Since agapic concern directs itself above all to the weak and vulnerable, children ought most to be protected against consequentialist incursions. Although self-sacrifice is mandatory for the Christian, it has moral significance and justifiability only when its subject is a volunteer, a status impossible of attainment by the fetus, child, or mentally incompetent person.

McCormick attempts to highlight the essential and natural sociality of persons-in-community while not denigrating their dignity. Rather than stressing the inviolability of noncompetent research subjects, McCormick locates them within the fabric of the "common good," in whose benefits they share. One ought reasonably to consent in social justice to contribute to the good of others, if at little or no risk to oneself. In such circumstances, consent of noncompetents may be presumed and their participation enlisted as obligatory, not supererogatory.

Though Ramsey has been branded an individualist and McCormick caricatured as a utilitarian, more profit might be gained by appreciation of the theological commitments conserved in the conclusions of each. Backing Ramsey's insistence on respect for the individual is his affirmation of steadfast concern for the "neighbor." By framing this concern deontologically, he ensures its vitality and imperviousness to the imperatives of long-range social ideals in whose light is contemplated the exclusion of those deemed less useful or less able to protect their interests. He does not leave communal needs (those of "all God's other children" [Ramsey 1968b, p. 151]) completely out of account, but here responds to a perceived immediate threat to one pole of the individual-community dialectic. McCormick's perceptions of imminent danger may lie in the opposite direction; in addition, his theological tradition makes available a relatively coherent method for balancing both individual rights and the welfare of the whole community (e.g., social encyclicals of nineteenth- and twentieth-century popes). The method's controlling concept is that of the "common good," a notion inclusive of persons, of their association in community, and of the totality itself, as more than a simple aggregate of individuals. This notion is distinctive in its comprehension of all persons equally and by its ordering to a transcendent communion, that of persons in God. McCormick defines justifiable experimentation on the premise that communal interaction is an essential component of the realization of values, and proposes it with the conviction that those values persons "tend toward" or seek are common ones.

From this exchange, it becomes evident that the links McCormick and Ramsey build between Christian presuppositions and moral conclusions are determined largely by the authors' particular ethical concerns, and that while these concerns and conclusions are defended within a teleological or deontological vision of moral agency, neither vision is entailed by Christian faith or necessarily conducive to some moral judgments rather than others. While on the problem at hand and generally, Ramsey defends the inviolability of individual freedom as a requirement of agape, he has sometimes (on justifiable warfare, on conscientious objection to civil law) defended strictures of social existence. While McCormick presently and characteristically endorses the reasonableness of exacting from all individuals their minimal social obligations, his natural law framework allows an occasional shift to the interests of individuals (e.g., on neonatal care, on contraception). For both of these ethicists, theology provides a court within which to hear a moral case but the outcome is decided only with the assistance of *amici curiae* (e.g., philosophy, the social and empirical sciences).

MORAL NORMS AND EXCEPTIONS

The justification of moral norms is a burden which theologians of the past two decades have shared with philosophers, and which has been borne in rather different directions by Paul Ramsey and Richard McCormick. Their recent joint effort to light the path, *Doing Evil to Achieve Good* (McCormick and Ramsey 1978), discloses tenacious differences. The effort of each to account for rules and delimit their function within his respective theological tradition evinces distinct historical concerns. Ramsey decried a Protestant "relativism" in ethics as long ago as *Basic Christian Ethics* (1951, p. 77) and devoted *Deeds and Rules in Christian Ethics* to a cure for the "professional allergy" to rules which he diagnosed among contemporary theologians (1967, p. 3). Ramsey pursues a definition of rules consistent with biblical agape. An unmistakable evolution occurs from *Basic Christian Ethics* (1951) through *Deeds and Rules* (1967) and an important article, "The Case of the Curious Exception" (1968a), to the *Ethics at the Edges of Life* (1978a); however, tracing the genealogy of the latest offspring is no easy matter.

The neo-Thomism of the moral manuals spawned a notorious Catholic legalism which it has been incumbent upon ethicists critically loyal to that tradition to reduce if not dismember. In the 1960s and 1970s, continental theologians challenged the notions of "intrinsic evil" and absolute norms; McCormick's "Ambiguity in Moral Choice" (1978b) both summarized the state of the question and broke new ground through a deepened understanding of the relation of norms to values. That attempt precipitated *Doing Evil to Achieve Good* (McCormick and Ramsey 1978), a collection of exchanges on norms which prohibit or permit acts having both a positive and negative relation to values (via "the principle of double effect"). The Catholic effort, however, is not simply to overturn the dictates of an absolutist morality; more broadly, it is an attempt to come to terms both with the real insights of the tradition and with an element that tradition neglected, that is, the centrality of Scripture and its normative imperative for any "Christian" ethics.

For Ramsey, rules indicate the continuity of covenant obligation. However, the primary meaning of covenant fidelity has shifted from a Christian love freely transforming every situation, even beyond prior rules (1961c, pp. 179, 190: "in the instant agape controls"), to the enactment of stable social institutions which protect the individual, albeit also as a requirement of agape (1978a, p. 217: "What rule of practice best expresses covenant fidelity?"). Early on, Ramsey developed the phrases "love-transformed-justice" and "in-principled-love" (1961a, 1961b) to signify that norms are consonant with Christian love itself, whether responsive to the one or many neighbors. The first indicates love building on the orders of natural justice, the second the intrinsic specification of love within covenant. Recently, for example, on medical ethics, Ramsey concentrates on the derivation of rules from love itself, though both themes continue.

His formal definition of rule Ramsey draws from John Rawls's "classic article," "Two Concepts of Rules" (Rawls 1955; cf. Ramsey 1967, chap. 4). Rawls's own intention is to outline a more defensible utilitarian theory by pointing out the distinction between justifying a "practice" and justifying an action falling under it. A practice as an institutionalized structure of activity is justified by utilitarian (or, for Ramsey, agapic) considerations. Once the practice is established, each act included under it is not reconsidered independently. Ramsey assimilates Rawls's terms to the language of theological ethics, though he is more interested in their function in his own system than in consistency with their original meaning. He proposes exceptionless general rules in Christian ethics, and derives their content from three sources. The first is Christian discernment of the individual and of what love requires toward the individual, for example, nontherapeutic research on children is prohibited generally and unexceptionably. The second source is discernment of the most loving social practice, or the practice that most adequately and generally embodies agape (Ramsey adverts to Robert Veatch's "red light rule" [Veatch and Branson 1976]; see Ramsey 1978a, p. 217). For example, the rule which prohibits inducing death delimits the most generally loving acts, and to admit exceptions would weaken it. Third, "a natural sense of justice and injustice" penetrates to the good for persons and formulates it in binding principles (Ramsey 1967, p. 127; see also Ramsey 1977b, p. 59). The first two sources represent Christian love's intrinsic requirements, captured in its perception of essential humanity and of the best possible social existence (Ramsey 1967, p. 143). The third is an independent source, presumed to be congenial with the first two, for any or all of the three reasons mentioned earlier in this essay.

Nevertheless, Ramsey formulates Christian rules of practice with a view to individual rights within a larger society conducive to encroachments. His denunciations of "atomistic individualism," which echo through *Ethics at the Edges*, therefore are surprising until one realizes that what Ramsey condemns is the refusal of individuals to make or keep covenant with others and to acknowledge that some requirements of covenant bind all and always (e.g., Ramsey 1967, p. 44; 1978a, p. 13). Far from sacrificing individual interests to social goods, those who enjoin compelling rules "would build a floor under the individual fellowman by minimum faithfulness-rules or canons of loyalty to him that are unexceptionable" (Ramsey 1968a, p. 133). A pressing question is whether the universalization of requirements for moral relations among individuals is adequate as "social" ethics, or whether it is finally a more equalitarian individualism. In attending to "rules of practice" as instruments of individual rights, Ramsey leaves aside the question of community as more than a mechanism for reconciling claims of individuals, and of the role and responsibility of persons within and to it.

Although whether rules can be absolute is not an issue for theological ethics alone, McCormick and Ramsey handle it with theological concerns in mind. McCormick undertakes a "reasonable" analysis of human moral agency as value actualization. While Ramsey is interested in the logical character of exceptions, he asks primarily if they are consistent with covenant fidelity, especially for the Christian. "The Case of the Curious Exception" (Ramsey 1968a), an article to which Ramsey continues to refer the reader (see Ramsey 1978a, p. 212, n. 37), explains the logical relation of the "exception" to the "exceptionless rule." The distinctive insight is that "exceptions" to norms veritably disappear when properly considered. If an exception has specifiable features, then it must be repeatable; and if repeatable, it is no exception at all, but an act falling under a different principle. In this case, some "exempting-condition" is present which destroys the exception's "singular" character. In other cases, what seems to be an exception to a rule is really another qualification of the rule-generating principle, based on a deepened understanding of it. If so, "qualifying conditions" are present which turn violation into fulfillment. For example, telling a falsehood to save life might be construed as form of serving truth, rather than as "lying." In such instances, exceptions are not created by consequence features of acts, but by a deeper understanding of the covenant faithfulness expressed in those acts. Ramsey thereby provides some flexibility to moral rules without resorting to consequentialism. Ultimately, these two types of exceptions converge (see Ramsey 1976a). The more precisely defined and universalizable "exception" to a prior rule is justified in relation to the same principle that generated the original rule. For example, just as proxy consent to hazardous research is ruled out by the standard of care, so such research becomes "exceptionally" justified if it is a last resort for therapy.

Sometimes, though, Ramsey seems to disallow even duty-generated exceptions. In one of his responses to McCormick on pediatric experimentation (Ramsey 1976b), he advises that when neglect of research is as immoral as the infringement of rights it requires, the Christian, at least, might better "sin bravely." This phrase captures nicely a Protestant acknowledgment of moral gray areas and even paradox, to be contrasted with the Catholic drive to reconcile values in rationally perspicacious choices.

EXCEPTIONABLE NORMS IN AN ETHICS OF REASONABLE VALUES

Doing Evil to Achieve Good is an enormously complex discussion of an equally complex principle, that of "double effect." I will confine my remarks to the collection's central subject, Richard McCormick's revisionist justification of norms.[3] The Catholic tradition of ethics, appealing for a reasoned consideration of moral agency, has generated rule absolutely prohibiting some acts as "intrinsically evil." By this principle it has permitted others, despite morally objectionable aspects. In the justifiable act, the associated evil is described as "tolerated" or "indirectly intended," not desired in itself or even the means of producing the good effect. Thus destruction of a fetus in utero to save the mother was not permitted, though removal of a cancerous and pregnant uterus for the same purpose was.

Originally written 1973, "Ambiguity in Moral Choice" (in McCormick and Ramsey 1978) was McCormick's first extended attempt to reinterpret this principle by focusing on "proportionate reason," rather than "indirectness" of action and intention. McCormick showed that there can be teleologically justified exceptions to moral norms forbidding "physical," "premoral," "nonmoral," or "ontic" evils (synonymous terms for disvalues such as error, pain, death) and that, in fact, the norms themselves are justified on the same grounds. A "premoral" value is precisely one which is not absolute. Premoral values and disvalues are relevant to moral judgments insofar as they are in general either to be sought (life) or avoided (death); however the obligation to actualize them concretely depends upon the weight of other values simultaneously at stake. *Moral* values, on the other hand, ought never to be violated since they do not in principle conflict. Moral norms specify the relation of acts to values in the *ordo bonorum;* acts can be enjoined or prohibited generally, because and to the extent that they affirm or deny values. Exceptions occur because goods per se to be realized conflict concretely with equal or higher goods. In conflict situations, the commendable act is the act which realizes the highest value then possible. The only "absolute" norms enjoin moral values (fidelity, truthfulness, justice); norms cannot specify material acts which always or never embody these values. Killing might be "unjust" in most circumstances, but "just" in exceptional ones, while "Never act unjustly" is an unconditional prohibition. It is *proportionate reason,* observes McCormick, that justifies killing at all. One may kill to preserve one's life but not one's purse. *Moral* evil is precisely to do avoidable (disproportionate) concrete harm, that is, to do premoral evil deliberately, and without adequate cause (see McCormick 1978a, pp. 255–260). A premoral evil may be directly done if the value promoted outweighs the disvalue caused, if no less harmful alternative is available, and if the greater value will not "in the long run" be undermined by the manner of its protection now (McCormick 1978b, p. 45). Only moral evil ought never be intended directly. Direct intention of a moral evil would entail approval, since moral values are not mutually exclusive (honesty and fidelity); the difficulty is rather to determine which acts best concretize them by appropriately reconciling premoral values (telling a lie to save a friend).

Ramsey's chapter does not alter considerably his own position on rules or that of his adversary. It is largely an attack upon consequentialism and a defense of the requirement of "indirectness" as part of the principle under discussion. If values in conflict, either moral or nonmoral, are incommensurable, he insists, one may not justifiably be sacrificed for the other except indirectly. McCormick's reply is that indirectness does not resolve incommensurability (1978a, p. 227) and, further, that even "incommensurables" must be commensurated approximately and the due trepidation—as is often done in moral choices (1978a, pp. 229–230, 251–253). This assessment, of course, relies on a confidence not shared by Ramsey, namely, trust in a providentially ordered moral universe, where conflicts are permeable and resolvable by reason, however falteringly (McCormick 1978a, pp. 217, 222).

A more substantial objection may be Ramsey's resistance to the inclusion of charity within the domain of proportionate reason (Ramsey 1978b, pp. 131–137). Given his starting point, McCormick is pressed to incorporate a distinctively Christian self-understanding, and a Christian norm, charity, as more than superfluous appendages to ethics. Some lack of success in doing so to the satisfaction of his non-Catholic peers is a liability shared with the rest of natural law moral theology. In "Ambiguity in Moral Choice," McCormick remarks that "self-sacrifice to save the neighbor can truly be proportionate" (1978b, p. 48), a statement open to the inference that which is obligatory precisely at cost to oneself. McCormick has proposed also that organ donation or participation in therapeutic experimentation may be "personally good for" the subject and that this good is "the good of expressed charity" (1974, p. 220). Yet McCormick himself undoubtedly agrees that "charity" in the New Testament sense is not commended because of "sticky benefits." Although the virtue of the agent justifies an act of sacrifice in a general sense, the dominant and immediate motivation is the neighbor's good (McCormick 1975b, p. 508). Nevertheless, there apparently remains here, as in Ramsey's covenant ethics, an impermeable tension between rational discourse and the biblical norm of sacrifice.

By this revised theory of proportionate reason, McCormick claims to repudiate crude consequentialism. He names himself a "moderate teleologist" (McCormick 1978a, pp. 239–255) because, besides consequences, "proportionate reason" refers to an intrinsic relationship of acts to goods sought. Or, citing Louis Janssens, "'the principle which has been affirmed in the end must not be negated by the means'" (McCormick 1978a, p. 202; cf. Janssens 1972, p. 142).

Having defined teleology to include consideration both of consequences and of "feature-dependent" norms, McCormick enfolds the goats with the sheep by insisting that "all of the contributors to this volume are teleologists in the sense just explained." Some, indeed, are "crypto-teleologists (e.g., Ramsey) who remain in the closet" (McCormick 1978a, p. 200). Ramsey as well as McCormick generally maintains the separation between teleology and deontology, asserting that only one is an adequate model for Christian ethics; at the same time, both struggle to define the chosen model inclusively. In Ramsey's frequent deontological apologiae, teleology consistently is reduced to utilitarianism ("producing *teloi*") and rejected (e.g., Ramsey 1967, p. 108). Yet, in the same paragraph in which he brands McCormick a consequentialist, Ramsey affirms, "Traditional Christian ethics assumed that the greatest good for persons is friendship with God and that this is not measurable at all" (1978b, p. 70). McCormick's arguments are approved to the extent that they incorporate nonteleological elements (Ramsey 1978b, p. 117); however, when Ramsey issues his own imperatives, "duty" can demand efforts to "stem the tide" toward harmful effects of present legislative or to other social decisions (1978a, p. 329). Ramsey makes the effort to demonstrate that both "consequential" and "intrinsic" moral considerations are required in a deontological model ("mixed agapism"); McCormick's effort is to demonstrate that the same is true in a teleological one ("moderate teleology").

It might be concluded from this that the controversy over these models is to a large degree unnecessary.[4] The issue is not whether either model inadequately accounts for moral experience by minimizing or excluding one of these factors. The issues are rather (1) which model more appropriately portrays the fundamental quality of that experience, given the shape of one's "metaethical" (e.g., religious and theological) convictions, symbols, and communal self-understanding; and (2) how the diverse more specific elements of moral theory and decision can be defined coherently within that model (e.g., a fulfillment of duties, accountability for consequences, a sense of moral purposiveness, justification of rules and exceptions, etc.).

NOTES

1. Variations of the phrase "love for every man for whom Christ died" are numerous (see esp. Ramsey 1961c, pp. xvi, xviii, xx, 54, 114, 305; 1968b, pp. 150–151). All indicate that any individual must be regarded as redeemed by the grace of Christ. Ramsey also cites Karl Barth's affirmation that covenant is "the inner meaning and purpose" of creation, inferring that natural and Christian morality are complementary (see Ramsey 1961a, p. 28; 1967, p. 67; 1970b, p. xii).
2. The controversy has been prolonged and sometimes acerbic; see, e.g., Ramsey (1968a, 1970b, 1975, 1976b, 1977a); McCormick (1973b, 1975a, 1976); McCormick and Walters (1975).
3. Helpful analyses of this work, especially the exchanges of McCormick and Ramsey, are provided by Allen (1979) and Langan (1979).
4. Other authors agree, albeit for varied reasons, e.g., Maguire (1978). See also Broad (1944, p. 207); Ramsey (1967, p. 108); and McCormick (1978a, pp. 197–200).

REFERENCES

Allen, Joseph L. "Paul Ramsey and His Respondents Since *The Patient as Person.*" *Religious Studies Review* 5:89–95, 1979.

Broad, C. D. *Five Types of Ethical Theory.* New York: Harcourt, Brace & Co., 1944.

Carney, Frederick S. "On McCormick and Teleological Morality." *Journal of Religious Ethics* 6:81–107, 1978.

Evans, Donald. *The Language of Self-Involvement.* London: SCM Press, 1963.

Janssens, Louis. "Ontic Evil and Moral Evil." *Louvain Studies* 4:115–156, 1972.

Langan, John. "Direct and Indirect—Some Recent Exchanges Between Paul Ramsey and Richard McCormick." *Religious Studies Review* 5:95–101, 1979.

McCormick, Richard A. "Proxy Consent in the Experimentation Situation." In *Love and Society*, edited by James Johnson and David Smith. Missoula, Mont.: Scholars Press, 1973(b).

McCormick, Richard A. "To Save or Let Die." *America* 30:6–10, 1974.

McCormick, Richard A. "Fetal Research, Morality, and Public Policy." *Hastings Center Report* 5 (No. 3):41–46, 1975(a).

McCormick, Richard A. "Transplantation of Organs: A Commentary on Paul Ramsey." *Theological Studies* 36:503–509, 1975(b).

McCormick, Richard A. "Experimentation in Children: Sharing in Sociality." *Hastings Center Report* 6, (No. 6):41–46, 1976.

McCormick, Richard A. "Notes on Moral Theology: 1976." *Theological Studies* 38:57–114, 1977.

McCormick, Richard A. "A Commentary on the Commentaries." In McCormick and Ramsey; 1978(a).

McCormick, Richard A. "Ambiguity in Moral Choice." In McCormick and Ramsey; 1978(b).

McCormick, Richard A. "Notes on Moral Theology, 1977: The Church in Dispute." *Theological Studies* 39:76–138, 1978(c).

McCormick, Richard A. "Notes on Moral Theology, 1978." *Theological Studies* 40:59–112, 1979.

McCormick, Richard A., and Ramsey, Paul, eds. *Doing Evil to Achieve Good*. Chicago: Loyola University Press, 1978.

McCormick, Richard A., and Walters, Leroy. "Fetal Research and Public Policy." *America* 132:473–476, 1975.

Maguire, Daniel. *The Moral Choice*. New York: Prentice-Hall, 1978.

Ramsey, Paul. *Basic Christian Ethics*. New York: Scribner's, 1951.

Ramsey, Paul. *Christian Ethics and the Sit-In*. New York: Association Press, 1961(a).

Ramsey, Paul. "Faith Effective Through In-Principled Love." *Christianity and Crisis* 20:76–78, 1961(b).

Ramsey, Paul. *War and the Christian Conscience: How Shall Modern War Be Conducted Justly?* Durham, N.C.: Duke University Press, 1961(c).

Ramsey, Paul. *Deeds and Rules in Christian Ethics*. New York: Scribner's, 1967.

Ramsey, Paul. "The Case of the Curious Exception." In *Norm and Context in Christian Ethics*, edited by Gene Outka and Paul Ramsey. New York: Scribner's, 1968(a).

Ramsey, Paul. *The Just War: Force and Political Responsibility*. New York: Scribner's, 1968(b).

Ramsey, Paul. *Fabricated Man*. New Haven, Conn.: Yale University Press, 1970(a).

Ramsey, Paul. *The Patient as Person*. New Haven, Conn: Yale University Press, 1970(b).

Ramsey, Paul. "The Ethics of a Cottage Industry in an Age of Community and Research Medicine." *New England Journal of Medicine* 284:700–706, 1971.

Ramsey, Paul. *The Ethics of Fetal Research*. New Haven, Conn.: Yale University Press, 1975.

Ramsey, Paul. "Conceptual Foundations for an Ethics of Medical Care: A Response." In Veatch and Branson 1976(a).

Ramsey, Paul. "The Enforcement of Morals: Nontherapeutic Research on Children." *Hastings Center Report* 6 (No. 4):21–30, 1976(b).

Ramsey, Paul. "Children as Research Subjects: A Reply." *Hastings Center Report* 7 (No. 2):40–41, 1977(a).

Ramsey, Paul. "Kant's Moral Philosophy or a Religious Ethics?" In *Knowledge, Value and Belief*, edited by H. Tristram Englehardt, Jr., and Daniel Callahan. Hastings-on-Hudson, N.Y.: Hastings Center, 1977(b).

Ramsey, Paul. *Ethics at the Edges of Life*. New Haven, Conn.: Yale University Press, 1978(a).

Ramsey, Paul. "Incommensurability and Indeterminacy in Moral Choice." In McCormick and Ramsey 1978(b).

Ramsey, Paul. "On in Vitro Fertilization." Testimony before the Ethics Advisory Board, Department of Health, Education and Welfare. Chicago: Americans United for Life, 1979.

Rawls, John. "Two concepts of Rules." *Philosophical Review* 64:3–32, 1955.

Veatch, Robert M., and Branson, Roy, eds. *Ethics and Health Policy.* Cambridge, Mass.: Ballinger Publishing Co., 1976.

The religious ethical traditions are not the only alternatives to the Hippocratic ethic for medical decisionmaking. Schools of thought in secular philosophy offer coherent ethical systems that can be applied to medical ethical problems. The most important challenge to Hippocratic ethics in the mid-to-late twentieth century has come from secular liberal political philosophy. Liberalism, in the philosophical sense of the term, offers an ethic that focuses on the individual as an autonomous agent. The key ethical focus shifts from the benefits and harms of Hippocratism to rights. The right of the patient to consent, to refuse treatment, to confidentiality, and to knowledge all flow from this focus on the individual. In the following essay John Hallowell outlines the primary characteristics of liberalism.

Liberalism: The Political Expression of Individualism

JOHN HALLOWELL

Liberalism is premised upon the assertion of the absolute moral worth of each individual. It is the political expression of a comprehensive Weltanschauung, of an intellectual climate of opinion that has pervaded all realms of thought since the Renaissance. It is the theory of political order based upon individualism.

The individual seemed the proper starting point for many reasons. First of all, the early liberals lived in a cultural climate that was essentially Christian. The idea of the supreme worth of the individual, of all individuals everywhere, was contributed by Christianity through the notion of the salvation of individual souls. Each man was equal in the sight of God. When the Reformation posited the Church as "a fellowship of believers, each the direct concern of God, each directly responsible to God, each guided by the illumination of God in his own heart and conscience," responsibility for salvation devolved directly upon the individual.

This notion of the absolute value of human personality, of human dignity and worth, was coupled with the belief that all creativity springs from the individual. Ever since the Renaissance, when man rediscovered his ego, he has been conscious, as he never was in the Middle Ages, of his own will and of his power to create things for their own sake and for his own pleasure. As men turned from a theistic concept of God to a deistic concept (in which God was conceived as the Creator but no longer as the Regent of the universe), it was possible to ascribe greater freedom of will to individuals. And when deism gradually gave way to pantheism and God became absorbed in the material world, still greater emphasis could be placed upon individual autonomy. As God was conceived less and less as a Creator, man was conceived as having more and more powers of creation.

Liberalism, as the political expression of individualism, espoused freedom for the individual from all personal arbitrary authority. Starting from the premise of the absolute value and dignity of human personality, liberals necessarily demanded freedom for each individual from every other individual, from the state, from every arbitrary will. Only when liberalism coupled the contract theory with the belief in objective truth and value, transcending all individuals and binding upon each without promise, could it reconcile freedom from arbitrary authority with the idea of an ordered commonwealth.

Liberalism in its integral form, therefore, starting from the premise of the absolute value of human personality, demands freedom for each individual from all personal, capricious, and arbitrary authority. Since freedom degenerates into license without some notion of responsibility and since submission to any individual will is incompatible with the postulate of human dignity and equality, it follows that freedom can only be secured through an impersonal authority, through a law that is found and not made. Integral liberalism, therefore, espouses freedom for each individual under the law, the law being conceived as embodying certain substantive and eternal truths transcending all individuals and binding upon each without promise.

All modern thinkers, with the exception of the functionalists, have agreed in placing the individual at the center of their thought. Most of them have posited a free-willed, autonomous, rational individual through whom alone creative forces could be put to work. Progress, until recently, has been considered as inevitable and as proceeding through the perfection of individuals. Progress, moreover, has been measured in terms of individual values, and although the socialists emphasize reform through the group, rather than by private initiative, the success of their endeavor is measured in terms of benefits to individuals. The betterment of individual conditions, spiritual and economic, is an essential aim of socialism. It does not abandon the individual but seeks rather to bring about conditions under which it believes the individual will be able to realize himself more fully, share more fully in material goods, and attain the economic security and well-being requisite to human dignity.

Individual values have found their place in conservative Hegelianism and in

Marxian socialism, as well as in liberalism. Some writers have emphasized the collectivity, rather than the individual, but they have been able to do so only by accepting as fundamental the antimony between the one and the many. They have focused their attention on one side of a "two-headed coin" but they have been able to do so only by positing a "two-headed coin" to start with. Some writers have emphasized nature, rather than man, but they have been able to do so only by first presupposing a fundamental antimony between man and nature. Some writers have emphasized man as a physical entity, rejecting his spirituality, but again they have been able to do so only by accepting a fundamental antimony between soul and body. With the exception of the functionalists, all modern thinkers have started from this dichotomy. The differences between schools of thought have been differences in emphasis, not in conceptual presuppositions. These conceptual presuppositions are those of individualism, and it is in this perspective that all modern thinkers have endeavored to explain and understand their physical, spiritual, and social environment.

In the realm of political theory, too, the individual was placed at the center of thought. Professor Sabine sums it up well when he says:

> The individual human being, with his interests, his enterprise, his desire for happiness and advancement, above all with his reason, which seemed the condition for a successful use of all of his other faculties, appeared to be the foundation upon which a stable society must be built. . . . Not man as a priest or a soldier, as the member of a guild or an estate, but man as a bare human being, a "masterless man," appeared to be the solid fact. . . . Society is made for man, not man for society; it is humanity, as Kant said, that must always be treated as an end and not a means. The individual is both logically and ethically prior. To the philosophy of the seventeenth century relations always appeared thinner than substances; man was the substance, society the relation. It was this assumed priority of the individual which became the most marked and the most persistent quality of the theory of natural law, and the clearest differentia of the modern from the medieval theory. Developed especially by Hobbes and Locke, it became a universal characteristic of social theory down to the French Revolution and maintained itself far beyond that date. It persisted, moreover, as a presumption in Bentham's School long after David Hume had destroyed the methodology of natural rights.

Perhaps one of the most ardent individualists among German political thinkers was Wilhelm von Humboldt. He wrote:

> Reason cannot desire for man any other condition than that in which each individual not only enjoys the most absolute freedom of developing himself by his own energies, in his perfect individuality, but in which external nature even is left unfashioned by any human agency, but only receives the impress given to it by each individual of himself and his own free will, according to the measure of his wants and instincts, and restricted only by the limits of his powers and his rights.

His individualism was as extreme as that of Spencer and Mill (who was greatly influenced by von Humboldt) in England. But his belief in the moral uniqueness of individuals, his desire to treat each individual as an end in himself, was shared by many Germans and particularly by Kant and Fichte.

As a basic law of all human conduct Kant adopted the principle: "so act as to treat humanity, whether in thine own person or in that of any other, in every case as an end withal, never as a means only." And Fichte declared: "Whatsoever does not violate the rights of another, each person has the right to do and this, indeed, constitutes each person's right. Each one, moreover, has the right to judge for himself what is, and to defend, by his own powers, what he so judges to be, the limit of his free actions."

We have seen that the concept of individuality permeated the whole fabric of thought which emerged with the Renaissance. It is found in science, in theology, in economic and political theory; it is found in England, in France, and in Germany.

INDIVIDUALISM AND NATURAL RIGHTS

From the presupposition that individuals are moral entities it followed logically that they must have some inviolable rights as human beings, that they are entitled as human beings to do certain things and to possess certain things if they are to realize their potentialities as individuals. Although there was some idea of rights peculiar to corporations and groups in the Middle Ages, the idea of natural rights peculiar to individuals first emerged as a definite concept in the seventeenth century. Since by that time the concept of God was gradually being replaced by the concept of nature, as deism replaced theism and in turn was giving way to pantheism, men called the immutable rights which they believed to be inherent in individuals by virtue of their humanity, *natural* rights.

By the thinkers of the seventeenth and eighteenth centuries "natural rights were felt to rest on the same basis as Newton's discoveries; and reason discerned these rights despite their daily violation, just as reason discerned the true movement of the earth despite its apparent immobility." These rights were generally stated to consist of the right to life, liberty, and property. As gradually codified, they included such rights as freedom of worship, of speech, of press, and of assembly. By most of writers of the age the existence of these rights was considered to be more or less self-evident, inherent in the nature of man and demonstrable by reason.

Belief in natural rights was essentially "an assertion that certain human desires have greater validity than, and must therefore prevail over, force of circumstances or mere beings." And the fact that they were said to be grounded in human nature, that they were deduced in a sense from the nature of things, gave them "something of the prestige of physical, earthly existence" and the doctrine "could claim to be both a standard and a fact."

Many writers, in endeavoring to prove the existence of natural rights, posited the existence of a "state of nature" antecedent to civil society in which individuals lived in a "natural" state and possessed rights which were peculiar to them as human beings. Locke, for example, posited a "state of nature" in which reason rules supreme, and he believed that it taught those who would consult it "that being all equal and independent, no one ought to harm another in his life, health, liberty, or possessions." It is important to realize that the early liberals did not conceive of the right to property as did the nineteenth-century liberals. Property was defined by Locke, for example, as that with which one had mixed his labor. It was not the right to receive dividends from stocks and bonds that the early liberal demanded, nor the right of impersonal business corporations to do with "their property" what they liked, but rather the right of a man to make himself economically secure by his own labor. The early liberal appreciated the fact that liberty without economic security was meaningless, and it was for that reason that he linked the right to property (to the fruits of one's own labor) with life and liberty.

To seek to explain seventeenth-century liberalism in terms of nineteenth-century conceptions of property and individual rights, as many writers do, is to mistake a distorted form of liberalism for integral liberalism. In an over-zealous attempt to "explain" everything in terms of economic determinism, some writers, in effect, credit the seventeenth-century liberal with the ability to foresee social and economic developments of the nineteenth century, and, further, attribute to him the ulterior motive of providing a rationale for what was to take place two hundred years later! If liberal concepts were used in the nineteenth century to justify economic license, this is no indictment of integral liberalism, but more properly of those nineteenth-century "liberals" who perverted original concepts to their own advantage.

Locke presupposed that men were equal in the sense that each individual was a moral entity, an end in himself, and he posited the existence of rights deduced rationally from this premise. "Every one," he wrote, "as he is bound to preserve himself, and not to quit his station willfully, so by the like reason, when his own preservation comes not in competition, ought he as much as he can to preserve the rest of mankind, and may not, unless it be to do justice on an offender, take away, or impair the life, or what tends to the preservation of the life, the liberty, the health, limb, or goods of another."

These rights to life, liberty, and property Locke regarded as inalienable, as attributes of personality, as essential to human dignity. They were binding, he believed, on both society and government, and should the government attempt arbitrarily to dispose "of the lives, liberties, or fortunes of the people" he thought that the people were justified in dissolving the old government and acquiring a new one, by revolution if necessary.

So strong was this belief in rights peculiar to individuals as human beings that it survived attacks made on the rationalistic basis upon which those rights had been originally posited. Even when the rights were no longer regarded as "natural," their existence was not questioned. Belief in a system of rights peculiar to individuals, although "explained" and justified differently, extended into the nineteenth century. Men like Bentham and Mill, for example, thought that individual rights were simply a matter of historical fact, that Englishmen had always possessed such rights. They justified them on the grounds of history, utility, heredity, and so forth. However they explained and justified these rights, few thinkers in the eighteenth century and the early part of the nineteenth centuries doubted that individuals did possess inalienable rights peculiar to them as human beings. This was true not only in England but also in France, in Germany, and, indeed, throughout most of the Western world.

INDIVIDUALISM AND FREEDOM

Starting, then, from the assumption that each individual is a moral entity possessing certain substantive rights by virtue of his humanity, it follows logically that each individual ought to be free to develop all his potentialities as a human being. And since arbitrariness is incompatible with human dignity any subjection to the will of another individual, to the will of any personal, capricious authority, is incompatible with the idea that each individual is an autonomous being, equal in moral value with every other individual.

Freedom, however, logically implies responsibility. In order for each individual to have freedom, all individuals must recognize some common authority, some common responsibility. This authority, moreover, must be impersonal, calculable, and objective. Only through the acceptance by the individual of a common, impersonal, rational, and objective authority can the individual be said to be free.

LAW AS THE BASIS OF FREEDOM

The central problem with which liberalism is concerned is the relation between the individual and authority. Liberalism holds that the individual should be free, but realizes that freedom demands the common acceptance of an impersonal authority if it is to be freedom and not license. Accordingly, liberalism espoused freedom from every form of social control except law. As Voltaire succinctly put it: "Freedom exists in being independent from everything but law."

The authority, which necessarily had to be impersonal, objective, and independent of will, could be nothing else than law. Law, moreover, had to be conceived as eternal, immutable, and rational. If the authority was not to be arbitrary, it could not emanate from any will that was capable of acting capriciously; it could not change from day to day or place to place; it must be rational and predictable. It was found, but not made, by reason and by conscience.

Implicit in this reasoning is the assumption that positive law will conform to certain norms and values secured transcendentally, and the further assumption that the enforcement of law is purely impersonal and technical. In this assumption concerning the enforcement of the law there is already an element of formalism, a quantitative conception of justice, but the notion of natural rights is a qualitative conception, and in the beginning this latter conception overshadowed the former.

Accordingly, two essential elements are found in liberalism in its integral form: first, the belief that society is composed of atomic, autonomous individuals; and second, the belief that there are certain eternal truths transcending individuals and independent of either individual will or desire. These eternal truths are referred to by the writers of the seventeenth and eighteenth centuries as natural law or natural rights, but writers of the early nineteenth century arrived at a similar conception in somewhat different terminology. Positive law, in either view, is legitimate and capable of commanding obligation if its content conforms to the content of these transcendental truths.

Positive law is not binding simply because it emanates from the legitimate sovereign, for the sovereign, like all individuals, is under a higher law. He cannot act arbitrarily and cannot make his will binding on other individuals unless his acts fall within the limits set by the higher law. The individual can know if the sovereign is acting justly—if his acts fall within the limits set by law—only through con- science, for it is by objective reason that the individual recognizes the content of law and conscience alone bids him reason objectively. Obligation, accordingly, rests essentially upon individual conscience. The contract does not bind the individual to obey blindly all the commands of the political sovereign, for if the sovereign acts unjustly, if he oversteps the limit set by law, the contract is void and his subjects may legitimately depose him.

It is the duty of individuals to reason objectively, to subordinate passion and desire, in order to recognize the limitations upon will which alone make freedom possible. The content of law is discovered by dispassionate reason, but only con- science obligates the individual so to reason. The link, therefore, between transcen- dental norms, which constitute the only limitation upon will, and individual will is conscience.

For the liberals, human conscience is the source of law and order. They start "from the conviction that man (is) not only a physical being, subject to natural laws, but also a moral being subject to his conscience. . . . Freedom (is) not arbitrariness but subjection to the moral nature of man, which is governed by the moral law. Freedom is accordingly only to be found in subjection to reason, that is to say, man is free only when all his actions are determined by reason."

The immediate followers of Grotius in the seventeenth and eighteenth centuries differed somewhat from him in describing the content of natural law, but few, if any, doubted its existence and most agreed on defining it as the dictate of right reason. This law of nature was thought to be binding upon all individuals, and although the concept of sovereignty which emerged in the sixteenth century might seem at first, by its definition, to contradict this principle, actually it did not.

There was no idea that the monarch was not bound by natural law; on the contrary, he was as much bound by it as any other individual. The test of freedom was whether or not the legislator was subject to limitation, whether or not there was some limitation upon arbitrary will. If there were no such limitation, there could be no freedom. Freedom meant concrete and substantive limitations upon will, whether the individual will of a monarch or the collective will of a legislature. It did not mean a formal limitation but a *substantive* limitation.

When legislative assemblies emerged and began to transfer to themselves the concept of sovereignty which had first been espoused for absolute monarchs, they too were thought of as subject to certain definite limitations imposed by a higher law. Locke made this particularly clear. Tyranny, for Locke as for other liberals, was not synonymous with autocracy but rather with despotism. A government might be highly centralized and autocratic but so long as it recognized substantive limitation to its will it was legitimate. "Wherever law ends, tyranny beings," Locke declared. It was not the form of government which determined its legitimacy, though one form might be preferred to another, but whether there was personal, arbitrary rule or the impersonal rule of law.

The idea of the liberal political philosophers that "the law" was a natural order filled with substantive content was shared by the economists of the seventeenth and eighteenth centuries, finding early expression particularly among the Physiocrats. According to one of them: "The natural order is merely the physical constitution which God Himself has given the universe." "Its laws," according to another, "are irrevocable, pertaining as they do to the essence of matter and the soul of humanity. They are just the expression of the will of God." The idea of a natural order is carried over from the Physiocrats into classical economics by Adam Smith and perpetuated by his followers.

The theologians were similarly abandoning a theistic concept of authority and accepting more and more an immanent authority in the form of certain principles. As one writer has expressed it, although they gave up "the belief in God's extraordinary and miraculous intervention in human affairs" they "laid all the more stress upon God's regular and orderly government." For the pessimistic outlook of orthodox Christianity they substituted an optimistic outlook. Whereas the orthodox Christian looked upon sin as the root of all evil, the liberal theologians tended to regard ignorance as the root of evil. Sin could be removed only by God and by grace; ignorance could be overcome by man through education. Orthodox theologians did not believe the world could be freed from evil, liberal theologians did. This optimistic belief in inevitable progress by education was shared by classical economists and liberal political philosophers.

Thus, in the fields of political philosophy, economics, and theology, emphasis was placed in the seventeenth and eighteenth centuries upon an impersonal natural order which could be rercalized by human reason and conscience. On the one hand, there was the autonomous individual, on the other, the potential order objectified in eternal and universal principles with conscience and reason as the link between the two.

One of the most important manifestations of the emphasis on rights in medical ethics is the American Hospital Association's statement articulating a bill of rights for patients. It demonstrates the shift to the perspective of Western liberal political philosophy. Note that rights are taken primarily as "liberty rights," that is the right to noninterference or "entitlement rights" focusing on noneconomic issues such as the right to considerate and respectful care. This rights focus does not yet address the more entitlement rights claims with more direct economic implications, the claims summarized in the phrase "the right to health care."

A Patient's Bill of Rights

AMERICAN HOSPITAL ASSOCIATION

The American Hospital Association Board of Trustees' Committee on Health Care for the Disadvantaged, which has been a consistent advocate on behalf of consumers of health care services, developed the Statement on a Patient's Bill of Rights, which was approved by the AHA House of Delegates February 6, 1973. The statement was published in several forms, one of which was the S74 leaflet in the Association's S series. The S74 leaflet is now superseded by this reprinting of the statement. The American Hospital Association presents a Patient's Bill of Rights with the expectation that observance of these rights will contribute to more effective patient care and greater satisfaction for the patient, his physician, and the hospital organization. Further, the Association presents these rights in the expectation that they will be supported by the hospital on behalf of its patients, as an integral part of the healing process. It is recognized that a personal relationship between the physician and the patient is essential for the provision of proper medical care. The traditional physician-patient relationship takes on a new dimension when care is rendered within an organizational structure. Legal precedent has established that the institution itself also has a responsibility to the patient. It is in recognition of these factors that these rights are affirmed.

1. The patient has the right to considerate and respectful care.
2. The patient has the right to obtain from his physician complete current information concerning his diagnosis, treatment, and prognosis in terms the patient can be reasonably expected to understand. When it is not medically advisable to give such information to the patient, the information should be made available to an appropriate person in his behalf. He has the right to know, by name, the physician responsible for coordinating his care.

3. The patient has the right to receive from his physician information necessary to give informed consent prior to the start of any procedure and/or treatment. Except in emergencies, such information for informed consent should include but not necessarily be limited to the specific procedure and/or treatment, the medically significant risks involved, and the probable duration of incapacitation. Where medically significant alternatives for care and treatment exist, or when the patient requests information concerning medical alternatives, the patient has the right to such information. The patient also has the right to know the name of the person responsible for the procedures and/or treatment.

4. The patient has the right to refuse treatment to the extent permitted by the law and to be informed of the medical consequences of his action.

5. The patient has the right to every consideration of his privacy concerning his own medical care program. Case discussion, consultation, examination, and treatment are confidential and should be conducted discreetly. Those not directly involved in his care must have the permission of the patient to be present.

6. The patient has a right to expect that all communications and records pertaining to his care should be treated as confidential.

7. The patient has the right to expect that within its capacity a hospital must make reasonable response to the request of a patient for services. The hospital must provide evaluation, service, and/or referral as indicated by the urgency of the case. When medically permissible, a patient may be transferred to another facility only after he has received complete information and explanation concerning the needs for and alternatives to such a transfer. The institution to which the patient is to be transferred must first have accepted the patient for transfer.

8. The patient has a right to obtain information as to any relationship of his hospital to other health care and educational institutions insofar as his care is concerned. The patient has the right to obtain information as to the existence of any professional relationships among individuals, by name, who are treating him.

9. The patient has the right to be advised if the hospital proposes to engage in or perform human experimentation affecting his care or treatment. The patient has the right to refuse to participate in such research projects.

10. The patient has the right to expect reasonable continuity of care. He has the right to know in advance what appointment times and physicians are available and where. The patient has the right to expect that the hospital will provide a mechanism whereby he is informed by his physician or a delegate of the physician of the patient's continuing health care requirements following discharge.

11. The patient has the right to examine and receive an explanation of his bill regardless of source of payment.

12. The patient has the right to know what hospital rules and regulations apply to this conduct as a patient.

No catalog of rights can guarantee for the patient the kind of treatment he has a right to expect. A hospital has many functions to perform, including the prevention and treatment of disease, the education of both health professionals and patients, and the conduct of clinical research. All these activities must be conducted with an overriding concern for the patient, and, above all, the recognition of his dignity as a human being. Success in achieving this recognition assures success in the defense of the rights of the patient.

The shift in focus in medical ethics to the perspective grounded in liberal political philosophy is not without its critics. In addition to those who attempt to defend the more traditional Hippocratic alternative, the American Hospital Association's Patient's Bill of Rights has been criticized by those who argue that the AHA proposal does not go far enough. Some criticize the provision that information can be withheld from a patient "when it is not medically advisable," claiming this is a reversion to the older paternalistic Hippocratic perspective. Others, including Willard Gaylin in the following essay, question the authority of an association of hospitals to "bestow" certain rights on patients. If these are "natural rights," as the liberal tradition has held, then they have their foundation in sources other than a hospital association.

The Patient's Bill of Rights

WILLARD GAYLIN

A stay in a hospital exposes an individual to a condition of passivity and impotence unparalleled in adult life, this side of prison. You are dressed in an uncomfortable garment, leaving you exposed and ludicrous; told when you must sleep and when you must rise; informed of what you may eat and when you have to eat it; notified as to when you can have visitors, who they shall be, and how long they can stay. You are discussed in the third person in your presence as though you were some idiot child or inanimate object. If you are unfortunate enough to have an interesting case, you will be presented to a group of strangers who may take the invasion of your privacy as their privilege. Your chart, at the foot of the bed, will contain all the vital information that you would seem to be entitled to have; yet, should you attempt to examine it, you will be treated like a prepubescent caught with a copy of *Portnoy's Complaint*.

Some of this may be necessary for health and some for convenience, but most of it is simply the inevitable result of an authoritative person dealing with people who unquestionably accept his authority.

Hospital regulations are endured by a patient conditioned to seeing his physician as a benevolent father in whose reassuring presence he is prepared to play the role of the child. Beyond this, however, more serious rights are violated under the numbing atmosphere of the same paternalism.

Modern scientific medicine, as exemplified in complex teaching hospitals, has advanced technical skill at the cost of personal warmth. Often there is no one physician rendering care, rather a battery of specialists, and while "treatment" may be superior, "care" is absent. This depersonalization of medicine is having a predictable effect on the patient, causing him to abandon his tendency to romanticize the physician, and, by extension, the medical community. For this and other reasons the patient is now pressing for a reevaluation of the medical contract.

In response to this, the American Hospital Association recently presented, with considerable fanfare, a "Patient's Bill of Rights." It is a document worth examining, for nothing indicates the low estate of current hospital care (as distinguished from treatment) more graphically than the form of the proffered cure.

The substance of the document is amazingly innocent of controversy. It affirms that "the patient has the right to considerate and respectful care" and, beyond that, the right to "reasonable continuity of care." He is told that he may expect a modicum of personal privacy; that the usual medical concern for confidentiality should be respected; that he has a right to expect "a reasonable response" to his request for service: and, as in any other commercial transaction, that he has a right to receive an explanation of his bill.

In addition, he will be relieved to hear that, as a patient in a hospital, knowledge of the "rules and regulations" that apply to him is manifestly his due—just as it would be if he were a participant in a poker game. Similarly, the right to obtain information "concerning his diagnosis, treatment and prognosis" seems perfectly straightforward—no more than the minimum required of any standard commercial transaction. On the other hand, the patient's right to "obtain information as to any relationship of his hospital to other health care and educational institutions in so far as his care is concerned" is disquieting, for it anxiously suggests that while his exclusive reason for being in the hospital is his personal health, the hospital may have multiple, unstated other reasons influencing its treatment of him.

Finally, when the bill affirms the patient's right to "give informed consent prior to the start of any procedure," his "right to refuse treatment to the extent permitted by law," and his right to be advised "if the hospital proposes to engage in or perform human experimentation" on him, it seems to be merely belaboring the obvious. It says no more than that the hospital is subject to the same laws concerning assault and battery as any other institution or member of society.

The objection to this well-intended, though timid, document is that it perpetuates the very paternalism that precipitated the abuses. But presenting its considerations as a "Patient's Bill of Rights," it creates the impression that the hospital is "granting" these rights to the patient. The hospital has no power to grant these rights. They were vested in the patient to begin with. If the rights have been violated, they have been violated by the hospital and its hirelings. The title a "Patient's Bill of Rights" therefore seems not only pretentious but deceptive. In effect, all that the document does is return to the patient, with an air of largess, some of the rights hospitals have previously stolen from him. It is the thief lecturing his victim on self-protection—i.e., the hospital instructs the patient to make sure that the hospital treats him according to the rules of decency and law to which he is entitled. It would be more appropriate if the association addressed its 7,000 member hospitals, cautioning them that for years they have violated patient rights, some of which have the mandate of law, and warning them they must no longer presume on the innocence of their customers or the indifference of judicial authorities.

Since this is a patently decent document, the fact that the American Hospital Association takes the circuitous route of speaking to the patient of his rights, rather than to the hospital of its duties, reveals the essential weakness of such professional organizations. The AHA, like the American Medical Association and similar groups, is designed to be the servant of its constituent members—and not of the general public. A servant does not lay down the law to his master. In this regard the AHA can only state that it "presents these rights in the expectation that they will be supported" by the member hospitals. The fact that it feels the need to alert the patient indicates how insecure that "expectation" is.

A reevaluation of patient rights—one that goes beyond the old rights affirmed in this bill—is greatly needed. The public should not look to the professional association for leadership here. It is not for the hospital community to outline the rights it will offer, but rather for the patient consumer to delineate and then demand those rights to which he feels entitled by utilizing all the instruments of society designed for that purpose—including the legislature and the courts.

3

Medical Ethical Theories Outside the Anglo-American West

INTRODUCTION

The religions of Judaism and Christianity and the secular thought of the political philosophy of liberalism in the Anglo-American West are not the only alternatives to a Hippocratic medical ethic. Outside of the Anglo-American West there are a number of religious and philosophical alternatives. Most of them build their medical ethics on a more general underlying philosophical or religious foundation. Some of the medical ethical expressions are only fragmentary. Others are quite richly developed systems.

Socialist countries have medical ethics that reflect the broad philosophical commitments of socialism. Some of these are manifest in the democratic socialist states of Western Europe. Others, such as those of the Soviet Union, Eastern Europe, and contemporary China, reflect the Marxism upon which those societies are based. This chapter presents the Oath of the Soviet Physician as well as descriptions of medical ethics in the Soviet Union, Eastern Europe, and China.

Another major alternative to Hippocratic ethics is found in the moral-legal system of Islam. Islam, having common roots with Judaism and Christianity, grounds its ethics in the Quran, the book composed of writings of Muhammad accepted by Muslims as the revelations of Allah. A detailed system of medical ethical positions is derived from the Quran. Presented here is a summary of Islamic medical ethics and the code of ethics for medical professionals of the Islamic Medical Association of the USA and Canada.

Eastern cultures have medical ethical systems closely related to and derived from the teachings of their major religious/philosophical traditions. Indian cultural is dominated by the complex tradition of Hinduism. The ethics of the tradition reflects the important philosophical doctrines such as karma. A summary of the major positions together with one of the ancient Oaths, the Oath of Initiation from the Caraka Samhita, are presented here.

Chinese medical ethics draws on its major traditions as well: Confucianism, Buddhism, and Taoism. The dominant Confucian orthodoxy was challenged by Taoist and Buddhist variants. T'ao Lee's summary reveals the interplay of these traditions.

In Japan Buddhist influences from China and Korea began to penetrate and intermix with indigenous Japanese beliefs (the system called

Shintoism in Western scholarship). Space permits only one example of the product of that intermixing: a sixteenth-century code revealing strong Buddhist influence called the Seventeen Rules of Enjuin. The samples presented here only hint at the richness of the diversity of medical ethical systems in cultures outside the Anglo-American.

Contemporary Marxist cultures, whether they be in China, Cuba, or Eastern Europe, ground their ethical judgments in Marxism and its twentieth-century variants. Benjamin Page begins his essay on medical ethics in eastern Europe by surveying the philosophical and contextual background of such professional ethics. He reveals the links among ethical norms, the working class, and the party or state. He shows how positions on particular medical ethical problems, like genetics and transplantation, are related to underlying socioethical norms.

Eastern Europe in the Twentieth Century

BENJAMIN B. PAGE

Most areas of biomedical research and health care in Eastern Europe that involve ethical issues are similar to those in other technologically advanced countries. The ways in which they are expressed and approached differ as a consequence of Marxist philosophy and the resulting socioeconomic and political context in which they arise. Thus the context and philosophy must be considered first.

PHILOSOPHICAL AND CONTEXTUAL BACKGROUNDS

Marx held that the culture, laws, and ethics of any society reflect the interests of the ruling class, the class that owns the means of production. Thus, Marxism denies the existence of universal ethical principles. Under socialism, the working class is considered the ruling class, and all who work in a socially owned industry or service are members of that class. The ethical norms of a socialist society correspond to the interests of the working class as interpreted by its party and state. The ultimate interest of a Marxist working class is the attainment of communism, of a society in which each and all, liberated from exploitation and economic determinism, are free to develop their full human potential. The final test of the morality of a law, behavioral norm, or action is the degree to which it is believed to contribute to communism.

Similarly, Marxism rejects the existence of autonomous professional ethics. Professionals are regarded first of all as citizens of a socialist society and, like all others who are employed, as members of the working class. Their interests are—or should be—those of the working-class movement toward communism. One task of ethics is to help individual professionals overcome discrepancies in this regard.

The full development of science and technology, in mutual interaction with the socioeconomic and political changes already initiated by socialism, is seen as the means by which communism will eventually be achieved. Thus, science acquires a special moral sanction.

Man and Medicine in Marxist Philosophy

The Marxist view of man rejects any sort of dualism. Man is considered a unity of biochemical and genetic factors, of social factors, and as a result of their interaction, of psychological factors. It is untenable for medicine to abstract man from his environment and treat him in terms of biochemical processes or organ systems alone. Although medicine draws from the natural, it is more closely related to the social sciences and, in its ultimate concern for the welfare of man, is part of the humanities. Its humanistic mission is believed capable of full realization only on the basis of socialism.

The Socioeconomic and Political Context

The protection of health is considered a vital interest of the working class and is included in most socialist constitutions as a basic right. This and other social rights have more recently been extended to collective farmers, independent artisans, and the like. Marxism considers it irresponsible idealism to proclaim a right without providing means for its realization. Thus the constitutional proclamation makes the state responsible for training, equipping, distributing, and paying for all personnel and facilities—including those research—needed to make health protection and medical care universally available.

Prevention of accidents and illnesses and, more recently, the promotion of healthful living and working environments receive special priority. Considered more in keeping with the goals of Marxist humanism than is therapy, they are also more economically efficient when the state pays for both. Hence the many programs, some mandatory, to supervise the health of expectant mothers, of children and workers, especially those in health-hazardous environments or occupations, and of people with identified medical or genetic problems. This priority influences priorities in research and the selection of new technologies for further development. Finally, since the mid-1960s most countries have enacted laws placing legal responsibility for health promotion on managers of work places, agencies of public administration, and designers of housing, factories, etc. (e.g., Czechoslovakia's Law on the Health Care of the People). When standards cannot be met, fines are imposed, from which funds those people who are negatively affected, especially children and workers, are compensated by preferential treatment in access to summer camps, spa treatment, and the like.

Thus the constitutional right to the protection of one's health implies a continuum from education, promotion, and prevention, through care, to rehabilitation.

In addition to providing the means for this, the government is responsible for eliminating socioeconomic factors that, among other things, have a negative influence on health: e.g., unemployment, economic insecurity, the effects of differences in income, lack of cultural opportunities, inadequate housing, etc.

Health-Care Organization

In Soviet-based systems, health care is organized geographically. Citizens are assigned to neighborhood and work place clinics administered by the various levels of elected agencies of public administration. The latter receive budgets from the government for this purpose. Ministries of Health establish the norms that public administrations must follow, provide professional direction, undertake research and in some countries the manufacture of medications and medical equipment, and administer specialized facilities.

Neighborhood or industrial clinics staffed by general practitioners, gynecologists, pediatricians, and dentists are the primary points of contact with the health-care system; all other services are referral. Dissatisfied patients may appeal to the appropriate level of public administration for a change of physician or clinic. Free choice of medical providers is seen as conflicting with the community system and the possibilities it offers for coordinated work in prevention and health promotion. It would also undermine what is considered a positive feature of socialized medicine—the elimination of economic interest on the part of providers in the treatment of patients.

Patients may refuse recommended treatment only by signing a statement releasing the institution in which it was offered from legal responsibility. However, if a physician believes a treatment to be necessary for maintaining the patient's life, he is expected to treat, if possible, anyhow. The institutions, rather than individual providers, are legally responsible for damage to patients.

MAIN AREAS OF ETHICAL CONCERN

The Physician-Patient Relationship

In addition to sharing some of the problems found in non-Marxist societies, including those of the effects of technology and paperwork, socialist countries face other problems based on the changed social role of physicians.

Physicians are considered the salaried agents of socialist society's interest in the health of its citizens, agents of official health policy, and representatives of socialist humanism, as well as the personal physicians or ill or injured patients. However, it is felt that there are problems in the actual behavior of some physicians and other health workers towards patients, including the elderly. The natural dependency of a patient on one who can help is complicated by the fact that the only link between the two is the patient's need—which is not always enough to ensure the physician's continuing interest—and that patients can turn elsewhere only on the basis of lengthy appeals processes. Thus the conduct of health workers can become bureau-cratic. In turn, some patients occasionally try to use such illegal means as bribes in the hope of obtaining improved treatment or medically unwarranted services, medi-cation, or time releases from work. Physicians also complain that their services are sometimes taken for granted and that even those performed outside the scope of normal duties or hours go unnoticed and unthanked.

Truth-Telling and Confidentiality

The main considerations in the questions of truth-telling and confidentiality are to obtain patients' cooperation and to do nothing that might harm them or deprive them of hope. Patients are generally told only such information as fits within these parameters. In some case, e.g., when surgery or dialysis is indicated or when a patient or parents balk at recommended treatment, the whole truth may have to be told, but no a priori obligation is felt in this regard. Similarly, confidentiality is neither an end in itself nor an a priori commitment. Under normal circumstances, it is adhered to. However, health-care providers have obligations to society and to the prevention of harm to others, as well as obligations to particular patients. If a provider believes a patient has been involved in criminal activity or activity dan-gerous to others, he must notify the proper authorities and cooperate with them in seeking such individuals.

Team Approach and a Physician's Broader Obligation

The team approach is considered indispensable in modern medicine. To be effec-tive, it presupposes harmony, collegiality, and democracy among team members. For all of this the physician is responsible.

As citizens of a socialist society, physicians cannot be medical experts alone. They are expected to act, even in free time, in ways that reflect favorably on the health-care system and the society that provides it. They are also expected to be actively involved in the future of their country and of socialism. The social prestige still popularly attached to medicine only heightens these obligations.

Research and Experimentation

Research projects in any area are selected and funded in the context of national five-year planning processes. Theoretically research planning is kept within the frame-work of national priorities, resources, needs, and sociopolitical considerations. Gen-eral research priorities follow those established for health-care delivery. There is occasional tension, however, between these priorities and the interests of particular researchers or institutions.

Such is the context in which research involving human experimentation is permitted. Informed consent is required of all subjects except those used as control groups. The latter must be treated with the means currently considered the most effective. Although those damaged are compensated, participants are not rewarded.

Prisoners and the mentally incompetent may not be used as subjects. Fetuses are not considered the property of the "parents," and a limited amount of fetal research is quietly done. In most countries, unless a witnessed statement of opposition is included in one's identity papers, consent to autopsy for research purposes and to postmortem removal of organs or tissues for transplantation is assumed.

Genetics

Nazism and Lysenkoism were responsible for a considerable delay in the development of genetics. Today the main priorities include genetic counseling, efforts to remove genetically dangerous chemical agents from the environment and attempts to make genetics an integral part of medical education and practice. Counselors stress that even in connection with efforts to prevent genetic defects in future generations, a socialist society can go no farther than information and advice. People have the right to know whatever medicine can tell them about themselves; consideration is being given to requiring couples planning marriage to tell each other anything known about their health or genetic status that might place the partner or any children at risk. However, decisions about marriage and children are seen to belong to only those involved. The state is responsible for providing the means to support people in whatever decision they make: abortion, free if for medical reasons; artificial insemination; economic and other supports for parents of genetically defective children; institutional care facilities, and so on. Efforts to "improve the species" are focused on planned improvement of the physical, cultural, and sociopolitical environments in which people live, and on making parents and teachers sensitive to expressions of special talent on the part of children. The place for positive eugenics is in the improvement of food crops.

Unofficially, concern has been expressed about the growing numbers of genetically defective children in institutions. Like everyone else, they are given gratis whatever medical care they need. The concern is about the increasing burden the institutional approach places on the resources of the health system and about the quality of life the genetically expect.

Transplantation

Most East European countries have facilities for kidney transplantation, with an organ exchange program among themselves. Some concern has been expressed that the costs involved might better be spent in improving the prevention of conditions requiring transplantation.

Selection of recipients for kidneys is seen as presenting no ethical problem: people over fifty are not accepted because their success rate is too low; immunological and compatibility requirements are so stringent that, reportedly, no case of more than one appropriate candidate for a particular kidney has yet arisen in the exchange program. Living donors known to recipients are not desired because of possible psychological complications. The laws permitting also automatic postmortem removal of the organs suitable for transplantation also stipulate that removal may be done only in hospitals with resuscitation facilities, and only after the resuscitation team has certified brain death. (Some countries, e.g., the USSR, use cardiological criteria for death, with somewhat less transplantation activity.) To prevent conflicts of interest, resuscitation and transplantation teams must be separate. Recipients are not told the name of the donor, nor is the latter's family informed that the procedure has been done. Selection of recipients for dialysis and other scarce medical resources is a problem on which a definitive approach has not yet been established.

Euthanasia, Aging, and Dying

Legally, euthanasia is out of the question. At the same time, physicians are required to make every effort to save every life. The technologies for doing so are making dysthanasia ("ugly death") an ever more frequent problem. The fact that only patients themselves can refuse recommended treatment frees relatives from the burdens of decision and responsibility. Since physicians are required to treat, if possible, in what they consider life-threatening conditions—even over patient opposition—they alone are left with the final decision. Little in their training or the literature to date offers them norms or guidelines except individual conscience and what has been called "the ethics of the moment". The liberation of the physician from personal legal responsibilities and financial risk vis-a-vis patients' families, and of families from the economic consequences of continued treatment, removes these two secondary issues from consideration but hardly makes the physician's task much easier.

Thus far the aged have been assigned relatively low priority in the gradual development of socialist medical and social benefits. However, recent Party congresses and national legislation have mandated the development of a much wider range of programs and services for them. Additionally, the number of articles and conferences dealing with the aged and their special problems has markedly increased, urging people, including those in health care, to be patient and considerate of the aged and cognizant of their needs to feel wanted, needed, and loved. The implication seems to be that such attitudes are too frequently absent. However, the only reasons offered as to why the young should so act are that the aged, when younger, helped build socialism and that the young, too, will one day be old.

The area of dying and death is little developed in Marxist philosophy or socialist health-care practice. The literature increasingly recognizes it as an area health-care workers will have to take more seriously, because more people are dying in institutions while fewer are practicing believers with clergy to help them or their families. Recent articles, television programs, and the like call for more attention to the dimension of human existence that death represents. Health education has been called upon to prepare both the general public and health-care professionals better for death—their own and those of friends, family, and patients. However, very little of this discussion differs in essence from the kinds of things heard in recent years in the West.

Other Issues

There are two further areas of ethical significance that merit attention, even though neither is currently a topic of discussion in the official medical press of Eastern Europe. One of these, abortion, is significant because of the ethical debate surrounding it in the United States. The other, the political use of psychiatry, is significant because of reports of the practice in the USSR.

At present, abortion is not an area of public debate, nor is it seen as involving questions of humanhood or the right to life. It is legal, but not thereby a woman's right, and, except when done for medical reasons, there is usually a fee. Abortions are granted only after mandatory case reviews. Review committee decisions reflect current state abortion policy, which varies over time within, and differs considerably among, the countries of Eastern Europe.

Officially, Soviet psychiatrists deny that their profession has ever been misused for political purposes. As Western observers have commented, if true, this would be an enviable situation. Psychiatrists and jurists in many countries have traditionally been concerned over the problem of the possible role of external interests or factors in cases where authorities seek the involuntary confinement of people for non-criminal offenses. The number of stories of Soviet citizens reportedly so treated is great enough for concern to be warranted, particularly in view of the fact that Soviet legal practice denies those whose sanity is in question what would otherwise be due process or even basic information about the charges against them or the findings of psychiatrists consulted. It would seem, however, that, to the extent that psychiatry is misused for political purposes, the practice is related more to internal Soviet conditions than to the application of Marxist philosophy; there have been few reports of such practices elsewhere in Eastern Europe.

THE TEACHING OF BIOMEDICAL ETHICS AND THE OATH OF SOVIET PHYSICIANS

Except in the USSR there is as yet little coordinated work done in the teaching of ethics in biomedical research or health-care delivery contexts. Most efforts are at the level of articles, films, symposia, and the like. Individuals sensitive to the issues have, however, begun integrating them into their courses and grand rounds, and they are occasionally the topic of the regular political education seminars required of all health-care professionals. The Czech Ministry of Health has recently established a research team on "philosophical and ethical issues in medicine," one of whose projects is a study of the awareness of Marxist-Leninist methodology on the part of medical practitioners. Conclusions for teaching may follow from its findings.

In the USSR a new discipline, medical deontology, has emerged around the 1971 physicians' oath. Part of the curriculum of medical schools, it includes the duty of physicians, the history and psychology of medicine, and the moral relationships of physicians with patients, other health workers, and their own families. The 1971 physicians' oath has become the basis on which physician performance and patient grievances are evaluated. The oath taken by Russian physicians under Tsarism was abolished shortly after the Revolution; none was in effect until 1971.

SUMMARY

The similarity of most of the biomedical issues concerning which there is ethical debate in Eastern Europe and in the West suggests that they may be indigenous to scientifically based, technologically oriented medicine. The ways these issues are formulated reflect the socialist economic and political context in which health care is provided, but influence of Marxist philosophy is more strongly evident in that context, and in the ways in which the issues are handled, than in the issues themselves. Socialism has resolved some of the ethical and practical problems faced by the United States in financing and distributing care and research but has not thereby rendered care always more humane or considerate. The Party congresses held in much of Eastern Europe during 1976 stressed that, with quantitative problems largely under control, improving the quality of health care is to become an official priority.

Medical ethics in the Soviet Union reflects a complex history. Early Russian culture had historical links with Greece. It is not surprising that Czarist Russia traced its medical ethical roots to the Hippocratic Oath as did other European cultures. The exclusive individualism of the Oath, however, is not compatible with the system of political philosophy in the contemporary Soviet Union. In 1971 the Supreme Soviet Presidium adopted an oath that was meant to reflect an understanding of the duties of the physician consistent with the philosophical commitments of the society. The term "deontology" is used in the description of the medical ethics of the Soviet Union that follows. It is a term roughly meaning "ethics" that appears in many European discussions. The term traces back to the Greek word for duty. It should not be confused with the same term used in a much more narrow and technical sense in contemporary Anglo-American analytical ethics in which deontology is the name for one particular theory of normative ethics. While in Anglo-American analytical philosophy "deontology" refers only to one position in normative ethical theory, the position that there are inherent right-making characteristics of actions other than consequences (the position often contrasted with consequentialism of which utilitarianism is a major example), in European discussion "deontology" refers simply to ethical and philosophical discussion particularly regarding professions such as medicine. What follows is a description of the contemporary situation in medical ethics in the Soviet Union and an analysis of the Oath of the Soviet physician. Note that in the United States the dominant professional code of ethics, the Principles of the American Medical Association, is simply adopted by the professional association without any official government or other lay involvement. In the Soviet Union, the physician's Oath is officially adopted by the Supreme Soviet Presidium.

Medical Deontology in the Soviet Union

RALPH CRAWSHAW

Scholars are men of peace, they bear no arms, . . . for these are the men, that, when they have played their part and had their exits, must step out and give the moral of their scenes, and deliver unto posterity an inventory of their Virtues and Vices.

Thomas Browne *Religio Medici*

Medical deontology in the USSR is important to the medical profession throughout the world as an example of a concerted attempt to meet some fundamental problems assailing modern medicine. Succinctly, deontology is the study of duty, and medical deontology, necessarily, is the study of the physician's duty.

My interest in Soviet deontology antedates a recent visit, since in 1971 when the Supreme Soviet Presidium endorsed a new medical oath for Soviet physicians, I began an analysis of the structure and dynamic meaning of the oath. Correspondence with Professor V. Varakin of the Soviet Ministry of Health, produced a copy of the oath and encouragement to study further.

The Soviet definition of medical deontology includes much more than simply the delineation of the physician's duty. In the USSR, medical deontology has become the study of the profession as a living institution and includes not only the duty of the physician but the history of the profession, its psychology, its philosophy, and all of the relationships physicians may have with ancillary medical personnel, the patient, and his family.

HISTORY

The father of Russian deontology, though he never used the word, was M. Y. Moodroff (1776–1831). He founded a school of medicine that placed the doctor-patient relationship at the fulcrum of all therapeutic action. Later, Dr. Banilevsky systematized medical deontology for the first time with his book, *The Doctor: His Education and Calling.* This volume covered most of a physician's background, ranging from the physician's intellectual endowment, his personal well-being, his attitude toward society, and his successes and failures with patients, to his ultimate responsibility—his patient, a responsibility Banilevsky called, "the doctor's secret."

More recently, Professor K. A. Skoftoff has studied the psychological relationship of the patient and his disease. "The patient first thinks that he is above his disease, then filling with fear, runs from it, labeling it evil. As the disease persists, he becomes oppressed by it, first as the servant of his disease, and then its slave. Only then does he come to look at it in its every part" (B. D. Petrov, MD, oral communication, November 1973). As recently as 1969, Dr. R. Zagarnick summarized the role of the doctor as follows: "The doctor should understand the personality of the patient, his peculiarities, his suffering. Thus, he develops his tactic of treatment. The doctor should be capable of mobilizing all the strengths of the patient against disease, and develop this attitude of strength in the patient."

From this anlage of professional concern, deontological knowledge has gradually evolved in the Soviet Union. However, it was not until 1969 that thinking crystallized into a unified approach. In that year the first All Soviet Union Conference on Deontology was held in Moscow.

THE SOVIET OATH

The two most immediate and perhaps important, developments from the first conference have been the new Soviet Medical Oath and curriculum of medical deontology.

Dr. B. V. Petrosky, the Minister of Health, commissioned a group headed by

Dr. N. N. Blokhin to develop the oath. They met over 100 times during the course of eight months, and eventually produced the Soviet Medical Oath.

Dr. B. D. Petrov, Director of the Institute of Social Hygiene, emphasized, in contrasting the present oath with the Hippocratic Oath administered in Czarist Russia, that the Soviet Oath places more emphasis on the social relationships of the physician, particularly those with the State. The oath links the physician to the Soviet nation by his promise to devote his entire personality to the highest Soviet ethic, communist morality.

In Moscow, the oath is administered at a special ceremony during the student's final year, and reportedly, it is an emotional experience with tears, handshakes, and much camaraderie. Apparently, genuine emotion cements the oath and the man together, as only passion can do.

One of the immediate benefits resulting from the new oath has been a better review of grievances. With the oath as a standard, the Ministry of Health can now analyze the behavior of a physician whom patients complain about and it has been revealed that some physicians are rough, uncooperative, and at times, frankly unjust with patients.

One example of how the oath uncovered an unjust complaint against a physician occurred when a young boy dove into a shallow river and sustained severe injuries, which left him a paraplegic. The attending physician did everything possible to save the boy's life, staying at the bedside for the last 24 hours of his life, but to no avail. After the boy died, the bereft mother was informed by a busybody aide that if there had been a senior staff member "a professor" present the boy would have survived. For the mother this was the truth, and nothing would placate her. She brought a malpractice charge against the physician but the case was dismissed from court for lack of evidence. The mother then raised her friends and neighbors to a pitch of righteous indignation that led to 300 separate complaints against the doctor being sent, including a petition to L. I. Brezhnev, General Secretary of the Communist Party. Under the impact of this assault, the doctor became emotionally disturbed and suicidal and a medical deontologist was consulted. He traced the difficulty to its source, revealing how the spirit of the oath had been misunderstood by some of the medical staff through poor communication. Then, together with the staff, the deontologists began a group process of working through the difficulty. Presumably, this gave the staff sufficient insight and strength to work the conflict through with the mother's friends, one of whom eventually cleared the air and settled the uproar, by telling the mother, straight out that "You are a sad and unhappy woman but what is to be gained by making fifty more people unhappy?"

MOSCOW CURRICULUM

The second recent development is a curriculum of deontology for the medical students. Dr. Z. A. Bondar, member of the Academy of Medical Sciences of the USSR, and Director of the First Medical Institute of Moscow, was given the task of developing this curriculum. Incidentally, unlike medical schools in this country that operate as colleges under the aegis of universities, Soviet medical schools were divorced from their university affiliation in 1930 and have since operated as independent institutions under the Academy of Sciences.

It is anticipated that the curriculum will begin with a series of lectures for the first and second year students. However, their concept of professional life is so amorphous that much of the information, particularly the nuances of professional relationships, may slip by them, and therefore medical deontology is continued as an elective in the senior year, here focusing on student discussions of ward experiences.

Soviet medical deontology is an ethical theory based on communist morality. Medical deontology is divided into social hygiene and medical psychology, structure and process. Social hygiene is directly concerned with the organization and administration of medical services of the USSR while medical psychology is concerned with the general behavior of the physician and his practice of medicine. Medical psychology studies the physician's difficult position in mediating between patient demands and the complex of medical organizations. Nor are the details overlooked, for whether it is a matter of clean fingernails, the odor of alcohol on the breath, or fear of getting close to patients, the faculty is prepared to help the student. Dr. Bondar, incidentally, forbids students from smoking anywhere on the medical institute grounds, and, as she conducted me through the hospital, we had the amusing experience of looking in on the student lounge only to discover a surprised and unhappy student attempting to conceal his glowing cigarette behind his book. Kindly, ever so kindly, but with disciplined firmness, Dr. Bondar reminded him that his behavior was out-of-bounds.

Studying the curriculum is not limited to medical students, but includes all personnel who have any contact with the patient. All members of the staff are expected to consider the patient in the broadest perspective, and in Russian fashion, these details are made explicit. The patient's age, surroundings, experience, personality, training, the character of his disease and its possible complications, as well as his prognosis are to be considered by each person who has contact with the patient.

LENINGRAD CURRICULUM

In many ways, Leningrad and Moscow have a friendly yet pointed academic rivalry similar to that between Boston and New York. Vice Chancellor G. A. Dunaevsky was kind enough to conduct me through the First Institute of Medicine in Leningrad. At present, the Institute has a clinical base of 2,000 beds and trains approximately 5,000 pre-med, medical, resident, and postgraduate students.

The Leningrad faculty takes an active interest in finding the best candidates for medical school, and here, as in Moscow, the basic goal of medical deontology was characterized as selecting "men of character" for the medical profession. The Leningrad program begins with radio and television programs beamed to the public that outline goals and difficulties of the medical profession. In addition, a small medical academy for prospective medical students gives lectures detailing the specific work of physicians, acquaints them with the medical institute grounds, the anatomical theaters, physicians in training, and admits them to some medical lectures. As in our country, the number of applicants far exceeds the available positions in medical school and strenuous efforts are made to eliminate those simply interested in a lifetime of study or looking for a secure position.

Repeatedly, Dr. Dunaevsky emphasized that the spirit of medicine must be engendered in the student from the start, and the first official act of a student at the Leningrad Institute is a deontological one. Freshmen, on their first day, assemble outside the anatomical museum where a faculty member, dressed in the costume of Hippocrates, speaks to them about the seriousness of their undertaking. The first year students are given an oath of indoctrination, which, according to Dr. Dunaevsky, is "to study, study, study, and study."

Throughout his medical education the student deals with deontology. Each course has a specific portion devoted to the deontological implications of the subject. In the first and second years, it is the deontological problems of the basic sciences; while in the third and fourth years, problems of the relationship between doctor and patient are examined, with the emphasis on viewing the patient as a human being rather than a collection of organs. In the fifth and sixth year, the focus shifts to theoretical considerations, including those of forensic medicine.

At the completion of his formal training the student takes the Soviet Medical Oath in the presence of the entire faculty, who are robed in white. When questioned about costumes, Dr. Dunaevsky quickly responded, "Yes, the classical forms are preserved, simply because they make sense." Dr. Dunaevsky, like Dr. Petrov in Moscow, emphasized that the Soviet oath is not just a document, but an organic part of the State, approved by the Supreme Soviet Presidium. Through the oath the student relates not only to his profession, but to all of his society.

FURTHER DEVELOPMENTS

Present thinking on Soviet medical deontology is not limited to Moscow and Leningrad. Professor Levioff in Kiev has inaugurated a series of lectures through the Ukranian Institute of Social Hygiene, which are available to the local medical faculties as source material for the study of medical deontology. The medical faculty in the Iranian Republic has developed a Board of Medical History and Deontology to inculcate deontological principally among physicians. Many, if not all the Republics of the USSR are experimenting with various approaches. So far the outstanding ending is but the essential need of the professors is for "people of fire," ie, men and women of character, to carry on medical tradition.

COMMENT

This account of two weeks in the USSR is reportive, perhaps analytic but not prescriptive. During the course of my stay, I had an opportunity to talk with many serious scholars who have concerned themselves with the goals and development of the medical profession, the problems of ethical education, the conceptualization of the doctor-patient relationship, and with intraprofessional relationships of moment. Sometimes our sessions ended with caviar and cognac, sometimes with sugar cakes and tea, but always with a deep sense of comradeship engendered by our mutual respect for our profession.

Only on one point of medical care was there a patent difference of opinion, and that was the curiously compulsive attitude of optimism displayed by Soviet physicians toward patients. I was told that a physician must be optimistic to help his patient but in my limited judgment this optimism may sometimes exceed reality. To illustrate, regardless of the circumstances, no moribund patient in the Soviet Union is ever informed of his impending death. It was emphasized that this policy is universally observed throughout the country. Such firmly established policy of "optimism" appears to me to be more an expression of faith than a belief arrived at by examined doubts. Unfortunately, I had no way of examining this deeply and simply report the phenomenon as I saw it.

CONCLUSION

It is abundantly clear that there are physicians in the Soviet Union interested in more than just delivering medical service; they seek to deliver humane medical service and are open-minded in considering the moral authority of physicians. By taking a holistic view of their profession building on their strongest traditions and organizing as best they can to serve the spiritual needs of their patients, they address one of, if not the cardinal problem of our times, the loss of individual identity in mass capture. Perhaps limitations of time, resources, or politics will, in whole or in part, impede them and perhaps the task is as impossible as that of Sisyphus, yet to the degree that they sincerely devote themselves to their fellow man they are worthy of our admiration.

Soviet Medical Oath

Upon having conferred on me the high calling of physician, and entering medical practice I do solemnly swear:

To dedicate all my knowledge and strength to the preservation and improvement of the health of mankind and to the treatment and prevention of disease, and to work in good conscience wherever it is required by society;

To always be ready to provide medical care, to relate to the patient attentively and carefully, and to preserve medical confidences;

To constantly perfect my medical knowledge and clinical skill and thereby in my work to aid in the development of medical science and practice;

To refer, if patient's better interest warrant it, for advice from my fellow physicians and never myself to refuse to give such advice or help;

To preserve and develop the noble conditions of Soviet medicine, to be guided in all my actions by the principles of communist morality, and always to bear in mind the high calling of a Soviet physician and my responsibility to the people and the Soviet state.

I swear to be loyal to this as long as I live.

> Medical ethics in contemporary China provides another example of a Marxist socialist society's alternative to Hippocratic and liberal Western medical ethics. China adds a different dimension, however, in offering a culture with historical influences quite different from those of Eastern Europe. The Chinese concern for resource allocation and the theme "serve the people," for example, can be found in the ancient Confucian Chinese medical writings no matter how differently it is manifest in contemporary post-revolutionary thought. The essay provided here offers a Western philosopher-physician's observations about medical ethics in contemporary China.

Bioethics in the People's Republic of China

H. Tristram Engelhardt

From August 22 to September 5, 1979, I travelled throughout the People's Republic of China with a group of lawyers, philosophers, physicians, and theologians organized by the Kennedy Institute of Ethics. We traveled to Canton, Peking, Jinan, Qufu, and Shanghai, visiting not only communes and hospitals, but also academic centers like Peking University, the Medical College of Jinan, and Fudan University (Shanghai). We also met with government officials: Vice Premier Yau Yi-Lin; Dr. Huang, Director of the Academy of Medicine; the members of the Ministry of Education; and Judge Li, Chief Justice of the Shanghai court.

No one becomes an expert on any country's views, on any matter, in a period of two weeks. This is emphatically true in the case of China, and therefore, what I offer here are scattered reflections concerning biomedical ethics in China. These are drawn from our meetings and discussions with physicians, philosophers, judges, and others in China who were willing to explore topics in biomedical ethics.

The discussions were open and for the most part frank. At no time did I feel barred from exploring any particular issues, though on occasion it was difficult to distinguish evasion from failure to communicate. This was the case even though, in addition to two translators supplied by the China International Travel Service, two members of our group were fluent in Chinese. On one occasion, questions went unanswered because they purportedly touched on state secrets (the number of executions in China). However, in all circumstances I found our hosts to be friendly, eager to pursue scholarly issues, and interested in open exchange, even on matters that one might have thought somewhat sensitive, such as the state of academic freedom during the Cultural Revolution in the late sixties and early seventies. In fact, their patience with our perseverance on some issues was exemplary.

BACKGROUND ASSUMPTIONS

Attempts to discuss bioethical issues often led to some confusion because our hosts had little experience discussing ethical issues outside of a commitment to a particular moral viewpoint. That is, for many of them ethics was a mode of moral indoctrination or of exegesis of a single moral viewpoint, in this case Maoist-Leninist-Marxism. Consequently, consternation and puzzlement accompanied our efforts to identify their conceptual foundations. The Chinese failed to distinguish principles that would intellectually justify a moral point of view, the grounds that would likely motivate one to be faithful to such a view, and the causal influences that would tend to make a particular moral point of view the prevailing one.

Their resistance to these efforts was likely rooted in: (1) their lack of extended experience with a variety of moral viewpoints; (2) unfamiliarity with discussions focused primarily on discovering the comparative intellectual merits of varying moral viewpoints apart from any immediate concern to establish or maintain a single one; and (3) their overriding tendency, because of dialectical materialism, to hold that all ethical reflections are reducible to economic forces. As a result, questions directed to discovering the conceptual assumptions underlying a particular moral policy were likely to evoke: (1) a homily extolling the virtues of revolutionary humanitarianism; (2) an explanation of how moral views are determined by economic forces and reflect the interests of particular classes; or (3) both of the above. On the other hand, senior academicians recognized the intent of our questions and at times explained us with a smile to their colleagues: we had idealistic interests and were disposed to act as if one could deal with ideas independently of their economic or material bases. Finally, many individuals were at times simply puzzled about our interest in, not only purely intellectual issues in ethics, but in particular policies.

For example, some expressed wonderment at our concern that there should be a definition of death to employ when removing organs from the obviously imminently dying, but not yet dead. This was also the case with questions about contraceptive advice to unmarried young people. After all, there is little or no promiscuity in China.

As a result, the distinctions ethicists make so regularly in the United States, such as the line between unjustified coercion and justified manipulation, the limits of paternalism, and the definition of death, were often seen as exotic. Yet our hosts had their own positions, replete with implicit subtle distinctions. It is simply that they had not attended with a conceptual, analytical interest to the nature of those distinctions. In this respect, their approach resembled much of the medical ethos prevalent not too long ago in the United States. There was a well-developed set of moral views, but no systematic regard for the justification of their presuppositions or for how they might at times be contradictory. Consequently, in this article, I have arranged the issues we discussed topically rather than systematically.

THE FAMILY

A perhaps startling fact about China is that family life remains intact. Indeed, it is a central social and political unit. Divorce is rare. Three generations regularly live together in the same crowded set of rooms. In addition, the family is the focus of social rewards and punishments, and it is also a unit for negotiation of disputed ethical issues. Children still have the accepted moral task of supporting their parents. In fact, there are legal mechanisms to ensure that such support will be forthcoming. As a result, the family has an importance in decision making that it does not possess in the United States.

CONSENT

As far as we could determine, consent to medical and experimental procedures involves a full presentation of the likely risks and benefits of the procedures to be used. Thus, a woman about to undergo a thyroidectomy was told the risks of severing the recurrent laryngeal nerve or of removing the parathyroids, with the possible consequences of impaired speech and of other problems. When consent is obtained in difficult cases the family becomes the focus. In a commune hospital we were told that the physician often went to the family and that everyone then spoke with the patient about the virtues of the treatment of choice. This approach reflects two aspects of the Chinese resolution of disputes. First, community social pressure is the first and usually very effective mode of obtaining agreement. Second, the family plays an important role in securing patient consent, even with adult patients. However, others, such as fellow-workers, are also involved.

For the most part, such means of persuasion appeared to be very successful. "What would happen," we asked, "if a patient were to refuse life saving treatment?" We were told repeatedly that that situation never occurs. This, of course, is true only up to a point. It was reported to John Collins Harvey, M.D., that physicians in a screening program for esophageal cancer were, on the one hand, easily able to obtain the consent of workers and peasants to the somewhat uncomfortable examinations involved. Communal social pressures were undoubtedly used to ensure that almost everyone came to the screening. However, those discovered to have cancer of the esophagus frequently refused treatment. As a consequence, there was a partial discontinuation of the program.

The Director of the Academy of Medicine stressed that fully free and informed consent was sought from all persons involved in research. But even prior to recruiting subjects from the general population, researchers or physicians served as research subjects themselves. For example, a new male contraceptive was being tested first on urologists, primarily researchers involved in the project. However, one might suspect that members of whatever class selected to be research subjects would confront considerable social pressures to agree to participate. Consent in medicine appears to be obtained without overt coercion, but in a social milieu where there are strong social pressures for agreement to worthwhile undertakings.

There is an increasing interest in transplantation in China. Inquiries regarding the sources for organs produced varying answers. John Collins Harvey was told by one individual that a fair number of organs are available as a result of executions. A question on the subject at Fudan University produced an explanation of how consent was obtained from the relatives of donors along with a denial that executions produced organs for transplantation. Since traditional Chinese mores militate against removing body organs, the transplantation team would frequently bring the family of the donor to see the recipient, and then explain to them the importance of allowing their relative's organs to be used to save the intended recipient. We were told that such discussions of social responsibility usually resulted in consent.

DEFINITION OF DEATH

When queried about the criteria used in defining an individual's death prior to removing organs for transplantation, the Chinese were initially puzzled. Their definition of death remains oriented toward heart and lung function and they were unacquainted with recent discussions of brain-oriented definitions of death in the United States. When pressed, one physician explained that when organs from living donors were used, the organs were removed only when individuals were clearly dying. They were asked whether it was important to pronounce someone dead prior to removing organs for transplantation. In reply, they stressed that great care was taken to select as donors only those who were really in a terminal state and were expected to die in the very near future, presumably within minutes.

SEXUALITY

An understanding of the contraceptive and abortive practices of the PRC requires at least some notion of the sexual ethos currently prevailing in China. The Chinese claim that there is very little sexual activity either before marriage or outside marriage; we were also told that there were few homosexuals in China. Strong social sanctions proscribe aberrant or deviant sexual activities; and there appears to be a mechanism for fining unmarried individuals who have a child out of wedlock. Individuals who persist in committing adultery are subjected to criminal sanctions under the rubric of sexual molestation or of bigamy. However, we were told privately that though there was less unsanctioned sexual activity in China than in the United States, things were not so puritanical as publicly claimed.

Sexual matters of strictly biological nature are openly and freely discussed. For family planning purposes the menstrual periods of women living in a commune will often be charted for all to see and their means of contraception publicly stated as well. Large street posters explain the use of nearly all forms of contraception. This frank and public discussion of contraception contrasts with an embarrassment in discussing sexuality as a source of pleasure. For example, individuals found masturbating are likely, so we were told, to be subjected to a communal discussion of their moral aberration.

CONTRACEPTION

Having more than two children in China is regarded as an irresponsible act. Having only one child or no children at all is viewed as a praiseworthy contribution to the life of the community and a proper way of improving one's standard of living. Considering the population level of China, this is a generally defensible proposition. In fact, an argument can be made that anyone reproducing beyond those limits in an underdeveloped country (or one with a growing population) may indeed take sufficiently from the common resources of the community so as to endanger the security and the quality of life of all its members. That is, over-reproduction can be seen as a form of assault that justifies the use of social pressure in self-protection.

This general argument appears to underlie contraceptive policies in China. Rather than enforcing these policies through the use of force, such as imposing a system of mandatory sterilization, the Chinese rely primarily upon concerted group pressure. In addition, they provide rations for only two children, and impose fines on those who have more than two. Thus, their approach lies somewhere between the mandatory sterilization policies imposed in India by the government of Indira Gandhi and those of the West that make having fewer children a more alluring choice on the basis of the positive benefits.

ABORTION

Abortion appears to be accepted without problem as the second procedure of choice for the control of unwanted pregnancies. Fetuses are not considered to be persons, either before the law, or as objects of revolutionary humanitarian concern. When unmarried and married women do become pregnant, they appear to have no difficulty in procuring an abortion. Indeed, pregnant women who have already had two children are confronted by their social group and advised of their moral duty to seek an abortion. They usually agree.

DEFECTIVE NEWBORNS AND THE RETARDED

Infants are regarded as objects of revolutionary humanitarian concern, though a general account of this ethical commitment was never articulated. When asked under what conditions a child born with Downs syndrome or with spina bifida would not be treated, the Chinese answer that all attempts would be made to preserve the life of such a child. What ethical principles would they appeal to in providing treatment for individuals who would not be productive members of society? In China, they replied, ethical views are a manifestation of economic forces and class interests; the mores of the proletariat includes concern for the life of all persons, even those who are not productive.

Repeated attempts to discover a more complete account of this view were futile. Such attempts failed not only in discussions with physicians, but even with philosophers. It seemed enough for them to assert the moral maxim of concern for all human life. Nor did they see any tension between this concern and other medical moral maxims, which they offered in the same or similar discussions: one should invest one's resources in prevention first and cure only later; or, there are some children so badly deformed that it is best that they simply die. That is, there had been no attempt made to see how one could integrate these different and even competing moral interests.

THE RIGHT TO MEDICAL CARE

The provisions of medical care to all Chinese citizens is a goal that is clearly embraced and pursued. Talk about a right to medical care, insofar as such language is used or understood, appears however, to be understood as an endorsement of this goal and not a claim of a fundamental right. As a consequence, free health care is provided only to a portion of the population. We were informed, for example, that members of communes and factories were completely covered out of the resources of the communes; others were usually not covered. We were also told that in many cases parents were required to pay at least half of the costs of their children's medical care, and the third or fourth child received no free care. However, medical care is provided at a cost that does not appear to limit access.

Moreover, there seemed to be an implicit judgement that concern for costs is salutary; communes and factories as units are required to consider the amount and nature of medical care and the conditions under which it will be provided. As a result, the general appointments of the commune hospitals we visited would have made any charity hospital in the United States appear luxurious in comparison. In addition, disease prevention through general public health measures is given the greatest emphasis. In sum, the Chinese system for the provision of medical care is tied to worker productivity, and marked by unequal obligations to pay for services. This system, however, functions in a society committed to major efforts in community control of infectious diseases and thus to general health promotion.

Finally, the sense of what counts as unnecessary procedures in China is striking. After a thyroidectomy on a woman in her mid-thirties the surgical wound on her neck was closed with no concern for the cosmetic effect. When the surgeons were asked why they did not close the incision with as much care as possible to avoid a scar their response was: she can always buy a high-collared blouse and keep it buttoned. When pressed further as to what would be her fate if styles change (I mentioned noting advertisements for Western-style blouses in China), the answer remained the same. She can always get a blouse that will cover the scar.

DIALECTICAL MATERIALISM

In all our discussions, dialectical materialism and its account of ethical ideas and of the direction of history provided the structure for the answers to our questions. When seeking a justification or foundation for a particular bioethical policy, we were repeatedly told that it expressed the interest of the proletariat or was part of the ideals of a revolutionary humanitarianism. At no point were we able to acquire an account of how the interests of the proletariat or the ideals of revolutionary humanitarianism were to be discovered, much less how such claims of discovery were to be verified. Nor were there any attempts to distinguish conceptually those viewpoints from other viewpoints, or indicate why they were preferable, given general cognitive interests or commitments.

Instead, we were offered cliches, or only given suggestions, how these claims could be grounded by an appeal to Marxism-Leninism. Such claims were never fleshed out in detail. The result was an impression that Marxist-Leninist doctrine and dialectical materialism were employed in a very wooden fashion, without any well-developed cognitive understanding. In this vein, scientists and researchers told me privately that they were happy that in reporting and publishing their research, they were no longer compelled to make perfunctory references to the importance of dialectical materialism for their work. Some volunteered, though, that they would rather make no references at all to Marxism's philosophy of nature: natural dialectics.

A classic illustration of the prevailing contradictory views about dialectical materialism was provided by a discussion with one group of Chinese philosophers. On the one hand, they were quite willing to agree that dialectical materialism was a set of high-level empirical generalizations drawn from the consideration of observable facts. On the other hand, they insisted that not only were no facts likely to falsify dialectical materialism, but that no facts could in principle falsify dialectical materialism.

CONCLUSION

One finds in China a number of very sincere, interested individuals dealing with issues that we in the United States would unquestionably see as bioethical. These issues in China, however, have not evoked the same intellectual scrutiny; they lack a tradition of criticism and debate about the intellectual bases of social and moral policies. As well, there is no well-developed philosophical tradition of questioning basic assumptions and of seeking the underlying justifications for claims in ethics and in the sciences. For example, when most philosophers were asked whether they were interested in exploring the foundations of bioethical policies, it appeared that they had never considered the possibility of such an applied use of philosophy. As a result, such questions to Chinese philosophers evoked a well-worn Marxist economic explanation of how policies developed. However, senior scholars as well as a number of younger scholars found interest and merit in such analyses and were sympathetic and open in discussing their significance. Because of this interest I am confident that continued scholarly exchange between the PRC and the West can be of mutual benefit.

Islam offers still another alternative to Hippocratic medical ethics or the liberal ethics of Western political philosophy. The style of contemporary Muslim writings on medical ethics is quite different from the secular medical ethical literature of either the East or West. It is much more explicitly religious in tone. Much more so even than the medical ethical writings of most contemporary religious commentators on medical ethical issues. It works very closely with the Quranic texts that it considers relevant to medical decisionmaking. In doing so it makes clear how different the moral reasoning is of one in the Muslim tradition from secular and Judeo-Christian medical ethical discussions. The following text is representative. It was originally written for an international conference on Islamic Medicine in Kuait in 1981. It concludes with a reprinting of the oath of the Islamic Medical Association of the USA and Canada.

Islamic Code of Medical Professional Ethics

Abdul Rahman, C. Amine, and Ahmed Elkadi

Medicine was defined by Muslim physicians such as Al-Razi (841–926 AD) and Ibn Sina (Avicenna, 980–1036 AD) as the art concerned with the preservation of good health, combating of diseases and restoration of health to the sick. For several centuries, the world has witnessed and benefited from the great advances made by Muslim physicians in the area of health sciences. These advances were not just based on technical skill or intellectual superiority. They were equally well founded on a clear understanding of the role of the Muslim physician as derived from Islamic teachings and philosophy. For thousands of years, ethics have been recognized as an essential requirement in the making of a physician. Although the ancient codes of ethics[1,2] have to some extent stressed this requirement, they were still deficient and contained grave errors[3]. Contemporary codes of ethics tend to be more liberal and less restrictive[3]. The Quranic ethics, on the other hand, stand out as a perfect model for all mankind, all professions and all time.

The medical ethical requirements proposed in this paper are primarily based on Quranic ethics. They include guidelines for the physician's behavior and attitude, both at the personal and professional levels. The same standard of moral and ethical values should guide the physician in his private life and while conducting his professional business as well. A person who lacks moral values in private life cannot be trusted in professional activities, even with the highest professional and technical qualifications. It is impossible for a person to have two different ethical standards. Truthful is God the Almighty when He says:

> God has not made for any man two hearts in his body.[4]

The following verses from the Quran are most suited as a guide for the personal characteristics of the physician:

> Luqman admonished his son: "My son" he said "serve no God besides God for idolatry is an abominable injustice." We have enjoined man to show kindness to his parents, for with much pain does his mother bear him and he is not weaned before he is two years of age. We said: Give thanks to Me and to your parents; to Me shall all things return. But if they press you to serve besides Me what you know nothing of, do not obey them, be kind to them in this world and follow the path of those who submit to Me: to Me you shall all return and I will declare to you all that you have done. "My son, God will know about all things be they as small as a grain of mustard seed, be they hidden inside a rock or in heaven or on earth, God is wise and all-knowing. My son, establish regular prayer, enjoin what is just and forbid what is wrong; endure with fortitude whatever befalls you, for this is firmness of purpose in the conduct of affairs. Do not treat men with scorn nor walk proudly on the earth; God does not love the arrogant boaster. Rather, let your gait be modest and your voice low; the harshest of voices is the braying of the ass."[5]

> . . . and those who restrain anger and forgive other men, verily God loves those who do good.[6]

God further states:

> It was the mercy of God that you have dealt with them gently and if you were severe and harsh-hearted they would have broken away from about you. Therefore, forgive them, pray for their forgiveness and consult them in the conduct of affairs; then, when you have decided to proceed, depend on God for support: verily God loves those who depend on Him.[7]

Based on the above, the Muslim physician must believe in God and in Islamic teachings and practice, both in private and public life. He must be grateful to his parents, teachers and elders. He must be humble, modest, kind, merciful, patient and tolerant. He must follow the path of the righteous and always seek God's support.

The physician equipped with the above-listed virtues is capable of complying with the needed professional requirements. The professional requirement is to acquire and maintain proper knowledge. God makes it clear in the Quran: ". . . Say: Are those equal, those who know and those who do not know? . . ."[8]

God also states:

> . . . Verily, those who fear God among His servants are those who have knowledge. . .[9]

Therefore, the believer is encouraged to always seek knowledge.

> . . . Say: O my Lord, advance me in knowledge.[10]

The physician must also abide by the legal rule regulating the profession provided they do not violate Islamic teachings. The need to respect law and order is reflected in the following verse:

> Oh you who believe: Obey God and obey the Apostle, and those charged with authority among you. . .[11]

Recognizing God as the maker and the owner of both patient and physician, it is only logical that the care provided to his patient must be in accordance with God's guidelines.

A subject of great importance is the subject of life. Life is given by God and cannot be taken away except by Him or with His permission. God says in the Quran:

> It is He who created death and life, that He may try which of you is best in deed. . .[12]

He also says: ". . . Nor can they control death nor life nor resurrection."[13] God further states:

> . . . Whoever kills a human being in lieu of another human being nor because of mischief on earth, it is as if he has killed all mankind and whoever saves the life of a human being, it is as if he has saved the life of all mankind. . .[14]

The physician therefore has no right to terminate any human life under his care. This also applies to the unborn baby since clear evidence indicates that human life starts at the time of conception. Consequently, the physician has no right to terminate the life of the unborn baby unless it constitutes a definite threat to the mother's life.

The physician must realize that God is watching and monitoring every thought and deed. This was clearly indicated in the verses quoted earlier from Sura 31 of the Quran.[5] The same verses also indicate that the parents' demands are not to be obeyed if they are in violation of God's orders, in spite if the fact that parents are considered to be the most important persons to their children after God. Following the same principles, the physician has no right to follow popular demand or his patient's wishes if they are in violation of God's orders.

Based on sound logic and clear Islamic teachings, the physician has no right to recommend or administer any harmful material to his patients. The most concise yet comprehensive guide in this matter is found in the following verse of the Quran:

> . . . and He makes for them good things lawful, and bad things forbidden. . .[15]

This implies that anything forbidden by God must be bad or harmful; anything proven to be bad or harmful must be forbidden.

The humanitarian aspect of the medical profession must never be neglected nor overlooked. The physician must render the needed help regardless of the financial ability or ethnic origin of the patient. A beautiful hint is found in the following Quranic verses:

> And they feed, for the love of God, the indigent, the orphan, and the captive, (saying) 'We feed you for the sake of God alone: no reward do we desire from you, nor thanks.'[16]

When entrusted with the care of a patient, the physician must offer the needed advice with consideration for both the patient's body and mind, always remembering his basic obligation to enjoin what is just and forbid what is wrong.

The physician must protect the patient's confidentiality, reflecting God's description of the believers: "Those who faithfully keep their trusts and their covenants."[17]

The physician must adopt an appropriate manner of communication and be reminded of the ethics of speech referred to in the Quranic verses quoted earlier in this paper.[5] God also describes the good believers in the Quran and says: "For they have been guided to the purest of speeches."[18]

Situations requiring the physician to examine patients of the opposite sex are always a test of his moral character and his strength. A basic instruction is found in the following Quranic verses:

> Say to the believing men that they should lower their gaze and guard their modesty; that will make for greater purity for them, for God is well acquainted with all that they do. And say to the believing women that they should lower their gaze and guard their modesty. . .[19]

God further says: "God does wish to lighten your burden, for man was created weak."[20]

It is, therefore, advisable that the physician examine patients of the opposite sex in the presence of a third person whenever feasible. This will be an added protection for the physician and the patient.

The physician must not criticize another physician in the presence of patients or health personnel, remembering the wise Quranic advice:

> O you who believe, let not some men among you make fun of others; it may be that they are better than them; nor let some women make fun of others; it may be that they are better than them; not defame, nor be sarcastic to each other, nor call each other by offensive nicknames. . .[21]

God further says:

> God does not love that evil be voiced in public speech, except where the person has suffered injustice. . .[22]

The physician must refuse payment for the treatment of another physician or his immediate family. There is no specific instruction regarding this particular matter in the Quran or Islamic tradition. However, reference is made to another situation which may be used in analogy. God says in regarding Zakat money: "Alms are for the poor, the needy and those employed to administer the funds. . ."[23]

Here is a situation where the persons providing a certain service are entitled to the use of the same service at the time of need. Applying the same principle, the physician who provides the health service to others is entitled to the use of the same service at the time of need.

Last, but not least, the physician must always strive to use wisdom in all his decisions and the reward will be great. Truthful is God almighty when He says: ". . . and he to whom wisdom is granted, is granted a great deal of good indeed. . ."[24]

In closing, reference is made to the Oath of the Muslim Physician adopted by the Islamic Medical Association in 1977(25), and which reflects the spirit and philosophy of the Islamic Code of Medical Professional Ethics proposed in this paper.

In summary, the Muslim physician must believe in God and in Islamic teachings and practice in private and public life; be grateful to his parents, teachers, and elders; be humble, modest, kind, merciful, patient and tolerant; follow the path of the righteous; and always seek God's support. The Muslim physician must stay abreast of current medical knowledge, continuously improve his skill, seek help whenever needed and comply with legal requirements governing his profession; realize that God is the maker and owner of his patient's body and mind, and treat him within the framework of God's teachings; realize that life was given to man by God, that human life starts at the time of conception, and that human life cannot be taken away except by God or with His permission; realize that God is watching and monitoring every thought and deed; follow God's guidelines as his only criteria, even if they differ with popular demand or the patient's wishes; not recommend nor administer any harmful material; render needed help regardless of financial ability or ethnic origin of the patient; offer needed advice with consideration for both the patient's body and mind; protect the patient's confidentiality; adopt an appropriate manner of communication; examine a patient of the opposite sex in the presence of a third person whenever feasible; not criticize another physician in the presence of patients or health personnel—refuse payment for treatment of another physician or his immediate family and strive to use wisdom in all his decisions.

The Oath of a Muslim Physician

Praise be to Allah (God), the teacher, the unique, Majesty of the heavens, the Exalted, the Glorious, Glory be to Him the Eternal Being who created the Universe and all creatures within, and the only Being who containeth the infinity and the eternity. We serve no other God besides Thee and regard idolatry as an abominable injustice.

Give us the strength to be truthful, honest, modest, merciful and objective.
Give us the fortitude to admit our mistakes, to amend our ways, and to forgive the wrongs of others.
Give us the wisdom to comfort and counsel all towards peace and harmony.
Give us the understanding that ours is a profession sacred that deals with your most precious gifts of life and intellect.

Therefore, make us worthy of this favored station with honor, dignity and piety so that we may devote our lives in serving mankind, poor or rich, wise or illiterate, Muslim or non-Muslim, black or white, with patience and tolerance, with virtue and reverence, with knowledge and vigilance, with Thy love in our hearts and compassion for Thy servants, Thy most precious creation.

Hereby we take this oath in Thy name, the Creator of all the Heavens and the earth and follow Thy counsel as Thou have revealed to Prophet Muhammad (*pbuh*).

Whoever killeth a human being, not in lieu of another human being nor because of mischief on earth, it shall be as if hath killed all mankind. And if he saveth a human life, it shall be as if he hath saved the life of all mankind. . .[25]

This Oath is adopted by the Islamic Medical Association of USA and Canada.

NOTES

1. Oath of Hippocrates
2. Oath of the Hindu Physician
3. "Professional Ethics; Ethics in the Medical Profession," by Ahmed Elkadi, MD. *Journal of the Islamic Medical Association,* (September):pp. 27–30, 1976.
4. Quran: 33/4
5. Quran: 31/13–19
6. Quran: 3/134
7. Quran: 3/159
8. Quran: 39/9
9. Quran: 35/28
10. Quran: 20/114
11. Quran: 4/59
12. Quran: 67/2
13. Quran: 25/3
14. Quran: 5/32
15. Quran: 7/157
16. Quran: 76/8–9
17. Quran: 23/8
18. Quran: 22/24
19. Quran: 24/30–31

20.   Quran: 4/28
21.   Quran: 49/11
22.   Quran: 4/148
23.   Quran: 9/60
24.   Quran: 2/269
25.   "Oath of the Muslim Physician," *Convention Bulletin of Islamic Medical Association,* October 1977.

Like Islamic medical ethics, Hindu medical ethics traces its origins back to the most sacred writings of the tradition. Unlike Islam, however, Hindu thought has a large set of texts dating over many centuries. The most ancient and most sacred texts are the Vedas—collections of hymns, prayers, and stories. K. R. Srikanta Murthy's discussion of ancient Indian medicine by contrasting the oldest Vedic collection the Rigveda, which has no uniquely professional ethic, with the Ayurvedic literature, a more recent collection containing two oaths, one in the Charaka Samhita, the other in the Sushruta Samhita. Portions of the Sushruta Samhita oath are contained in this essay. The full text of the Charaka Samhita oath appears as the next selection. The author makes clear his belief that the Indian oaths share in common much ethical content with the insights of Hippocrates and representatives of virtually all other great ethical traditions in medicine. Others have argued that the Indian codes, like all other ethical texts, reflect more specific ethical beliefs and values that are unique to the tradition upon which they are based.

Professional Ethics in Ancient Indian Medicine

K. R. SRIKANTA MURTHY

EVOLUTION OF ETHICS

Though medicine had become an independent profession as early as the period of Rigveda (3000–2000 BC) there does not, seem to have been any kind of professional ethics. The Atharvana Veda (2000–1000 BC) reveals the existence of many types of 'healers' practicing in society; the Rigvedic priest with his prayers and sacrifices to Gods of healing, the Atharvana priest with his magic spells, amulets and drugs, the Angirasa rituals of black magic and probably many others each claiming superiority over the other. Professional jealousy and public exploitation were rampant. Society had grown weary of these and there was necessity to infuse new vitality which was achieved by the Upanishads (800 BC–600 AD). They emphasized greater importance to man than to God, created faith and confidence in human efforts and capacity; asserted that prosperity and happiness can best be achieved by one's good conduct. The four principal pursuits of life Dharma, Artha, Kama and Moksha were enunciated as higher values of life. Every one—the king or commoner, philosopher or butcher, poet or professional—was required to follow certain rules of right conduct based on the sanctity of life of every creature, sympathy for the sufferer, service without expectation, contentment and efficiency in all activities. These great principles became the soul and spirit of all people. Each profession in turn, evolved its own rules of moral behavior, personal as well as professional codes of conduct.

Ayurvedic literature, which was composed during or just after the period of the Upanishads (800 BC–600 AD) reflect these views only. Medical ethics were formulated and insisted upon. Strict Charaka adherence and Sushruta Samhitas bear testimony to the importance of the subject.

NATURE AND SCOPE

Professional ethics in Ayurveda cover both aspects of medical activity namely education and practice, the latter having been considered more important than the former. In addition there was also a third set of rules to be followed during the last quarter of one's life in preparation for the 'hereafter.'

ETHICS OF EDUCATION

A student of good descent, endowed with good health with capacity for hard work, and keenly desirous of medical study after selecting a suitable preceptor approached him reverentially and took for instructions. The learned and experienced teacher, accepted the student only after careful examination. The pupil and the preceptor, then, swore before the sacred fire, the former to submit wholeheartedly to the master and the latter to teach the pupil to the best of his knowledge, lest evil may be fall him. The pupil stayed with the teacher under the same roof and learnt the science. Theoretical and practical training were given; the strident followed the teacher to the forest in search of herbs, to the sick man's house to study diseases and their treatment and to the wide world to learn etiquette and manners. The teacher-student relationship was intimate and affectionate, yet rigid and disciplined. Paternal care combined with the watchful eye, moral and noble behavior of the teacher molded the novice into an efficient physician, an ideal man and a model for others in the society.

ETHICS OF PROFESSIONAL CONDUCT

Having taught the science thoroughly, the teacher administered an Anushasana— an oath to the disciple, which contained many do's and dont's to be followed strictly during his professional career. Charaka Samhita contains one such Anushasana—the *Atreya Anushasana* (seventh century BC)—predating the famous Hippocratic oath by two centuries.* This oath not only bears valid testimony to the high level of professional ethics in ancient India but stands preeminently suitable for universal adoption by present day medicine.

Besides the injunctions embodied in the oath, Ayurvedic literature is full of advice, directions and warnings on different aspects of the professional and personal conduct of medical man.

1. The physician should first investigate the patient and his disease thoroughly and on correct diagnosis, should think of treatment. Treatment however efficient is bound to fail if the diagnosis is wrong.
2. Theoretical knowledge and practical experience together make for better knowledge.
3. Knowledge of any one science by itself is not enough to arrive at correct decision, the physician should learn many sciences.
4. Knowledge of any one part, cannot stand for the whole.
5. Careful observation of the different stages of the disease, discriminating the manageable and unmanageable—helps to undertake proper therapy. Lack of such knowledge leads to loss of reputation to himself and his science.
6. After diagnosis, the physician should adopt effective and appropriate therapy at the proper time; but should on no account delay suitable treatment nor adopt ineffective measures.
7. Physician who by his conduct allows the disease to progress or adopts hasty measures even before the right time is to be considered a 'sinner' and stands liable for punishment. (S.S. 1/17–1/11)
8. Drugs and recipes should be suitable and effective; no harmful therapy should be adopted however much it has been extolled.
9. If by single therapy no relief accrues, alternate therapy is to be adopted soon after. (S.S.1. 35/47)
10. Aim of treatment is not merely to relieve the suffering but to restore health; strive to maintain and promote health but do not undermine the natural strength of the patient.
11. The scope of medical science is merely to lend a helping hand to those who are sinking in the quagmire of disease; it is just an aid. Physicians should not assume too much either to himself or to his science in case of cure.
12. Physician is not the controller of life, (neither its saviour nor its remover) proper diagnosis and suitable therapy are the only two on which he has control.
13. It is impossible to guarantee life in all cases even by experts, even under ideal conditions nor death be predicted as certain when suitable conditions do not exist.

---

*Note that this dating differs from that of Ludwig Edelstein, who argues for the fourth century BC for the Hippocratic Oath. A full text of the Oath of Initiation from the Charaka Samhita may be found in the next selection. (*Editor's note.*)

14. Treatment is to be done to the last breath, for, many a hopeless patient recovers by the grace of God.

15. In case of grave emergency adopt all measures immediately just as redeeming a house from fire.

16. When death is certain if not intervened, and even if intervened success is doubtful, surgery or any other method of treatment is to be adopted, with due permission of the patient or his relatives.

17. No charity is greater than saving a life. Treatment never goes waste, in some it brings wealth, with some others fame, friendship with some others but with every one it brings experience to the physician.

18. Medical science should not be used for selfish gains nor for money, but should be for the service of all creatures.

19. Medical practice is quadri-facetted, viz., friendship with all, sympathy and compassion for the sick, utmost care and attention towards the manageable patient and connivance of the hopeless. (C.S 1/9–26)

20. He who makes medicine a merchandise shall only reap a heap of sand casting away a heap of gold.

21. He who bestows health and relieves the pain is worthy of every kind of worship and all the fruits of righteousness shall accrue him.

22. Physician by relieving the suffering attains heaven without performing sacrifices.

23. Practicing the profession on the principles of philosophy of life, looking after the health of the deserving and the needy, showing kindness and compassion to all beings is the Dharma for the medical man; accepting from the rich just enough money to meet the minimum needs, his life and his dependents is the Artha; respecting the elders, scholars, professional brethren and nobles and receiving honors from them, winning love and affection of all by sympathetic service is the Kama; by practicing thus the physician is sure to attain salvation Moksha.

Ayurveda further envisages that the medical man should spend the last years of his life in the pursuit of emancipation; to prepare himself to reach heaven. He is advised to gradually minimize contact with society, devote all his time to study and teaching, practice yoga, conquer his mind and senses, concentrate on higher goal, eat once to sustain life, pray for the well-being of all creatures, not to be carried away by desires and emotions, and lead a simple but noble living like the sages of yore.

This is how Bharadwaja, Atreya, Agnivesha, Divodasa, Sushruta, Charaka, Nagarjuna and Vagbhata lived in India. So did Inhotep, Akhetanon, Hippocrates, Avicenna, Celsus and Galen. Great men of medicine of present times like Pavlov, Osler, Shweitzer, Carrel were equally philosopher scientists who substantiated the ancient truth that sciences should merge with ethics and philosophy to bring peace and happiness to man. It is strict adherence to medical ethics that can make as efficient physician, an ideal man as well.

REFERENCES

Charaka Samhita (C. S.) Ed. Jadavaji Tricumji Acharya. Bombay: Nirnayasagar Press, 1941.
Sushruta Samhita, Ed. (S. S) Jadavaji Tricumji Acharya. Bombay: Nirnayasagar Press, 1931.
Asthanga Hridaya (A. S. H.), Ed. *Annamoreshwar Kunte Harishastry.* Bombay: Nirnayasagar Press, 1939.
Charaka Samhita (C. S.) *English Translation,* vol. I. P. M. Mehta et al. Jamnagar: Gulab Kunverba Ayurvedic Society, 1949.
Surgical Ethics in Ayurveda. G. D. Singhal et al. Banaras, 1971.

The ancient oath from the Charaka (or Caraka, as this translator spells it) Samhita of which K. R. Srikanta Murthy spoke deserves closer examination. The translation presented here is by A. Menon and H. F. Haberman. It reveals some uniquely Hindu elements such as the obligation to remain celibate, eat no meat, and carry no arms. Characteristic of Hindu thought, there is an explicit prohibition on causing another's death. There are some passages remarkably similar to Hippocratic commitments (the commitment to be devoted entirely to being helpful to the patient), but there are also some dramatic contrasts. Note especially the requirements that "No persons who are hated by the king or who are haters of the king or who are hated by the public or who are haters of the public shall receive treatment." An understanding of the Hindu doctrine of karma, of rebirth in a position based on the way one has led his previous life, may be necessary to understand the moral meaning of such a sentence.

Oath of Initiation

FROM THE CARAKA SAMHITA

1. The teacher then should instruct the disciple in the presence of the sacred fire, Brahmanas [Brahmins] and physicians.
2. [saying] "Thou shalt lead the life of a celibate, grow thy hair and beard, speak only the truth, eat no meat, eat only pure articles of food, be free from envy and carry no arms.
3. There shall be nothing that thou should not do at my behest except hating the king, causing another's death, or committing an act of great unrighteousness or acts leading to calamity.
4. Thou shalt dedicate thyself to me and regard me as they chief. Thou shalt be

subject to me and conduct thyself for ever for my welfare and pleasure. Thou shalt serve and dwell with me like a son or a slave or a supplicant. Thou shalt behave and act without arrogance, with care and attention and with un-distracted mind, humility, constant reflection and ungrudging obedience. Act-ing either at my behest or otherwise, though shalt conduct thyself for the achievement of thy teacher's purposes alone, to the best of thy abilities.

5. If thou desirest success, wealth and fame as a physician and heaven after death, thou shalt pray for the welfare of all creatures beginning with the cows and Brahmanas.

6. Day and night, however thou mayest be engaged, thou shalt endeavor for the relief of patients with all thy heart and soul. Thou shalt not desert or injure thy patient for the sake of thy life or thy living. Thou shalt not commit adultery even in thought. Even so, thou shalt not covet others' possessions. Thou shalt be modest in thy attire and appearance. Thou shouldst not be a drunkard or a sinful man nor shouldst thou associate with the abettors of crimes. Thou shouldst speak words that are gentle, pure and righteous, pleasing, worthy, true, wholesome, and moderate. Thy behavior must be in consideration of time and place and heedful of past experience. Thou shalt act always with a view to the acquisition of knowledge and fullness of equipment.

7. No persons, who are hated by the king or who are haters of the king or who are hated by the public or who are haters of the public, shall receive treat-ment. Similarly, those who are extremely abnormal, wicked, and of miserable character and conduct, those who have not vindicated their honor, those who are on the point of death, and similarly women who are unattended by their husbands or guardians shall not receive treatment.

8. No offering of presents by a woman without the behest of her husband or guardian shall be accepted by thee. While entering the patient's house, thou shalt be accompanied by a man who is known to the patient and who has his permission to enter; and thou shalt be well-clad, bent of head, self-possessed, and conduct thyself only after repeated consideration. Thou shalt thus prop-erly make thy entry. Having entered, thy speech, mind, intellect and senses shall be entirely devoted to no other thought than that of being helpful to the patient and of things concerning only him. The peculiar customs of the pa-tient's household shall not be made public. Even knowing that the patient's span of life has come to its close, it shall not be mentioned by thee there, where if so done, it would cause shock to the patient or to others.

Though possessed of knowledge one should not boast very much of one's knowledge. Most people are offended by the boastfulness of even those who are otherwise good and authoritative.

9. There is no limit at all to the Science of Life, Medicine. So thou shouldst apply thyself to it with diligence. This is how thou shouldst act. Also thou shouldst learn the skill of practice from another without carping. The entire world is the teacher to the intelligent and the foe to the unintelligent. Hence, knowing this well, thou shouldst listen and act according to the words of instruction of

even an unfriendly person, when his words are worthy and of a kind as to bring to you fame, long life, strength and prosperity."

10. Thereafter the teacher should say this—"Thou shouldst conduct thyself properly with the gods, sacred fire, Brahmanas, the guru, the aged, the scholars and the preceptors. If thou has conducted thyself well with them, the precious stones, the grains and the gods become well disposed towards thee. If thou shouldst conduct thyself otherwise, they become unfavorable to thee." To the teacher that has spoken thus, the disciple should say, "Amen."

Chinese medical ethics is as closely integrated with ancient Confucian, Buddhist, and Taoist teaching as Indian medicine is with Hindu texts. In China, however, there are no definitive religious texts as there are in Hindu and Muslim thought. Instead there exists compendia of codes or rules of conduct compiled by many Confucian medical scholars and critics of the classical Confucian positions. Note contrast in the Chinese texts with the Caraka Samhita oath regarding whom the physician should treat.

Medical Ethics in Ancient China

Tao Lee

The real foundation for medical ethics as understood in the west is laid in the grand Hippocratic Oath in fifth century BC. The Egyptian papyri of the second millennium BC also mentioned medical ethics. Medical ethics in China, however, were not established until the seventh century.[1] Sun Ssu-miao (581–673 AD), the father of medicine in China, first discussed the duties of a physician to his patients and to the public in his book, "The Thousand Golden Remedies." In content this is similar in certain respects to the Hippocratic Oath. The essential points may be translated as follows:

Medicine is an art which is difficult to master. If one does not receive a divine guidance from God, he will not be able to understand the mysterious points. A foolish fellow, after reading medical formularies for three years, will believe that all diseases can be cured. But, after practicing for another three years, he will realize that most formulae are not effective. A physician should, therefore, be a scholar, mastering all the medical literature and working carefully and tirelessly.

A great doctor, when treating a patient, should make himself quiet and determined. He should not have covetous desire. He should have bowels of mercy on the sick and pledge himself to relieve suffering among all classes. Aristocrat or commoner, poor or rich, aged or young, beautiful or ugly, enemy or friend, native or foreigner, and educated or uneducated, all are to be treated equally. He should look upon the misery of the patient as if it were his own and be anxious to relieve the distress, disregarding his own inconveniences, such as night-call, bad weather, hunger, tiredness, etc. Even foul cases, such as ulcer, abscess, diarrhoea, etc., should be treated without the slightest antipathy. One who follows this principle is a great doctor, otherwise, he is a great thief.

A physician should be respectable and not talkative. It is a great mistake to boast of himself and slander other physicians.

Lao Tze, the father of Taoism, said, "Open acts of kindness will be rewarded by man while secret acts of evil will be punished by God." Retribution is very definite. A physician should not utilize his profession as a means for lusting. What he does to relieve distress will be duly rewarded by Providence.

He should not prescribe dear and rare drugs just because the patient is rich or of high rank, nor is it honest and just to do so for boasting.

Another important work on medical ethics is "The Medical Talks" written by Chang Kao in 1189.[2] In a special chapter he collected twelve stories of retribution in order to warn physicians against professional faults. Gratuitous service was especially commended. Lusting after women and riches was considered to be immoral. The inducing of artificial abortion was severely denounced. The following story is cited as an example of gratuitous service.

Mr. Hsu Shu-wei in his youth prayed to the Gods that he might attain literary rank. One night he dreamed of a God who told him to perform some secret deeds of virtue in order to attain his ambition. Hsu was so poor that he could not help others financially. The only thing he could do was to become an doctor and then help the sick. He decided therefore to study medicine and soon mastered the art. He gave free treatment to all patients and responded readily to any request for his assistance without consideration whether the patient was of high or low rank. When he sat in the next examination, he passed with honors.

A story is told concerning artificial abortion as follows:

A woman called Pai Mu-tan, lived by selling drugs for artificial abortion. One day she suffered suddenly from headache and her head became swollen. Physicians were unable to cure her. After many days an ulcer appeared with an offensive odor. Her crying at night could be heard by all the neighbors. One day she asked her son to burn all the prescriptions for abortion, and warned him not to engage in such a vocation as hers. Her son asked her why she would not hand down the prescriptions to him. She answered, "I dreamed of hundreds of infants striking at my head every night. My illness is entirely due to my selling drugs for abortion." After saying this, she died.

Ancient Chinese laid great emphasis on the virtue of chastity. The following story from the same book is a good example.

> During the period of Hsuan-ho (1119–1125) a scholar was sick for many years. His wife requested the great doctor, Ho-cheng, to come to her boudoir and said to him, "My husband has been sick for a long time; everything we possess has been sold to pay the expenses of medical care. We have no more money. If you will kindly cure my husband, I will place my body at your disposal." The doctor rejected her offer sternly and said to her: "Don't insult me. I will cure your husband. If your suggestion should be spread abroad by any chance, my career would be spoiled and I would be condemned by man and by the spirits." Soon her husband was cured. One night the physician dreamed of a man taking him to a temple where a judge said to him, "You have the virtue of the medical profession. You did not lust after woman in time of danger. God grant you 50,000 strings of cash and an official rank." A few months later a prince of the Imperial family was sick. The court medical official could not cure him. An Imperial decree was then issued to summon the physicians in the country. Ho-cheng presented himself and cured the prince. The court thereupon granted him 3,000 strings of cash and an official rank.

In the Ming Dynasty the question of medical ethics was discussed by many physicians. Hsu Chun-fu[3] in 1556 compiled a section on this subject under a special title "The Medical Way." At the same time Kung Hsin[4] wrote a maxim for reputable physicians. The maxim, which was instructive and concise, has been used as a motto in the baccalaureate service of the Peiping Union Medical College since 1939. It reads:

> The good physician of the present day cherishes kindness and righteousness. He reads widely and is highly skilled in the arts of his profession. He has in his mind adequate methods of treatment, which he adapts to different conditions. He cares not for vainglory, but is intent upon relieving suffering among all classes. He revives the dying and restores them to health: his beneficence is equal to that of Providence. Such a good physician will be remembered through endless generations.

Kung Ting-hsien,[5] son of Kung Hsin, set ten requirements for physicians in 1588, in content very similar to the maxim given above. About thirty years later Chen Shih-kung[6] in his book *An Orthodox Manual of Surgery*, stated five commandments and ten requirements for physicians. These included the duties of a physician to his patients, such as professional secrecy, responsibility, deportment and compensation. Attention was also given to the obligations of a physician to other physicians. The importance of advancement of medical knowledge was pointed out and rules for social intercourse were also suggested. This is really the most comprehensive statement on medical ethics in China. It reads as follows:

FIVE COMMANDMENTS

1. Physicians should be ever ready to respond to any calls of patients, high or low, rich or poor. They should treat them equally and care not for financial reward. Thus their profession will become prosperous naturally day by day and conscience will remain intact.
2. Physicians may visit a lady, widow or nun only in the presence of an attendant but not alone. The secret diseases of female patients should be examined with a right attitude, and should not be revealed to anybody, not even to the physician's own wife.
3. Physicians should not ask patients to send pearl, amber or other valuable substances to their home for preparing medicament. If necessary, patients should be instructed how to mix the prescriptions themselves in order to avoid suspicion. It is also not proper to admire things which patients possess.
4. Physicians should not leave the office for excursion and drinking. Patients should be examined punctually and personally. Prescriptions should be made according to the medical formulary, otherwise a dispute may arise.
5. Prostitutes should be treated just like patients from a good family and gratuitous services should not be given to the poor ones. Mocking should not be indulged for this brings loss of dignity. After examination physicians should leave the house immediately. If the case improves, drugs may be sent but physicians should not visit them again for lewd reward.

TEN REQUIREMENTS

1. A physician or surgeon must first know the principles of the learned. He must study all the ancient standard medical books ceaselessly day and night, and understand them thoroughly so that the principles enlighten his eyes and are impressed on his heart. Then he will not make any mistake in the clinic.
2. Drugs must be carefully selected and prepared according to the refining process of Lei Kung. Remedies should be prepared according to the pharmaceutical formulae but may be altered to suit the patient's condition. Decoctions and powders should be freely made. Pills and distilled medicine should be prepared in advance. The older the plaster is the more effective it will be. Tampons become more effective on standing. Don't spare valuable drugs; their use is eventually advantageous.
3. A physician should not be arrogant and insult other physicians in the same district. He should be modest and careful towards his colleagues; respect his seniors, help his juniors, learn from his superiors and yield to the arrogant. Thus there will be no slander and hatred. Harmony will be esteemed by all.
4. The managing of a family is just like the curing of a disease. If the constitution of a man is not well cared for and becomes over-exhausted, diseases will

attack him. Mild ones will weaken his physique, while serious ones may result in death. Similarly, if the foundation of the family is not firmly established and extravagance be indulged in, reserves will gradually drain away and poverty will come.

5. Man receives his fate from Heaven. He should not be ungrateful to the Heavenly decree. Professional gains should be approved by the conscience and conform to the Heavenly will. If the gain is made according to the Heavenly will, natural affinity takes place. If not, offspring will be condemned. Is it not better to make light of professional gain in order to avoid the evil retribution?

6. Gifts, except in the case of weddings, funerals and for the consolation of the sick, should be simple. One dish of fish and one of vegetable will suffice for a meal. This is not only to reduce expenses but also to save provisions. The virtue of a man lies not in grasping but rather in economy.

7. Medicine should be given free to the poor. Extra financial help should be extended to the destitute patients, if possible. Without food, medicine alone can not relieve the distress of a patient.

8. Savings should be invested in real estate but not in curios and unnecessary luxuries. The physician should also not join the drinking club and the gambling house which would hinder his practice. Hatred and slander can thus be avoided.

9. Office and dispensary should be fully equipped with necessary apparatus. The physician should improve his knowledge by studying medical books, old and new, and reading current publications. This really is the fundamental duty of a physician.

10. A physician should be ready to respond to the call of government officials with respect and sincerity. He should inform them the cause of the disease and prescribe accordingly. After healing he should not seek for a complimentary tablet* or plead excuse for another's difficulty. A person who respects the law should not associate with officials.

In 1695, Chang-Lu[7] wrote *Chang-shih-iitung*, a book on general medicine, with ten commandments for physicians in the first chapter. The physician's self control and his duties to his patients and to the public are emphasized. The essential features are to abstain from the following: 1. acquiring evil habits; 2. over self-confidence; 3. strong prejudice; 4. imitation or lack of initiative; 5. making careless diagnosis; 6. practicing magic healing; 7. treating the nobility and commoners similarly†; 8. neglecting poor patients; 9. extorting high compensation from critical cases; 10. criticizing or slandering other physicians.

In the early nineteenth century Huai Yuan[8] also stated six maxims for physicians in his book. They are very much the same as those above cited, and will not be quoted here.

---

*A wooden board inscribed with complimentary words, hung in the physician's office for propaganda.
†It was believed that the physique of the nobility was delicate while that of a commoner was tough. They should, therefore, be treated differently.

COMMENT

Medical ethics is a body of rules compounded from idealism and practicality which physicians accept as their moral standard. Its purpose is to promote the prime object of the medical profession, service to humanity, and also to assist the regulation of medical practice by the government. The standard of medical ethics varies according to races, habits, customs and times. An action considered moral by one people may not be so considered by others. On the other hand, conduct once regarded as a great fault may not be so in our times. Medical ethics has no permanent single standard. From the Chinese medical literature cited above we may recognize several differences in the ideals of oriental and western peoples on medical ethics. Several points should be noted:

1.   Treatment of Female Patients

Mencius[9] said, "Men and women, in giving and receiving, must not touch each other." The influence of this proverb on the medical profession is very great. As the female patient could not expose any part of her body to the male physician, a model, the so-called "medicine lady" was used for illustration during the medical examination. For the same reason palpation was not considered proper for women. The examination of the female sex organs was a great offence to the ancient Chinese custom. It was also not proper for a physician to lay his fingers on a woman's wrists to examine her pulse. This last inconvenience was ingeniously avoided by physicians in the Imperial family of the Ming Dynasty.[10] A long string was tied to the patient's wrists while another person held the other end. The doctor then laid his fingers in the middle of the string to examine the pulse, a method based on the principle of the transmission of waves through the string. But since the transmission was too weak to be effective, this fantastic method was not generally adopted.

2.   Gratuitous Service

Most of the prominent physicians in Chinese medical history were either retired government officials or scholars who had failed in the Imperial examination. They disliked to think of the practice of medicine as their profession. They all endeavored to encourage gratuitous services and looked on the practice of medicine as a philanthropic undertaking or a benevolent act. As a result a good tradition has come down among physicians. All, with few exceptions, are pledged to serve the community by the alleviation of suffering without caring much for financial return.

3.   Retribution

The idea of retribution played an important part in medical ethics. Most Chinese believed that disease and distress were retribution for past sins while health and happiness were rewards for past virtues. This is probably attributable to Buddhist influence in China. The practice of medicine was considered a benevolent act and observance of professional ethics would be rewarded with rich harvest of blessing. For this reason ancient Chinese physicians dared not to do anything unethical or unprofessional.

4. Complimentary Tablets

Chinese patients used to present wooden boards with complimentary inscriptions to doctors who had cured them, as an expression of appreciation. This was also intended to announce the skill of the doctor to others who might suffer from the same disease. This good custom can be traced back to ancient times. Later, however, it was abused as a means of propaganda. Physicians began to ask patients to present tablets. Some even made tablets themselves and claimed that they were presented by their patients.[11] The wrong use of this good custom made Chen Shih-kung consider it vainglory and he warned physicians against it in his ten requirements in the early seventeenth century.

5. Relationship Between Social Problems and Medical Problems

Many patients cannot be cured of their illness unless their financial pressure or other social problems are also relieved. Therefore, a social service has been established in many modern hospitals. Chen Shih-kung, in the early seventeenth century, noticed the close connection between medicine and social problems and made the utmost effort to provide relief work for the poor.

6. Difference Between the Physique of the Nobility and Commoners

Chang Lu believed that the physique of a noble was delicate while that of a commoner was tough and they should be treated differently. He also classified physicians into two groups, one specialized in curing those of high rank, and the other, the common people. Although this idea, very similar to the four temperaments in Greek medicine,[12] overestimates the difference between individual constitutions, it is not altogether without scientific basis.

7. Secret Prescriptions

The dispensing of secret prescriptions was never considered to be unethical in China. Some even deemed it an honor for a physician to know a secret formula. Even today secret remedies still prevail. The public generally believes that such prescriptions will become ineffective if popularly used. This attitude is probably due to the lack of formal medical organization before the introduction of western medicine.

CONCLUSION

The important writings on medical ethics in ancient China have been briefly mentioned and commented upon. One of the good features of Chinese medical ethics is the encouragement of gratuitous service to the poor. This custom is well established in China and should continue to be followed by modern physicians. Fortunately the Chinese Medical Code promulgated by the Chinese Medical Association in 1932 already has given a great emphasis to this point.[13]

The chief weakness in Chinese medical ethics is the lack of opposition to patients and secret remedies. This is probably due to there being no medical guilds in China. Another shortcoming is that no reference is made to the teaching of medicine such as that found in the second sentence of the Hippocratic Oath, where the pledge is given to teach without fee or stipulation to all who are bound by a stipulation and Oath according to the law of medicine. This places all medical knowledge at the disposal of all physicians. The Chinese adhere rather to the Hippocratic injunction to restrict the teaching of medicine to the sons of physicians and to disciples bound by a stipulation and Oath.

NOTES

1. Sun Ssu-miao, *The Thousand Golden Remedies,* vol. 1, pp. 1–3.
2. Chang Kao, *Medical Talks,* vol. 10, 1189, pp. 31–39.
3. Hsu Chun-iu, *General Medicine of the Past and Present,* vol. 3, 1556, pp. 11–14.
4. Ch'un Meng-lei and others, *A Compilation of Ancient and Modern Books: Section of Medicine,* vol. 518, 1723–1734, p. 6.
5. Kung Ting-hsien, *Ten Thousand Diseases Are Cured,* vol. 8, 1587, p. 59.
6. Chen Shih-kung, *An Orthodox Manual of Surgery,* vol. 4, 1617, pp. 125–128.
7. Chang Lu, Chang's *General Medicine,* vol. 1, 1695, pp. 1–4.
8. Huai Yuan, *Medical Drill,* vol. 4, 1808, pp. 43–47.
9. Mencius, *The Four Books,* vol. 7, p. 56.
10. Lee, T., *History of Medicine,* 1940, p. 99.
11. Li Chia-jui, *Classified Literatures of Peiping Topography,* vol. 1, 1927, p. 160.
12. Singer, C., *A Short History of Medicine,* 1928, p. 97.
13. *The Chinese Medical Directory* (Chinese text), 1934.

Traditional Japanese medical ethics draws both on Buddhist thought and indigenous Shinto tradition. One example comes from the sixteenth century when an approach to disease commonly known as the *Ri-shu* school was widely practiced. A code known as the Seventeen Rules of Enjuin was drawn up by practitioners of this medical art. Note that similar to the Hippocratic Oath, there is a notion that medical knowledge can be very dangerous. It is desseminated only to members of the school and to no others. These rules even go so far as to require that if a practitioner dies or ceases to practice, he must return his books to the school so that they will not fall into the hands of untrained persons. The view of knowledge, quite consistent with the Hippocratic tradition, stands in dramatic contrast with the ethics of Protestantism, which places great emphasis on entrusting the texts to the lay person, and with secular liberalism, which insists that lay persons should be reasonably informed about the nature of treatments and the consequences thereof.

The 17 Rules of Enjuin
(For Disciples in Our School)

1. Each person should follow the path designated by Heaven (Buddha, the Gods).
2. You should always be kind to people. You should always be devoting and loving.
3. The teaching of Medicine should be restricted to selected persons.
4. You should not tell others what you are taught, regarding treatments without permission.
5. You should not establish association with doctors who do not belong to this school.
6. All the successors and descendants of the disciples of this school shall follow the teachers' ways.
7. If any disciples cease the practice of Medicine, or, if successors are not found at the death of the disciple, all the medical books of this school should be returned to the SCHOOL OF ENJUIN.
8. You should not kill living creatures, nor should you admire hunting or fishing.
9. In our school, teaching about poisons is prohibited, nor should you receive instructions about poisons from other physicians. Moreover, you should not give abortives to the people.
10. You should rescue even such patients as you dislike or hate. You should do virtuous acts, but in such a way that they do not become known to people. To do good deeds secretly is a mark of virtue.

11. You should not exhibit avarice and you must not strain to become famous. You should not rebuke or reprove a patient, even if he does not present you with money or goods in gratitude.

12. You should be delighted if, after treating a patient without success, the patients receives medicine from another physician, and is cured.

13. You should not speak ill of other physicians.

14. You should not tell what you have learned from the time you enter a woman's room, and, moreover, you should not have obscene or immoral feelings when examining a woman.

15. Proper or not, you should not tell others what you have learned in lectures, or what you have learned about prescibing medicine.

16. You should not like undue extravagance. If you like such living, your avarice will increase, and you will lose the ability to be kind to others.

17. If you do not keep the rules and regulations of this school, then you will be cancelled as a disciple. In more severe cases, the punishment will be greater.*

---

*William O. Reinhardt provided this translation.

II

The Basis of Medical Ethics

4

The Source and Justification of Medical Ethics

INTRODUCTION

In the previous chapters different systems or traditions of medical ethics were presented including the Hippocratic tradition, various Western religions, ethical systems derived from secular philosophical thought, and ethics grounded in philosophical and religious systems of non-Western cultures. Once it is apparent that there are many different possible systems of medical ethics, the natural question is how one ought to establish an ethic appropriate for medical decisionmaking. The selections in this chapter present some of the critical thinking on how an ethic for medicine should be grounded.

The most obvious, traditional approach is to turn to medical professional groups. The Hippocratic group of physicians in ancient Greece articulated an ethical perspective in a number of writings including, most importantly, in the Hippocratic Oath. The Oath makes clear that the knowledge of medicine, including knowledge about the ethics of medicine, was believed to be available only to members of the Hippocratic group. Naturally, this meant that only Hippocratic physicians were in an appropriate place to articulate the moral norms of medical practice.

Members of modern professional medical groups have often shared this assumption that the profession itself is the group that should articulate the moral norms for medicine. Professional groups have traditionally written codes of ethics that are applied to their members. In fact, sociologists sometimes define a profession, in part, as an occupational group that articulates its own code of ethics, enforces its ethical norms upon its members, and adjudicates ethical disputes that may arise over the ethical conduct of its members.

It is not clear exactly what is being claimed by groups of professionals who write their own codes of ethics. On the one hand they may believe that they create the ethical standards for members of the group. Some other kinds of groups outside the professions may make such claims. Fraternal organizations, for example, may claim to create rules of behavior that members should follow: oaths of secrecy, ritual practices, and so forth. In such cases, the rules of conduct have no foundation beyond what the group agrees to. Sometimes professionals claim that the professional organization actually creates the norms that define the practices of the group.

In other cases professional groups take a slightly different perspective. This is especially true regarding ethics. Ethical norms are normally thought of as more than the mere invention of a group. They are thought to be grounded in more than agreement of the group's members. They might, for example, be derived from more general ethical systems: religious systems or philosophical systems. They might have their foundations in natural moral law or in reason, either of which is more universal than mere group consensus. For example, a physician may hold that physicians should preserve life and that abortion or active mercy killing are violations of the natural moral law. One who takes such a view could articulate the rule: physicians ought not to actively kill even for mercy. Such a physician would see the rule governing physician conduct as grounded in a moral law that is not just the invention of the medical profession.

Someone who holds that the ethical norms for medicine are grounded in something beyond the mere invention of the professional group could still believe that only members of the group can have the knowledge of what the norms are as they apply to physician conduct. Such moral norms or rules could be "role-specific," that is, even though they come from moral law that is universal, the specific rules could govern only people in certain specific roles. It is possible, for example, to hold that the natural moral law forbids physicians from participating in active killing, but still hold that other people in other roles, such as military roles, could morally kill under certain circumstances.

One position regarding the grounding of medical ethics is that even though the moral norms are grounded in a universal ethical foundation, when it comes to articulating the rules for physicians, only the profession can know what is required. Someone might hold this because of the belief that great experience in a profession is necessary to know the moral norms for that profession or that knowledge is revealed only through professional circles. Thus it is possible to hold that professional groups either invent the norms or that they alone have the capacity to discover what the norms are even though they come from a more basic, universal source.

There are problems with either of these views. Many people hold that ethics for something as fundamental as medicine cannot be the mere invention of a group. Furthermore, there is no reason necessarily to believe that only members of the group can have moral knowledge about the professional role. (Many hold, for example, that one does not need to be a military officer in order to know what is morally appropriate conduct for military officers. Some would even go so far as to say that being a military officer biases one's perspective so that officers' claims about what constitutes moral conduct of officers may be even less reliable than other people's claims.)

People who are skeptical about the claim that only members of the professional group can invent or discover the norms for conduct of the group must turn to some other way of knowing what is morally appropriate. The same must be said for people who want to know what is morally acceptable in aspects of medicine not involving health professionals. Lay people often have to make morally important decisions having to do with medicine. Couples decide whether to use contraceptive techniques, some of which do not involve any connection with a health professional. Legislators and public officials must decide about spending of public resources on research and therapy. It seems odd that the medical ethical norms for these decisions would be decided by members of medical professional groups.

People who see ethics as coming from outside professional groups have several alternatives. They can ground their ethics in basic religious and philosophical systems using their methods of determining the norms. Jewish bioethics, for example, would reasonably come from Old Testament study and rabbinical scholarship. Catholic medical ethics would be derived from scripture and tradition using the ways of knowing established within Catholicism. Secular philosophical schools have their own ways of knowing what is ethical using reason, empirical observation, intuition, and so forth.

Recently, one important way of grounding ethics has been through a group of methods collectively referred to as contract methods. Contract theorists hold that if one wants to determine what the moral norms are, either in general or for a particular role such as the medical roles, one asks, either figuratively or in actuality, a group of people what norms they would agree to. Most contract theorists at this point want to distinguish what actual people would agree to (which will be influenced by personal biases, differences in power and intelligence, and other idiosyncratic characteristics) and what hypothetical people would agree to.

Most people hold that what is ethical can be distinguished from what is prudent or merely self-serving. According to this view if one wants to know what is ethical (rather than merely what is prudent), one asks what people would agree to who are not self-serving, but rather, have the characteristics necessary for ethics. Generally this might include making the contractors unbiased by self-interest, committed equally to the welfare of others, as knowledgeable as possible, and so forth. The idea is that if you want to know what is ethical try to find out what people would agree to under circumstances as close as possible to these. Since real contractors do not have these characteristics, this view is often referred to as a hypothetical contract position. By definition, the correct ethical norms are what such hypothetical contractors would agree to.

These theories differ among themselves in explaining why hypothetical contractors would agree. Some people say that they would agree because this is what it takes to know what is moral—either because such people would be ideal observers of the moral reality or would be perfectly capable in their ability to reason. Others hold that, simply by definition, whatever people would agree to under these circumstances is what we would consider to be moral. Regardless, contract theories share the notion that in order to know ethical norms one should try to get people together who approximate the ideal conditions and see what they agree to. Assuming that the knowledge that is relevant includes a very wide range of areas including psychological, social, economic, religious, etc., as well as medical, there is no reason to assume that having special medical expertise will also make one good at knowing what is moral in medicine.

Much of Judeo-Christian religious ethics is built on the notion that there are basic covenants that spell out moral obligations. These covenants are between God and human moral communities. They are, according to one way of thinking, a variant on the contract idea. Furthermore, in order to know the content of the convenant, there may have to be something like the gatherings of humans to try to discern the content. Thus, some would hold that religious convenant theories of ethics are part of the broader contract tradition with an added emphasis on the special nature of the agreements that take place.

Some people reject the hypothetical contract position. One reason is that they are uninterested in what hypothetical people might agree to. They see ethics as more a strategy for living together peaceably. They prefer to find out what actual people would agree to within a particular moral community. Some, such as H. Tristram Engelhardt, hold that the actual agreements determine what is ethical for that community. Engelhardt insists on only one exception. In order to live together peaceably, he argues, there must be an underlying mutual respect for the autonomy of all persons in the community. This autonomy is the one underlying moral principle that governs all actual contracts. The codes of ethics for health-care professionals that derive from either hypothetical or actual contracts may be quite different from those that are invented by or articulated by medical professional organizations. The essays in this chapter examine these different approaches to grounding an ethic for medicine.

The medical profession is where many people turn to determine the moral norms for medicine. Historically, professions have defined what is ethical for members of professional groups. In the following essay by Russell Roth, once the Speaker of the House of Delegates of the American Medical Association, the claim is made that the medical profession has "imposed upon itself certain proscriptions." According to Roth these are not always understood by those outside the profession. Roth wants to defend this way of generating ethical norms. He contrasts it to what he calls authoritarianism, by which he apparently means the state-dominated system of defining what is ethical, which he sees as characteristic of the way medical ethical duties are established in the Soviet Union. He holds that it is better to rely on the ethical commitments made by the profession. He sees that the main reason why persons might not rely on the profession to generate the norms of medical ethics is that the profession can be perceived as self-interested. He does not consider the possibility that medical lay persons may simply differ from physicians over what is ethical when it comes to advertising or other practices. For him, the professional group is most qualified to evaluate the standards of medical care.

Medicine's Ethical Responsibilities

RUSSELL B. ROTH

An interesting question arises at formal conferences, where the nature of physicians' activities is discussed under the general heading of ethics. Time was when the physician graduated from medical school, gave testimony to his competence in passing assorted examinations for licensure or recognition as a specialist and then devoted himself rather exclusively to the business of exercising his talents and his skills on behalf of those who came to him as patients. So long as he dealt with his patients equitably and ministered to them with competence he was regarded as a paragon of ethical probity. Today it would appear that such professional isolationism is not so completely defensible. There is the implication that, when one undertakes a career in medicine, one at the same time, assumes responsibilities extending beyond a one-to-one physician-patient relationship. The interesting question is this: to what extent is this implication true?

In certain circumscribed circumstances, the answers appear to be relatively easy to reach. There have always been pressures upon physicians to behave as responsible members of their communities, and physicians have traditionally responded well, supporting—even initiating and developing—causes for the common good in civic enterprise and through a variety of agencies.

As physicians have become members of the staffs of hospitals or other professional organizations, it has become clear that institutional and organizational responsibilities go with this privilege. The physician must do his share of committee work, must contribute to such things as education and teaching efforts and must meet certain standards of involvement and performance beyond just devoting himself to his patients.

But I think that in this Congress on Medical Ethics we have tended to go far beyond these narrow confines. We have spoken of what medicine must do, what it is doing, and although we have talked in large part about the medical profession collectively, it must follow that the responsibilities of the profession can only be discharged by the actions of physicians individually, even though they act in concert.

A BROADER ASPECT OF MEDICAL ETHICS

I presume that one as perceptive as Edward Jenner was well aware of the fact that he had upon his hands, or upon his conscience, an ethical question of awesome proportions. He was reasonably sure that cow pox was a relatively benign disease. He had substantial reason to believe that an attack of cow pox provided protection against smallpox, which was clearly not a benign disease. He felt that he could transfer the benign disease from one person to another. But—in spite of all inference—should he really take the responsibility of giving a fellow human being a disease he didn't have?

I begin my discussion of the ethical responsibilities of the medical profession with this rhetorical question because I believe it epitomizes the import of the word "responsibility" as we use it today. Jenner was impelled to determine his responses to certain sets of surmises, conjectures, and bits of evidence. Today, in less well-circumscribed matters, our surmises, conjectures, and bits of evidence are even more difficult to assess. Our responses, and, therefore, our responsibilities, are correspondingly more difficult to crystallize clearly. I think the complexity arises from the many new and altered elements to which the profession must respond rather than from any need for change in our fundamental ethical principles. Scientific progress and socioeconomic adaptations create new problems almost daily. We shall undoubtedly always require the services of a Judicial Council in Adjudicating differences of opinion in regard to specific sets of circumstances. There has been a gradual and logical extension of this judicial process from pure physician-patient concerns to such diverse matters as the ethical considerations in organ transplantation and in computer technology. I would offer the opinion that we are in early phases of an even greater extension of the range of ethical responsibility for medicine and its organizations. I am speaking of ethical considerations in the provision of medical service as they may arise in matters of systems design, legislative mandates, consumer representation, and quality control, as internally imposed by the medical profession or externally imposed by government.

Perhaps my thought may be best explained by referring to the provision of medical service in czarist Russia, as contrasted to medical service in Russia today under the dictates of a highly evolved totalitarian regime. To what extent have there been, are there, or should there be ethical considerations for the medical profession in Russia? I assure you that this has been a much discussed subject—at least in Russia. Physicians, individually and collectively, and their convictions in the czarist days; as these convictions were carried over into the days of transition, they lead thousands to death or exile. Many individuals and groups fought losing battles to defend a concept of inherent ethical responsibility and a doctrine of self-determinism for medicine against engulfment by the dialectical materialism of Marxism and Leninism. The battles were all lost. To ensure that they do not need to be fought over again, there are courses in the principles of dialectical materialism as applied to medical practice which come early in the curriculum of the medical school and the paramedical course. There is no judicial council for the Russian medical profession, and there is no counterpart for the American Medical Association or for a state or county medical society. There is the union of medical workers and there is the state. On the other hand, there is an interesting element of the Russian system which deserves examination. Once the state, as represented by the supreme soviet, has determined the relative priority of medical care in respect to its demands for a share of the gross national product and the available manpower, the planning and the implementation of plans are turned over to the medical profession itself. There is, thus, the inherent possibility, indeed the necessity, for the medical profession itself to determine how best to use its available resources within the circumscriptions of the system.

AUTHORITARIANISM AS SUBSTITUTE FOR ETHICS

I do not intend to discuss with you the problems of the Russian physician, but I use him and the system under which he practices to suggest that there are substitutes for reliance upon a pervasive body of medical ethics. A nation may, under certain circumstances, choose to put its trust in authoritarianism, feeling that the ethical commitments of a profession are not good enough. Indeed, one might argue that when a nation loses its respect for the ethical principles of a profession, substituting external controls, it takes the first major step in converting the profession into a trade. The issue, I submit, is the basic matter of the survival of professionalism. It has long been the tradition of the medical profession, at least in this country, to guard jealously the position that it may be relied upon to act in the public interest. It has, of its own initiative, imposed rather rigid standards on medical education. It has insisted upon significant safeguards before one may represent himself to the public as a qualified specialist. It has established for its institutions and its facilities complex standards for self-evaluation, for approvals, and for internal quality controls. It has imposed upon itself certain proscriptions which are often poorly understood by the public, such as avoidance of any semblance of professional advertising, which is all right for almost everyone except physicians, or the strictures against the splitting of fees, which is an accepted part of many other competitive enterprises. Nonetheless, when the medical profession takes positions on major issues of legislation and public policy, it is suspected of being motivated by self-interest. One is far more likely to equate policy positions in such legislative and policy issues with partisanship and political ideology than with considerations of medical ethics. Programs and proposals are more readily characterized as conservative or liberal, or as democratic or republican, than as ethical or unethical. Yet it is possible to take the position that it is, or should be, unethical to promote a system of medical service which would not be in the best interests of the public, as adjudged by those most qualified to evaluate standards of medical care. Obviously, this is a highly judgmental matter, with sincere, honest, and generally ethical physicians aligned on each side of every debatable question.

It is because of this very lack of objective criteria that I suggest that we are involved only in the beginnings of the extension of ethical considerations in the area. It would be good for a heated argument to brand any one of the many proposals for the financing of medical care, or for the revision of the medical delivery system, as unethical. And yet, it seems apparent that those organizations of physicians which would defend the traditional patterns of medical care financing and delivery are seriously concerned with extending and improving those patterns in ways which will emphasize their ethical integrity.

MEDICAL ETHICS AND SOCIETAL NEEDS

Medical ethics have, over the years, acquired a rather firm philosophical character. This, it would seem to me, is bereft of any metaphysical element. It has its roots in a societal concept of summum bonum, with interesting modifications such as that expressed in the oft repeated maxim *primum non nocere*. Jenner's dedication to the greatest good created problems for the reason that the prosecution of his project required doing something at least mildly noxious to well people. Or ethical concerns stem from the great scientific, sociological, and cultural developments which have been more precipitous in our century, and which have extended our range of influence so far beyond the simple, or relatively simple, individual physician-patient relationship. It has become extraordinarily difficult—perhaps impossible—to crystallize ethical principles into any compact set of concise statements. This was the purpose of the AMA a few years back, when it decided that what is called its Principles of the ethics had become a set of rules of professional etiquette. It made a sincere and generally effective effort to replace these minor specifics with a series of ten governing principles. This, on balance, has been good. On the other hand, across the border in Canada, the Canadian Medical Association has developed, as a result of long study, a new code of ethics expressed in 48 rather specific precepts. As an aside, it may be noted that there have been expressions of pride in the fact that these are all positive precepts. There is not a "thou shalt not" among them, which might be interpreted as indicating the underlying suspicion that the Ten Commandments stand in need of amendment.

Be that as it may, we are at a point in societal development wherein the canons of medical ethics are difficult to express in a fashion addressed to the full range of potential specific applications, and in this country, we content ourselves with our expression of basic principles depending upon our Judicial Council to interpret their impact on both old and new variants in circumstance.

It is interesting to consider the ethical problems inherent in applying the underlying dedication to the greatest good to specific developments in science. For example, there is the intriguing fact that a physician whose last name is the same as mine discovered that a low-calorie food product containing cyclamates was being sent to southeast Asia—specifically Laos—because it could not be marketed in this country. He reasoned that since it had been banned as unsafe for Americans it would be immoral or perhaps unethical to send it to Indochina. We know that there has been an inference that cyclamates might possibly be carcinogenic, although they have never been shown to be so in human beings. We know that millions of people in other parts of the world are suffering from malnutrition or outright starvation. The question is, in pursuing the principle of greatest good, is it better to give a protein-rich, low calorie food stuff to people for whom any protein source is a plus, or is it better to withhold it because of a highly hypothetical risk of bladder cancer? I suppose we cannot bind an Ohio congressman who is not a physician to principles of medical ethics, but one might ask if it can be in accordance with any set of ethical principles for one to pontificate on matters in which he has no competence, and in effect, to force actions such as the denial of hundreds of tons of nutritive material to starving people. I cite this as an example of the complexities in which we may become involved as we pursue the general matter of applying our ethical standards.

In another area, the problems of determining ethical responsibilities can become even more diffuse. It is a general principle of the AMA that the medical profession has responsibilities in supporting and operating medical care systems which will serve the public best. As a corollary, it needs to oppose legislative alterations which it regards as adverse to the public interest.

Our expanded concept of concern with the greatest good becomes most difficult to apply in this field of social legislation. In some of its simpler aspects, there is little equivocation. A federal or state law which offers financial support to an inferior or dangerous substitute for scientific medical care is adverse to the support of the greatest good. Ethical integrity demands resistance to program which would give status and support to chiropractic. But what about the much more controversial matter of support to a system of medical care which has as its objective the elimination of fee for service, the substitution of prepaid comprehensive group for solo practice or other forms of group practice? Is such controversy just a matter of liberal vs. conservative, or democratic vs. republican, or are there elements of ethical vs. unethical? I do not believe that the Judicial Council is ready to rule on this. At the moment, there are sincere physicians on each side of the question. It seems to me, however, that a great deal of the activity of physicians and their medical organizations in support of such things as the perfection of peer review mechanisms, claims review procedures, and involvement in the operation of financing operations in conjunction with state and national programs have major ethical implications. These efforts would seem to be directed to giving survival value a system of care which the bulk of medical professionals sincerely believe to be in the interest of the greater good for society. It would seem possible to allege that many physicians feel that if our fundamental ethical principles are to prevail, we must fight for the preservation of the system which maintains the physician as a responsible professional rather than as a hired technician.

This, perhaps, brings us back to our initial concern with the ethical responsibilities of the medical profession. So long as a preponderance of the providers of medical service—particularly physicians—feel that the weight of the evidence favors the concept that the public may be better served—that the greatest good may be best accomplished—by a profession exercising its own responsibility to the state or to someone else, then the medical profession has an ethical responsibility to exert itself in making apparent the superiorities of the system which it supports.

The approach favored by Russell Roth of the American Medical Association in which professionals generate for themselves a set of moral norms gives rise to a code of ethics coming from only one side of the lay-professional relationship. It overlooks the possibility that some people on the other side of the relationship may have different conceptions of what is expected morally in the relation. Such questions as whether a physician should break confidence when it would serve the interests of society to do so are sometimes answered differently by different groups. Historically, the profession has insisted in such circumstances that confidences be kept while public bodies such as the courts and lay groups commenting on the ethics of medicine have insisted that when there are major risks to others, confidences should be broken. The differences probably cannot be explained entirely by the self-interest of the different groups.

An alternative way of resolving such conflict is to bring lay people and professionals together to see if they can jointly agree on some compromise set of principles. Contract theorists support such strategies. Hypothetical contractarians would hold that the agreement that emerges will tell us what is ethical to the extent that the contractors can approximate persons who have the characteristics of ideal contractors.

A variant on this approach is to talk about lay people and professionals forming a covenant together. The term covenant implies to some a less legalistic or business-like kind of agreement. In the essay that follows William May challenges the ethics of professional codes, supporting in their place an ethic of covenant between lay and professional.

Code, Covenant, Contract, or Philanthropy

WILLIAM F. MAY

Questions in medical ethics cannot be resolved apart from the professional matrix in which most decisions are made. What is the nature of the relationship between physicians and their patients? How best can we conceptualize professional ethics and understand its binding power? The times press these questions, while tradition offers us several starting points, alternative ways of interpreting professional obligations: the concepts of code and covenant, and the allied notions of philanthropy and contract.

The Hippocratic Oath, as Ludwig Edelstein notes in his unsurpassed study of that document,[1] contains two distinct sets of obligations—those that pertain to the doctor's treatment of his patients and those that are owed his teacher and his teacher's progeny. Edelstein characterizes the first set of obligations, those owed patients, as an ethical code and the second set, those toward the professional guild, as a covenant.

This distinction between code and covenant is extremely revealing and useful. Code itself, furthermore, may be divided into the unwritten codes of practical behavior, transmitted chiefly in a clinical setting from generation to generation of physicians, and into the written codes, beginning with the Hippocratic Oath and concluding with the various revisions of the AMA codes that have had wide currency in this country. Technical proficiency is the prized ideal in the unwritten and informal codes of behavior passed on from doctor to doctor; the ideal of philanthropy (that is, the notion of gratuitous service to humankind) looms large in the more official engraved tablets of the profession. Then, the notion of covenant stands in contrast not only with the ideals of technical proficiency and philanthropy but also with the legal instrument of a contract to which, at first glance, a covenant seems so similar. With these distinctions, then, let us begin.

THE HIPPOCRATIC OATH

As elaborated in the Hippocratic Oath, the duties of a physician toward his patients include a series of absolute prohibitions: against performing surgery, against assisting patients in attempts at suicide or abortion, breaches in confidentiality, and against acts of injustice or mischief toward the patient and his household, including sexual misconduct. More positively, the physician must act always for the benefit of the sick—the chief illustration of which is to apply dietetic measures according to the physician's best judgment and ability—and, more generally, to keep them from harm and injustice. These various professional obligations to the patient have a religious reference, as the physician declares, "In purity and holiness I will guard my life and art," and petitions, "If I fulfill this oath and do not violate it, may it be granted to me to enjoy life and art . . . ; if I transgress it and swear falsely, may the opposite of all this be my lot."

The second set of obligations, directed to the physician's teacher, his teacher's children and his own, require him to accept full filial responsibilities for his adopted father's personal and financial welfare, and to transmit without fee his art and knowledge of the teacher's progeny, to his own, and to other pupils, but only those others who take the oath according to medical law.

It will be the contention of this essay that the development of the practice of modern medicine, for understandable reasons, has tended to reinforce the ancient distinction between these two obligations, that is, between code and covenant; and that it has opted for code as the ruling ideal in relations to patients. The choice has not had altogether favorable consequences for the moral health of the profession.

THE CHARACTERISTICS OF A CODE

For the purposes of this essay, it can be said, a code shapes human behavior in a fashion somewhat similar to habits and rules. A habit, as Peter Winch has pointed out,[2] is a matter of doing the same thing on the same kind of occasion in the same way. A moral rule is distinct from a habit in that the agent in this instance understands what is meant by doing the same thing on the same kind of occasion in the same way. Both habits and rules are categorical, universal, and to this degree a historical: they do not receive their authority from particular events by which they are authorized or legitimated. They remain operative categorically on all similar occasions: Never assist patients in attempts at suicide or abortion; never break a confidence except under certain specified circumstances.

A code is usually categorical and universal in the aforementioned senses, but not in the sense that it is binding on any and all groups. Hammurabi's code is obligatory only for particular peoples. Moreover, inner circles within certain societies—whether professional or social groups—develop their special codes of behavior. We think of code words or special behaviors among friends, workers in the same company, or professionals within a guild. These codes offer directives not only for the content of action, but also for its form. In its concern with appropriate form, a code moves in the direction of the aesthetic. It is concerned not only with what is done but with how it is done; it touches on matters of style and decorum. Thus medical codes include directives not only on the content of therapeutic action, but also on the fitting style for professional behavior including such matters as suitable dress, discretion in the household, appropriate behavior in the hospital, and prohibitions on self-advertisement.

This tendency to more ethics in the direction of aesthetics is best illustrated in the work of the modern novelist most associated with the ideal of a code. The ritual killing of a bull in the short stories and novels of Hemingway symbolizes an ethic in which stylish performance is everything.

> . . . the bull charged and Villalta charges and just for a moment they became one. Villalta became one with the bull and then it was over.
> Hemingway, *In Our Time*

For the Hemingway hero, there is no question of permanent commitments to particular persons, causes, or places. Robert Jordan of *For Whom the Bell Tolls* does not even remember the "cause" for which he came to Spain to fight. Once he is absorbed in the ordeal of war, the test of a man is not a cause to which he is committed but his conduct from moment to moment. Life is a matter of eating, drinking, loving, hunting, and dying well. Hemingway writes about lovers, but rarely about marriage or the family. Catherine in *Farewell to Arms* and Robert Jordan in *For Whom the Bell Tolls* inevitably must die. Just for a moment, lovers become one and then it is over.

The bullfighter, the wartime lover, the doctor—all alike—must live by a code that eschews involvement; for each there comes a time when the thing is over; matters are terminated by death. But this does not mean that men cannot live beautifully, stylishly, fittingly. Discipline is all. There is a right and a wrong way to do things. And the wrong way usually results from a deficiency in technique or from an excessive preoccupation with one's ego. The bad bullfighter either lacks technique or he lets his ego—through fear or vanity—get in the way of his performance. The conditions of beauty are technical proficiency and a style wholly purified of disruptive preoccupation with oneself. Literally, however, when the critical moment is consummated, it is over; it cannot shape the future. Partners must fall away; only the code remains.

For several reasons, the medical profession has been attracted to the ideal of code for its interpretation of its ethics. First, a code requires one to subordinate the ego to the more technical question of how a thing is done and done well. At its best, the discipline of a code has an aesthetic value. It encourages a proficiency that is quietly eloquent. It conjoins the good with the beautiful. Since the technical demands of medicine have become so great, the standards of the guild are transmitted largely by apprenticeship to those who preeminent skills define the real meaning of the profession without significant remainder. All the rest is a question of disciplining the ego to the point that nervousness, fatigue, faintheartedness, and temptations to self-display (including gross efforts at self-advertisement) have been smoothed away.

A code is additionally attractive in that it does not, in and of itself, encourage personal involvement with the patient; and it helps free the physician of the destructive consequences of that personal involvement. Compassion, in the strictest sense of the term—"suffering with"—has its disadvantages in the professional relationship. It will not do to pretend that one is the second person of the Trinity, prepared to make with every patient the sympathetic descent into his suffering, pain, particular form of crucifixion, and hell. It is enough to offer whatever help one can through finely honed services. It is important to remain emotionally free so as to be able to withdraw the self when those services are no longer pertinent, when as Hemingway says, "it is over."

Finally, a code provides the modern doctor with a basic style of operation that shapes not only his professional but his free time, not only his vocation but his avocations. The self-same pleasure he derives from proficiency in his professional life, he transposes now to his recreational life—flying, skiing, traveling, daily in the precincts of suffering and death he learns that life is available only from moment to moment. As a hard-pressed professional, he knows that both his life and free time are limited—like the soldier's furlough. It makes sense to live by a code that operates from moment to moment, savoring pleasure in stylish action. Thus his code not only frees him from some of the awkwardness and distress that sentient beings are prey to in the midst of agony; but, when he is momentarily free of the battle, it provides him with a style and allows him to live, like most warriors who have tasted death, by the canons of hedonism, which money places specially within his reach.

THE IDEAL OF A COVENANT

A covenant, as opposed to a code, has its roots in specific historical events. Like a code, it may give inclusive shape to subsequent behavior, but it always has reference to specific historical exchange between partners leading to a promissory event. Edelstein is quite right in distinguishing code from covenant in the Hippocratic Oath. Rules governing behavior toward patients have a different ring to them from that fealty which a physician owes to his teacher. Loyalty to one's instructor is founded in a specific historical event—that original transaction in which the student received his knowledge and art. He accepts, in effect, a specific gift from his teacher which deserves his lifelong loyalty, a gift that he perpetuates in his own right and turn as he offers his art without fee to his teacher's children and to his own progeny. Covenant ethics is responsive in character.

In its ancient and most influential form, a covenant usually included the following elements: (1) an original experience of gift between the soon-to-be covenanted partners; (2) a covenant promise based on this original or anticipated exchange of gifts, labors, or services; and (3) the shaping of subsequent life for each partner by the promissory event. God "marks the forehead" of the Jews forever, as they respond by accepting an inclusive set of ritual and moral commandments by which they will live. These commands are both specific enough (e.g., the dietary laws) to make the future duties of Israel concrete, yet summary enough (e.g., love the Lord; thy God with all thy heart. . . .) to require a fidelity that exceeds any specification.

The most striking contemporary restatement of an ethic based on covenant is offered by Hemingway's great competitor and contemporary as a novelist—William Faulkner. While the Hemingway hero lives from moment to moment, Faulkner's characters take their bearings from a covenant event. Like Hemingway, Faulkner also writes about a ritual slaying, but with a difference. In "Delta Autumn," a young boy, Isaac McCaslin, "comes of age" in the course of a hunt:

> And the gun levelled rapidly without haste and crashed and he walked to the buck still intact and still in the shape of that magnificent speed and bled it with Sam Father's knife and Sam dipped his hands in the hot blood and marked his face forever. . . . Faulkner, "Delta Autumn"

The Hemingway hero slays his bull and then it is over; but young Isaac McCaslin binds the whole of his future in the instant.

> I slew you; my bearing must not shame your quitting of life. My conduct forever onward must become your death.

From then on, just as the marked Jew, the errant, harassed, and estranged Jew, recovers the covenant of Mt. Sinai through ritual renewal, Isaac returns to the delta every autumn to renew the hunt and to suffer his own renewal despite the alienation and pain and defeat which he as subsequently known across a lifetime. This covenant moreover looms over all else—his relationship to the land, to women, to blacks, to all of which and whom he is bound.

For some of the reasons already mentioned, the bond of covenant, in the classical period, tended to define and bind together medical colleagues to one another, but it did not figure large in interpreting the relations between the doctor and his patients. This gift establishes a bond between them and prompts him to assume certain lifetime duties not only toward the teacher (and his financial welfare), but toward his children. This symbolic bond with one's teacher acknowledged in the Hippocratic Oath is strengthened in modern professional life by all those exchanges between colleagues—referrals, favors, personal confidences, and collaborative work on cases. Thus loyalty to colleagues is a responsive act for gifts already, and to be received.

Duties to patients are not similarly interpreted in the medical codes as a responsive act of gifts or services received. This is the essential feature of covenant which is conspicuously missing in the interpretation of professional duties from the Hippocratic Oath to the modern codes of the AMA.

THE CODE IDEAL OF PHILANTHROPY VS. COVENANTAL INDEBTEDNESS

The medical profession includes in its written codes an ideal that seldom looms large in the ethic of any self-selected inner group—the ideal of philanthropy. The medical profession proclaims its dedication to the service of mankind. This ideal is implicitly at work in the Hippocratic Oath and the culture out of which it emerged;[3] It continues in the Code of Medical Ethics originally adopted by the American Medical Association at its national convention in 1847, and it is elaborated in contemporary statements of that code.

This ideal of service, in my judgment, succumbs to what might be called the conceit of philanthropy when it is assumed that the professional's commitment to his fellowman is a gratuitous, rather than responsive or reciprocal, act. Statements of medical ethics that obscure the doctor's prior indebtedness to the community are tainted with the odor of condescension. The point is obvious if one contrasts the way in which the code of 1847 interprets the obligations of patients and the public. On this particular question, I see no fundamental change from 1847 to 1957.

Clearly the duties of the patient are founded on what he has received from the doctor:

> The members of the medical profession, upon whom is enjoined the performance of so many important and arduous duties toward the community, and who are required to make so many sacrifices of comfort, ease, and health, for the welfare of those who avail themselves of their services, certainly have a right to expect a just sense of the duties which they owe to their medical attendants.[4]

In like manner, the section on the Obligations of the Public to Physicians emphasizes those many gifts and services which the public has received from the medical profession and which are basis for its indebtedness to the profession.

> The benefits accruing to the public, directly and indirectly, from the active
> and unwearied beneficence of the profession, are so numerous and impor-
> tant, that physicians are unjustly entitled to the utmost consideration and
> respect from the community.[5]

But turning to the preamble for the physician's duties to the patient and the
public, we find no corresponding section in the code of 1847 (or 1957) which
founds the doctor's obligation on those gifts and services which he has received from
the community. Thus we are presented with the picture of a relatively self-sufficient
monad, who, out of the nobility and generosity of his disposition and the gra-
tuitously accepted conscience of his profession, has taken upon himself the noble life
of service. The false posture in all this cries out in one of the opening sections of the
1847 code. Physicians "should study, also, in their deportment so as to unite tender-
ness with firmness, and condescension with authority, so as to inspire the minds of
their patients with gratitude, respect and confidence."

I do not intend to demean the specific content of those duties which the codes
set forth in their statement of the duties of physicians to their patients, but I am
critical of the setting or context in which they are placed. Significantly the code
refers to the Duties of physicians to their patients but to the Obligations of patients to
their physicians. The shift from "Duties" to "obligations" may seem slight, but in
fact, I believe it is a revealing adjustment in language. The AMA thought of the
patient and public as indebted to the profession for its services but the profession
has accepted its duties to the patients and public out of noble conscience rather than
a reciprocal sense of indebtedness.

Put another way, the medical profession imitates God not so much because it
exercises power of life and death over others, but because it does not really think
itself beholden, even partially, to anyone for those duties to patients which it lays
upon itself. Like God, the profession draws its life from itself alone. Its action is
wholly gratuitous.

Now, in fact, the physician is in very considerable debt to the community. The
first of these debts is already adumbrated in the original Hippocratic Oath. He is
obliged to someone or some group for his education. In ancient times, this led to a
special sense of covenant obligation to one's teacher. Under the conditions of modern medical education, this indebtedness is both substantial (far exceeding the
social investment in the training of any other professional) and widely distributed
(including not only one's teachers but those public monies on the basis of which the
medical school, the teaching hospital, and research into disease are funded).

In view of the fact that many more qualified candidates apply for medical
school than can be admitted and many more doctors are needed than the schools
can train, the doctor-to-be has a second order of indebtedness for privileges that
have almost arbitrarily fallen his way. While the 1847 codes refers to the "privileges" of being a doctor it does not specify the social origins of those privileges.
Third, and not surprisingly, the codes do not make reference to that extraordinary
social largesse that befalls the physician, in payment for services, in a society where

need abounds and available personnel is limited. Further, the codes do not concede the indebtedness of the physician to those patients who have offered themselves as subjects for experimentation or as teaching material (either in teaching hospitals or in early years of practice). Early practice includes, after all, the element of increased risk for patients who lay their bodies on the line as the doctor "practices" on them. The pun in the word but reflects the inevitable social price of training. This indebtedness to the patient was most recently and eloquently acknowledged by Judah Folkman, M.D., of Harvard Medical School in a Class Day Address.

> In the long run, it is better if we come to terms with the uncertainty of medical practice. Once we recognize that all our efforts to relieve suffering might on occasion cause suffering, we are in a position to learn from our mistakes and appreciate the debt we owe our patients for our education. It is a debt which we must repay—it is like tithing.
>
> I doubt that the debt we accumulate can be repaid our patients by trying to reduce the practice of medicine to a forty-hour week or by dissolving the quality of our residency programs just because certain groups of residents in that country have refused, through legal tactics, to be on duty more than every fourth or fifth night or any nights at all.
>
> And it can't be repaid by refusing to see Medicaid patients when the state can't afford to pay for them temporarily.
>
> But we can repay the debt in many ways. We can attend postgraduate courses and seminars, be available to patients at all hours, teach, take recertifications examinations; maybe in the future even volunteer for national service; or, most difficult of all, carry out investigation or research.[6]

The physician, finally, is indebted to his patients not only for a start in his career. He remains unceasingly in their debt in its full course. This continuing reciprocity of need is somewhat obscured for we think of the mature professional as powerful and authoritative rather than needy. He seems to be a self-sufficient virtuoso whose life is derived from his competence while others appear before him in their neediness, exposing their illness, their crimes, or their ignorance, for which the professional—doctor, lawyer, or teacher—offers remedy.

In fact, however, a reciprocity of giving and receiving is at work in the professional relationship that needs to be acknowledged. In the profession of teaching, for example, the student needs the teacher to assist him in learning, but so also the professor needs his students. They provide him with regular occasion and forum in which to work out what he has to say and to rediscover his subject afresh through the discipline of sharing it with others. Likewise, the doctor needs his patients. No one can watch a physician nervously approach retirement without realizing how much he needed his patients to be himself.

A convenantal ethics helps acknowledge this full context of need and indebtedness in which professional duties are undertaken and discharged. It also relieves the professional of the temptation and pressure to pretend that he is a demigod exempt from human exigency.

CONTRACT OR COVENANT

While criticizing the ideal of philanthropy, I have emphasized the elements of exchange, agreement, and reciprocity that mark the professional relationship. This leaves us with the question as to whether the element of gratuitous should be suppressed altogether in professional ethics. Does the physician merely respond to the social investment in his training, the fees paid for his services, and the terms of an agreement drawn up between himself and his patients, or does some element of gratuitous remain?

To put this question another way: is covenant simply another name for a contract in which two parties calculate their own best interests and agree upon some joint project in which both derive roughly equivalent benefits for goods contributed to each? If so, this essay would appear to move in the direction of those who interpret the doctor-patient relationship as a legal agreement and who want, on the whole, to see medical ethics draw closer to medical law.

The notion of the physician as contractor has certain obvious attractions. First, it represents a deliberate break with more authoritarian models (such as priest or parent) for interpreting the role. At the heart of a contract is informed consent rather than blind trust; a contractual understanding of the therapeutic relationship encourages full respect for the dignity of the patient, who has not, through illness, forfeited his sovereignty as a human being. The notion of a contract includes an exchange of information on the basis of which an agreement is reached and a subsequent exchange of goods (money or services); it also allows for a specification of rights, duties, conditions, and qualifications limiting the agreement. The net effect is to establish some symmetry and mutuality in the relationship between the doctor and patient.

Second, a contract provides for the legal enforcement of its items—on both parties—and thus offers both parties some protection and recourse under the law for making the other accountable for the agreement.

Finally, a contract does not rely on the pose of philanthropy, the condescension of charity. It presupposes that people are primarily governed by self-interest. When two people enter into a contract, they do so because each sees it to his own advantage. This is true not only of private contracts but also of that primordial social contract in and through which the state came into being. So argued the theorists of the 18th century. The state was not established by some heroic act of sacrifice on the part of the gods or men. Rather men entered in the social contract because each found it to his individual advantage. It is better to surrender some liberty and property to the state than to suffer the evils that would beset men except for its protection. Subsequent enthusiasts about the social instrument of contracts[7] have tended to measure human progress by the degree to which a society is based on contract rather than status. In ancient world, the Romans made the most striking advances in extending the areas in which contract rather than custom determined commerce between people. In the modern world, the bourgeoisie extended the instrumentality of contracts farthest into the sphere of economics; the free churches, into the arena of religion. Some educationists today have extended the device into the classroom (as students are encouraged to contract units of work for levels of grade); more recently some women's liberationists would extend it into marriage; and still others would prefer to see it define the professional relationship. The movement, on the whole, has the intention of laicizing authority, legalizing relationships, activating self-interests, and encouraging collaboration.

In my judgement, some of these aims of the contractualists are desirable, but it would be unfortunate if professional ethics were reduced to a commercial contract without significant remainder. First, the notion of contract suppresses the element of gift in human relationships. Earlier I verged on denying the importance of this ingredient in professional relations, when I criticized the medical profession for its conceit of philanthropy, for its self-interpretation as the great giver. In fact, this earlier objection should be limited to the failure of the medical profession to acknowledge those gifts and goods it has itself received. It is unbecoming to adopt the pose of spontaneous generosity when the profession has received so much from the community and from patients, past and present.

But the contractualist approach to professional behavior falls into the opposite error of minimalism. It reduces everything to tit-for-tat: do no more for your patients than what the contract calls for; perform specified services for certain fees and no more. The commercial contract is fitting instrument in the purchase of an appliance, a house, or certain services that can be specified fully in advance of delivery. The existence of a legally enforceable agreement in professional transactions may also be useful to protect the patient or client against the physician or lawyer whose services fall below a minimal standard. But it would be wrong to reduce professional obligation to the specifics of a contract alone.

Professional services in the so-called helping professions are directed to subjects who are in the nature of the case rather unpredictable. One deals with the sickness, ills, crimes, needs, and tragedies of humankind. These needs cannot be exhaustively specified in advance for each patient or client. The professions must be ready to cope with the contingent, the unexpected. Calls upon services may be required that exceed those anticipated in a contract or for which compensation may be available in a given case. These services, moreover, are more likely to be effective in achieving the desired therapeutic result if they are delivered in the context of a fiduciary relationship that the patient or client can really trust.

THE LIMITATIONS OF CONTRACT

Contract and covenant, materially considered, seem like first cousins; they both include an exchange and an agreement between parties. But, in spirit, contract and covenant are quite different. Contracts are external; covenants are internal to the parties involved. Contracts are signed to be expediently discharged. Covenants have a gratuitous, growing edge to them that nourishes rather than limits relationships. To the best of my knowledge, no one has put quite so effectively the difference between the two as the novelist already cited in the earlier discussion of covenant.

At the outset of Faulkner's *Intruder in the Dust,* a white boy, hunting with young blacks, falls into a creek on a cold winter's day. After the boy clambers out of the river, Lucas Beauchamp, a proud, commanding black man, brings him, shivering, to his house where Mrs. Beauchamp takes care of him. She takes off his wet clothes and wraps him in Negro blanket, feeds him Negro food, and warms him by the fire.

When his clothes dry off, the boy dresses to go, but, uneasy about his debt to the other, he reaches into his pocket for some coins and offers seventy cents compensation for Beauchamp's help. Lucas rejects the money firmly and commands the two black boys to pick up the coins from the floor where they have fallen and return them to the white boy.

Shortly thereafter, still uneasy about the episode at the river and his frustrated effort to pay off Lucas for his help, the boy buys some imitation silk for Lucas's wife and gets his Negro friend to deliver it. But a few days later, the white boy goes to his own backdoor stoop to find a jug of molasses left there for him by Lucas. So he is back to where he started, beholden to the black man again.

Several months later, the boy passes Lucas on the street and scans his face closely, wondering if the black man remembers the incident between them. He can't be sure. Four years pass, and Lucas is accused of murdering a white man. He is scheduled to be taken to jail. The boy goes early before the crowd gathers and ponders whether the old man remembers their past encounter. Just as Lucas is about to enter the jailhouse, he wheels and points his long arm in the direction of the boy and says, "Boy, I want to see you." The boy obeys and visits Lucas in the jailhouse, and eventually he and his aunt are instrumental in proving Lucas's innocence.

Faulkner's story is a parable for the relationship of the white man to the black man in the South. The black man has labored in the white man's fields, built and cared for his house, fed, clothed, and nurtured his children. In accepting these labors, the white man has received his life and substance from the black man over and over again. But he resists this involvement and tries to pay off the black man with a few coins. He pretends that their relationship is transient and external, to be managed at arm's length.

For better or for worse, blacks and whites in this country are bound up in a common life and destiny together. The problem between them will not be resolved until they accept the covenant between them which is entailed in the original acceptance of labor.

There is a donative element in the nourishing of covenant—whether it is the covenant of marriage, friendship, or professional relationship. Tit-for-tat characterizes a commercial transaction, but it does not exhaustively define the vitality of that relationship in which one must serve and draw upon the deeper reserves of another.

This donative element is important not only in the doctor's care of the patient but in other aspects of health care. In a fascinating study of *The Gift Relationship,* the late Richard M. Titmuss compares the British system of obtaining blood by donations with the American partial reliance on the commercial purchase and sale of blood.[8] The British system obtains more and better blood, without the exploitation of the indigent, which the American system has condoned and which our courts have encouraged when they refused to exempt non-profit blood banks from the anti-trust laws. By court definition, blood exchange becomes a commercial transaction in the United States. Titmuss expanded his theme from human blood to social policy by offering sober criticism of the increased commercialism of American medicine and society at large. Recent court decisions have tended to shift more and more of what had previously been considered as services into the category of commodity transactions, with negative consequences he believes for the health of health delivery systems.[9] Hans Jonas has had to reckon with the importance of voluntary sacrifice to the social order in a somewhat comparable essay on "Human Experimentation." Others have done so on the subject of organ transplants.

The kind of minimalism encouraged by a contractualist understanding of the professional relationship produces a professional too grudging, too calculating, too lacking in spontaneity, too quickly exhausted to go the second mile with his patients along the road of their distress.

Contract medicine not only encourages minimalism, it also provokes a peculiar kind of maximalism, the name for which is "defensive medicine." Especially under the pressure of malpractice suits, doctors are tempted to order too many examinations and procedures for self-protection. Paradoxically, contractualism simultaneously tempts the doctor to do too little and too much for the patient: too little in that one extends oneself only to the limits of what is specified in the contract; yet, at the same time, too much in that one orders procedures useful in protecting oneself as the contractor even though they are not fully indicated by the condition of the patient. The link between these apparently contradictory strategies of too little and too much is the emphasis in contractual decisions grounded in self-interest.

Three concluding objections to contractualism can be stated summarily. Parties to a contract are better able to protect their self-interest insofar as they are informed about the goods bought and sold. Insofar as contract medicine encourages increased knowledge on the part of the patient, well and good. Nevertheless the physician's knowledge so exceeds that of his patient that the patient's knowledgeability alone is not a satisfactory constraint on the physician's behavior. One must, at least in part, depend upon some internal fiduciary checks which the professional and his guild take on.

Another self-regulating mechanism in the traditional contractual relationship is the consumer's freedom to shop and choose among various vendors of services. Certainly this freedom of choice needs to be expanded for the patient by an increase in the number of physicians and paramedical personnel. However, the crisis circumstances under which medical services are often needed and delivered does not always provide the consumer with the kind of leisure or calm required for discretionary judgement. Thus normal marketplace controls cannot be fully relied upon to protect the consumer in dealings with the physician.

For a final reason, medical ethics should not be reduced to the contractual relationship alone. Normally conceived, ethics establishes certain rights and duties that transcend the particulars of a given agreement. The justice of any specific contract may then be measured by these standards. If, however, such rights and duties adhere only to the contract, then a patient may legitimately be persuaded to waive his rights. The contract would solely determine what is required and permissible. An ethical principle should not be waivable (except to give way to a higher ethical principle). Professional ethics should not be so defined as to permit a physician to persuade a patient to waive rights that transcend the particulars of their agreement.

TRANSCENDENCE AND COVENANT

This essay has developed two characteristics of conventional ethics in the course of contrasting it with the ideal of philanthropy and the legal instrument of contracts. As opposed to the ideal of philanthropy that pretends to wholly gratuitous altruism, covenantal ethics places the service of the professional within the full context of goods, gifts, and services received; thus covenantal ethics is responsive. As opposed to the instrument of contract that presupposes agreement reached on the basis of self-interest, covenantal ethics may require one to be available to the covenant partner above and beyond the measure of self-interest; thus covenantal ethics has an element of the gratuitous in it.

We have to reckon now with the potential conflict between these characteristics. Have we developed our notion of covenant too reactively to alternatives without paying attention to the inner consistency of the concept itself? On the one hand, we had cause for suspicion of those idealists who founded professional duties on a philanthropic impulse, without so much as acknowledging the sacrifice of others by which their own lives have been nourished. Then we had reasons for drawing back from those legal realists and positivists who would circumscribe professional life entirely within the calculus of commodities bought and sold. But now, brought face to face, these characteristics conflict. Response to debt and gratuitous service seem opposed principles of action.

Perhaps our difficulty results from the fact that we have abstracted the concept of covenant from its original context within the transcendent. The indebtedness of a human being that makes his life—however sacrificial—inescapably responsive cannot be fully appreciated by totaling up the varying sacrifices and investments made by others in his favor. Such sacrifices are there; and it is lacking in honesty not to acknowledge them. But the sense that one is exhaustibly the object of gift presupposes a more transcendent source of donative activity than the sum of gifts received from others. For the Biblical tradition this transcendent was the secret root of every gift between human beings, of which the human order of giving and receiving could only be a sign. Thus the Jewish scriptures enjoin: when you harvest your crops, do not pick your fields too clean. Leave something for the sojourner for you were once sojourners in Egypt. Farmers obedient to this injunction were responsive, but not simply mathematically responsive to gifts received from the Egyptians or from strangers now drifting through their own land. At the same time, their actions could not be constructed as wholly gratuitous. Their ethic of service to the needy flowed from Israel's original and continuing state of neediness and indebtedness before God. Thus action which at a human level appears gratuitous, in that it is not provoked by a specific gratuity from another human being, is at its deepest level but gift answering gift. This responsivity is theologically expressed in the New Testament as follows: "In this is love, not that we loved God, but that he loved us . . . if God so loved us, we also ought to love one another" (I John 4:10–11). In some such way, covenant ethics shies back from the idealist assumption that professional action is and ought to be wholly gratuitous, and from the contractualist assumption that it be carefully governed by quotidian self-interest in every exchange.

A transcendent reference may also be important not only in setting forth the proper context in which human service takes place but also in laying out the specific standards by which it is measured. Earlier we noted some dangers in reducing rights and duties to the terms of a particular contract. We observed the need for a transcendent norm by which contracts are measured (and limited). By the same token, rights and duties cannot be wholly derived from the particulars of a given covenant. What limits ought to be placed on demands of an excessively dependent patient? At what point does the keeping of one's covenant do an injustice to obligations entailed in others? These are questions that warn against a covenantal ethics that sentimentalizes any and all involvements, without reference to a transcendent by which which they are both justified and measured.

FURTHER REFLECTIONS ON COVENANT

So far we have discussed those features of a covenant that affect the doctor's conduct toward his patient. The concept of covenant has further consequences for the patients self-interpretation, for the accountability of health institutions, for the placement of institutional priorities within other national commitments, and, finally, for such collateral problems as truth-telling.

Every model for the doctor/patient relationship establishes not only a certain image of the doctor, but also a specific concept of the self. The image of the doctor as priest or parent encourages dependency in the patient. The image of doctor as skillful technician prompts the patient to think less in terms of his personal dependence, but still it encourages a somewhat impersonal passivity, with the doctor and his technical procedures the only serious agent in the relationship. The image of doctor as covenanter or contracter bids the patient to become a more active participant both in the prevention and the healing of the disease. He must bring to the partnership a will to life and a will to health.

Differing views of disease are involved in these differing patterns of relationship to the doctor. Disease today is usually interpreted by the layman as an extraordinary state, discrete and episodic, disjunct from the ordinary condition of health. Illness is a special time when the doctor is in charge and the layman renounces authority over his life. This view, while psychologically understandable, ignores the growth during apparent periods of health of those pathological conditions that invite the dramatic breakdown when the doctor "takes over."

The cardio-vascular accident is a case in point. Horacio Fabrega[10] has urged an interpretation of disease and health that respects more fully the processive rather than the episodic character of both disease and health. This interpretation, I assume, would encourage the doctor to monitor more continuously health/disease than ordinarily occurs today, to share with the patient more fully the information so obtained, and to engage the layperson in health maintenance.

The concept of covenant has two further advantages for defining the professional relationship, not enjoyed by models such as parent, friend, or technician. First, covenant is not so restrictively personal a term as parent or friend. It reminds the professional community that it is not good enough for the individual doctor to be a good friend or parent to the patient; that it is important also for whole institutions—the hospital, the clinic, the professional group—to keep covenant with those who seek their assistance and sanctuary. Thus the concept permits a certain broadening of accountability beyond personal agency.

At the same time, however, the notion of covenant also permits one to set professional responsibility for this one human good (health) within social limits. The professional covenant concerning health should be situated within a larger set of covenant obligations that both the doctor and patient have toward other institutions and priorities within the society at large. The traditional models for the doctor/patient relationship (parent, friend) tend to establish an exclusivity of relationship that obscures those larger responsibilities. At a time when health needs command 120 billion dollars out the national budget, one must think about the place held by the obligation to the limited human good of health among a whole range of social and personal goods for which men are compacted together as a society.

A covenantal ethic has implications for other collateral problems in biomedical ethics, some of which have been explored in the searching work of Paul Ramsey, *The Patient as Person.* I will restrict myself simply to one issue that has not been viewed from the perspective of covenant: the question of truth-telling.

Key ingredients in the notion of covenant are promise and fidelity to promise. The philosopher J.I. Austin drew the distinction, now famous, between two kinds of speech: descriptive and performative utterances. In ordinary declarative or descriptive sentences, one describes a given term within the world. (It is raining. The tumor is malignant. The crisis is past.) In performative utterances, one does not merely describe a world, in effect, one alters the world by introducing an ingredient that would not be there apart from the utterance. Promises are such performative utterances. (I, John, take thee, Mary. We will defend your country in case of attack. I will not abandon you.) To make or to go back on a promise is a very solemn matter precisely because a promise is world-altering.

In the field of medical ethics, the question of truth-telling has tended to be discussed entirely as a question of descriptive speech. Should the doctor, as technician, tell the patient he has a malignancy or not? If not, may he lie or must he merely withhold the truth?

The distinction between descriptive and performative speech expands the question of the truth in professional life. The doctor, after all, not only tells descriptive truths, he also makes or implies promises. (I will see you next Tuesday; or, Despite the fact that I cannot cure you, I will not abandon you.) In brief, the moral question for the doctor is not simply a question of telling truths, but of being true to his promises. Conversely, the total situation for the patient includes not only the disease he's got, but also whether others ditch him or stand by him in his extremity. The fidelity of others will not eliminate the disease, but it affects mightily the human context in which the disease runs it course. What the doctor has to offer his patient is not simply proficiency but fidelity.

Perhaps more patients could accept the descriptive truth if they experienced the performative truth. Perhaps also they would be more inclined to believe in the doctor's performative utterances if they were not handed false diagnoses of false promises. That is why a cautiously wise medieval physician once advised his colleagues: "Promise only fidelity!"

THE PROBLEM OF DISCIPLINE

The conclusion of this essay is not that covenantal ethics should be preferred to the exclusion of some of those values best symbolized by code and contract. If we turn now to the problem of professional discipline, we can see that both alternatives have resources for self-criticism.

Those who live by a code of technical proficiency have a standard on the basis of which to discipline their peers. The Hemingway novel, especially, *The Sun Also Rises,* is quite clear about this. Those who live by a code know how to ostracize deficient peers. Indeed, any "in-group," professional or otherwise, can be quite ruthless about sorting out those who are "quality" and those who do not have the "goods." Medicine is no exception. Ostracism, in the form of discreetly refusing to refer patients to a doctor whose competence is suspected, is probably the commonest and most effective form of discipline in the profession today.

Defenders of an ethic based on code might argue further that deficiencies in enforcement today result largely from too strongly developed a sense of covenantal obligations to colleagues and too weakly developed a sense of code. From this perspective, then, covenant is the source of the problem in the profession rather than the basis for its amendment. Covenantal obligation to colleagues inhibits the enforcement of code.

A code alone, however, will not in and of itself solve the problem of professional discipline. It provides a basis for excluding from one's own inner circle an incompetent physician. But, as Eliot Freidson has pointed out in *Professional Dominance,* under the present system the incompetent professional, when he is excluded from a given hospital, group practice, or informal circle of referrals, simply moves his practice and finds another circle of people of equal incompetence in which he can function. It will take a much stronger, more active and internal sense of covenant obligation to patients on the part of the profession to enforce standards within the guild beyond local informal patterns of ostracism. In a mobile society with a scarcity of doctors, local ostracism simply hands on problem-physicians to other patients elsewhere. It does not address them.

Code patterns of discipline not only fall short of adequate protection for the patient; they may also fail in collegial responsibility to the troubled physician. To ostracize may be the lazy way of handling a colleague when it fails altogether to make a first attempt at remedy and to address the physician himself in his difficulty.

At the same time, it would be unfortunate if the indispensable interest and pride of the medical profession in technical proficiency were allowed to lapse out of an expressed preference for a professional ethic based on covenant. Covenant fidelity to the patient remains unrealized if it does not include proficiency. A rather sentimental existentialism unfortunately assumes that it is enough for human beings to be "present" to one another. But in crisis, the ill person needs not simply presence but skill, not just personal concern but highly disciplined services targeted on specific needs. Code behavior, handed down from doctor to doctor, is largely concerned with the transmission of technical skills. Covenant ethics, then must include rather than exclude the interests of the codes.

Neither does this essay conclude with a preference for covenant to the total exclusion of the interests of enforceable contract. While the reduction of medical ethics to contract alone incurs the danger of minimalism, patients ought to have recourse against those physicians who fail to meet minimal standards. One ought not to be dependent entirely upon disciplinary measures undertaken within the profession. There ought to be appeal to the law in cases of malpractice and for breech of contract explicit or implied.

On the other hand, in the case of injustice a legal appeal cannot be sustained without assistance and testimony from physicians who take their obligations to patients seriously. If, in such cases, fellow physicians simply herd around and protect their colleagues like a wounded elephant, the patient with just cause is not likely to get far. Thus the instrumentation of contract and other avenues of legal redress can be sustained only by a professional sense of obligation to the patient. Needless to say, it would be better for all concerned if professional discipline and continuing education were so vigorously pursued within the profession as to cut down drastically on the number of cases that needed to reach the courts.

The author inclines to accept covenant as the most inclusive and satisfying model for framing questions of professional obligation. Covenant fidelity includes the code obligation to become technically proficient; it reenforces the legal duty to meet minimal terms of contract; but it also requires much more. This surplus of obligation moreover may be redound not only to the benefit of patients but also to the advantage of troubled colleagues and their welfare.

NOTES

1. Edelstein, Ludwig. *Ancient Medicine.* Baltimore: Johns Hopkins Press, 1967.
2. Winch, Peter. *The Idea of a Social Science and Its Relation to Philosophy.* New York: Humanities Press, 1958.
3. See P. Lain Entralgo, *Doctor and Patient* (New York: McGraw-Hill, 1969), for his analysis of the classic fusion of *techne* with *philanthropia;* skill in the art of healing combined with a love of mankind defines the good physician.
4. Chapter I, Article II, "Obligation of Patients to Their Physicians," *Code of Medical Ethics,* American Medical Association, May 1847. Chicago: AMA Press, 1987.
5. *Ibid.,* Chapter III, Article II.
6. *New York Times,* editorial and comment, 6 June 1975.
7. Sir Henry Summer Maine, *Ancient Law.* London: Oxford University Press, 1931.
8. Titmuss, Richard M. *The Gift Relationship: From Human Blood to Social Policy.* New York: Pantheon, 1971.
9. Titmuss does not observe that physicians in the United States had already prepared for this commercialization of medicine by their substantial fees for services (as opposed to salaried professors in the teaching field or salaried health professionals in other countries).
10. Fabrega, Horacio. Jr., "Concepts of Disease: Logical Features and Social Implications." *Perspectives in Biology and Medicine* 15: University of Chicago Press, Summer 1972.

Not everyone is convinced by the position of the hypothetical contractarians or by the covenant theorists. K. Danner Clouser, in the essay that follows, offers the first of the two objections we shall examine. He claims that ethical norms come in different forms. One form is expressed by a small number of rules that proscribe certain evils such as do not deceive, do not break promises, or do not cheat. On these he says all rational persons would agree. Insofar as he is grounding these rules in the claim that "all rational persons would agree" to what extent is his position different from the hypothetical contractor's, who grounds norms in agreement among hypothetical people who were impartial and knowledgeable?

Clouser goes beyond this set of rules, however. He says that professional codes that delineate certain duties of persons in the professional role. He goes on, however, to say that a "professional code cannot (morally) be simply a self-expression of some group toward any old 'goods' they see fit to pursue." It must be in accord with other basic moral rules. The profession can choose to promote various goods as long as they are not incompatible with more general moral rules. Clouser leaves us with the question of whether the profession can determine whether its self-defined goods are in conflict with more general moral rules. For example, would keeping a confidence when keeping it would benefit a patient but permit harm to others be compatible with or in violation of more general rules? Clouser seems to want to retain a role for professionals to define their special duties within the broader framework of social norms.

Models: A Critical Review and a New View

K. Danner Clouser

This is a critical review of two articles which, apparently, have become important and well-known in the literature of the physician-patient relationship. They are Robert Veatch's 'Models for Ethical Medicine in a Revolutionary Age'[1] and William F. May's 'Code, Covenant, Contract or Philanthropy'[2]. It is out of character for me to devote an article to criticizing others. It seems therefore appropriate to mention that I was enlisted in this task by the editor of the book, *The Clinical Encounter,* because of the role these two papers play in the unfolding discussion that has become that book's theme. I do it in the interests of continuing and advancing this discussion.

These two papers raise a great flurry of issues, any or all of which could be pursued. May's paper in particular—with its rich fund of historical, literary, and theological allusions—could lead a commentator in a multitude of directions. It is therefore important to say that this critique will focus rather single-mindedly on the ethical aspects of the articles. That is, the critique will be concerned with what these models have to do with ethics, what they assume, what they imply, how they deal with and relate to ethics.

Stressing that this critic will focus on ethics may strike many as being super-fluous. I suspect the two authors themselves would be so struck, replying something like "But of course these models have to do with ethics; the total issue is one having to do with ethics." Herein lies a crucial point for the understanding of the critique that follows.

'Ethics' is used to denote widely differing domains. For some it seems to include nearly everything—goals, ideals, goods, aesthetics, philosophies of life. For others it is very narrowly circumscribed. (One cannot help thinking that this issue lies at the basis of most disagreements in, at least, applied ethics, though it is seldom addressed head-on.) A lot is at stake in this matter. How we explicate such a concept makes a lot of difference as to what we can do with it. It can be so all inclusive it becomes meaningless; it can be so restricted that it becomes useless. Considerable work must be done to explicate a concept which has had a long and varied use with accumulating connotations. Each step of such conceptual trimming requires an argument. The reader will no doubt be relieved to know that the explication of 'ethics' will not be argued out as such in this critique, though I believe that our differing views of ethics lie at the base of our differences on the issues dealt with here. These differences should become clear as we proceed.

AN OVERVIEW

Veatch's account of physician-patient relationships is logically and chronologically prior to May's. That is, it is as if May picks up where Veatch leaves off, attempting to advance, widen, and deepen the morally ideal type of relationship. It unfolds some-thing like the following. Veatch briefly describes and subsequently rejects three 'models' of the physician-patient relationship. They are the engineering model, the priestly model, and the collegial model. They are, in a word: 'all facts, no values' (engineering), 'paternalistic' (priestly), and 'buddy-buddy' (collegial). The one, in the end, which Veatch approves of is the contractual model, which embodies the notion of 'contract or covenant'.

May picks up the theme at that point. Distinguishing two types of obligation found in the Hippocratic Oath, he elaborates on the meaning and connotations of each. One is the set of obligations that a physician takes on with respect to his patients and the other is that which he owes his medical mentors (and their chil-dren) for having taught the physician his craft. The first mentioned set (the code) is characterized by gratuitous, perhaps condescending, service rendered to patients (philanthropy). The second set of obligations (the covenant) is characterized as the recognition of a debt by virtue of favors received. It is this second (the covenant) to which May turns most of his attention. The thrust of his unfolding discussion is to show the richness of connotation of covenant and how much more appropriate it is for the physician-patient relationship than either code or contract. In a sense, then, May is picking up where Veatch left off. Veatch ends by recommending that contractual model; May finds the contractual models inadequate, and recommends the covenantal relationship. Very likely Veatch and May are not in substantial disagreement, if any at all. Veatch did not mean a legalistic contract; he even suggests that he means it more in the sense of the traditional religious or marriage 'contract' or 'covenant' ([1], p. 7). However, May explores the concept of covenant much more extensively, resulting in a greater distinction between contract and covenant, whereupon he then opts for the convenantal relationship as the most appropriate for the physician-patient relationship, by virtue of historical, sociological, theological, and—probably—ethical considerations.

VEATCH'S MODELS

It will be best to say at the outset that though these models are colorful, I find them too erratic, whimsical, and uneven to be helpful.

The Engineering Model

The Engineering Model is the one in which the physician sees himself as a 'pure' scientist dealing only with facts, apart from all consideration of value. This presumably must be rejected because the scientist "just cannot logically be value free" ([1], p. 5). That of course is an arguable point. But even assuming the truth of the point, exactly what is its moral relevance? The kinds of 'values' which affect the scientist's conclusion (choice of research design, perceptions, level of significance) are not necessarily moral values. They might be aesthetic or perhaps non-empirical commitments of one sort or another. But what then is the 'engineer's' moral failing? If values (of whatever sort) ineluctably taint scientific findings, then what is one to do? Very likely all one can do is to become as aware as possible of those values. But tracing them through medical theories, biochemical theories, microbiological theories and so on to the very foundation of science would be an enormous intellectual task. In fact it may be conceptually impossible, since that task itself would (ex hypothesi) be value-laden. Surely Veatch cannot be requiring such measures.

There must be a practical, down-to-earth edge to this issue. Perhaps Veatch is simply emphasizing that values enter into clinical decision-making and that the physician should bring these values to the attention of the patient. This would then be in accord with the good old basic, highly defensible, moral rule, 'Do not deceive.' In that case the Engineering Model would be seen as primarily involving deception, and its moral inadequacies would be obvious.

But apparently that is not what Veatch means to say. For he adds:

> . . . even if the physician logically could eliminate all ethical and other value considerations from his decision-making—it would be morally out-

rageous of him to do so. It would make him an engineer, a plumber
making repairs. . . . ([1], p. 5)

It is difficult to see what is morally wrong with this, let alone 'morally outrageous.'
Of course if the physician acts with respect to value assumptions without informing
or consulting the patient, then the physician (and also, incidentally, the plumber) is
morally wrong for either having deceived the patient or for having limited his
freedom. But if all value consideration could 'logically be eliminated,' where is the
moral failing?

In short, there is nothing in this rather abstruse 'engineering model' which
could not more clearly and more adequately be expressed in those time honored
and rationally based general moral rules "Do not deceive" and "Do not deprive of
freedom"[3]. There may be a specifically professional duty (as I shall discuss later)
beyond abstaining from deceit and from taking a decision out of the patient's hands,
but Veatch does not tell us what it is.

The Priestly Model

The sense of this model is one of paternalism, wherein the physician takes onto
himself the decision-making that is properly the patient's. Veatch sees this as 'the
opposite extreme' of the engineering model. Presumably the engineering type completely abstained from making value decisions, and the priestly type makes them all.
But we still are not sure whether the engineer did not make value judgments, or
only thought he did not. If he did not make them, it is not clear that he has been
immoral. If he did make them, but unwittingly, then he at least is cognitively
deficient, and also perhaps his actions are immoral because he has taken over the
decision-making that properly belongs to the patient. But now that sounds just like
the priestly type, rather than its 'opposite extreme.' Is there in fact a difference, or is
it only a difference in style?

There is further ambiguity as to the real difference between the engineering
and the priestly physician. It is not clear whether the priestly one makes value
decisions because he believes he has the expertise in values, or because he thinks
they are factual and not value decisions. If it is the latter, then he is the same as the
engineer. Is the 'generalization of expertise' unwitting or not?

However, the chief puzzler in the priestly model is Veatch's claim that the
admonition 'Benefit and do no harm' summarizes the priestly tradition and represents the tradition of paternalism. The puzzle may revolve around the ambiguity of
'harm.' I would think that a person is harmed when—among other things—he is
deceived, deprived of freedom, and deprived of opportunity. If value decisions that
are properly his are made by someone else, I would think he, as a person, is
harmed. (Though of course, like any moral infringement, there might be circumstances that would justify it.) Therefore, 'Benefit and do on harm' should exclude
paternalism, since paternalism would necessarily involve doing harm (or, at least,

the belief that one is doing harm), in the sense of 'harm' I have suggested.[4] 'Benefit and do not harm' seems like a sound moral principle, though perhaps too brief to avoid some ambiguity. Rather than incriminating it, Veatch should have focussed more specifically on 'Do not take decision-making away from the patient', for it is that which seems to be the essence of the priestly tradition which he wants to reject.

The Collegial Model

This model is characterized by patient and physician seeing themselves as colleagues, pursuing the common goal of the patient's health. Unfortunately for this to work we must assume that there would in fact be such mutual loyalty and goals. However, according to Veatch, there is no basis in reality for that assumption, and therefore by virtue of its utopian assumption, he rejected the collegial model.

The Contractual Model

This model's essence is as the name implies, though it is not to be "loaded with legalistic implications." Only in this model, says Veatch, "can there be a true sharing of ethical authority and responsibility" ([1], p. 7). The idea seems to be that patient and doctor would take out their 'basic value frameworks' in advance, and, if each one is acceptable to the other, they would 'contract' to honor these values on the other's behalf.

On the surface of it, one might wonder what will make this model any more secure than the collegial model. If breakdown of trust and confidence is inevitable on the collegial model, if mutual loyalty and goals are a baseless assumption on the collegial model, why aren't they similarly grounds for rejection of the contractual model? What makes human nature any different on one model than on the other? If trust and confidence are not justified in the collegial model because there is not reason to assume that the participants are truly committed to common goals, why would the contractual model be rejected for the same reason? It is hard enough to see how having a common goal is necessary, let alone sufficient, for trust and confidence, without having also to see how talking over 'value frameworks' in advance will guarantee a commitment of common goals. In short, it seems sheer whimsy to believe that there will be adherence to moral virtues in one case and not in the other. The real working difference between the collegial model and the contractual seems to be the explicitness with which each party makes known to the other his values and goals. That of course is an important point, but it is not the one on which these models have been accepted or rejected—at least not in any straightforward way. Rather they seem to have been accepted or rejected on whether or not the model itself somehow insures trust, confidence, moral behavior, and fulfillment of obligations. Yet, this is the very case that has not been made. No reason whatsoever is given as to why, if humans would be immoral in one case, they would not be in another. We can hardly be against an explicit and mutual understanding of values and goals (as in the contractual model) but it certainly is not a sufficient condition for moral behavior and it very likely is not even a necessary condition.

GENERAL REFLECTIONS OF MODELS OF PHYSICIAN-PATIENT RELATIONSHIPS

The central question concerning these models is: why bother? As in so much writing in medical ethics, matters are complicated and muddled beyond any redeeming value. The models are whimsical gestalts which obscure the crucial moral points that could have been made with clarity and crispness.

Given the implicit principles of construction we might have invented many more models: The 'bus driver' model (where the patient knows roughly where the doctor-driver is taking him, he gets on willingly, and he watches the passing scene until he reaches his destination or until something about the passing scene leads him to get off or transfer). The 'pin-ball machine' model (where the patient loudly expresses his emotions and goals and tries everything short of 'tilt' to influence the doctor-machine toward his ends). The 'back-seat driver' model (where there is general agreement about the destination and means of getting there but every inch of the way the patient is telling the doctor-driver how to handle every set of circumstances along the way). There might even be a plumber model—and this would be the ideal—wherein the plumber discusses with his client all the possible value-laden trade-offs within the constraints of the general building code: heat saving devices vs. appearances; less piping vs. slight structural changes; more expense vs. some living style inconveniences. (Why should we ever criticize a doctor for being 'nothing but a plumber'?)

The inventing of models could continue not only ad absurdum, but ad infinitum. The point is: what is the point of models?

One must assume from the title and subtitle that they have to do with ethics. Yet it is not really clear in any of the models precisely what the moral failing is. Moral points float about here and there but are lost in the miscellaneous details of the model. For example, we saw earlier that in some perfectly good ways of interpreting the engineering and the priestly models they are different only in morally irrelevant ways. At most it is a stylistic difference. That is, there are simple different reasons (and perhaps, causes) for their depriving the patient of his rightful decision-making. And to put the emphasis on the reasons rather than on the actions is to obscure the moral points. The moral point is that patients should not be deprived of freedom or opportunity, which is what happens when decisions affecting them are taken out of their hands.

That point emerges so much more clearly when abstracted from all the rest of the model's conceptual filigree. As they stand, it is not easy to say what is morally wrong with three of the models and what is morally right about the fourth. Mostly they seem to involve mistaken beliefs. (The engineer believes there are no values; the priestly believes he is an expert on values, and the collegial type believes he knows the patient's goals and values.) It would seem an empirical argument would the appropriate response in order to remedy mistaken beliefs, not veiled claims about moral shortcomings.

Consider the engineering model. So much could be inferred from it. If he does not acknowledge that values are intrinsically involved with and determinative of his facts, then he might simply be wrong about a matter of fact. If he knows it, but chooses to ignore it, then he is morally wrong because he is deceiving the patient about something relevant to that patient. But if he is straightforwardly factual with the patient, including such facts as where and how values have determined or influenced conclusions, then it is not clear that he is acting immorally. Indeed, many patients would prefer a physician exactly like that. The point is that the model is a very mixed bag. As such it is not clarifying, not helpful, and not clearly immoral. And I think that is true of all the models.

What would really be helpful is to be told what would be immoral to do to a patient. It is wrong to deceive a patient. It is wrong to deprive a patient of freedom or opportunity (as is done when the physician does not tell the patient of choices or options). These can happen on any of the models; it is mistaken to believe that the 'right' model could prevent it. With this kind of focus, we could let as many models develop as will—as long as no moral rules are broken with respect to the patient. Some patients will prefer the priestly type, and knowingly turn over all decision-making to him. In that case there is no apparent immorality. The physician-patient relationship would be better served if, instead of delineating models with all their complicated and ambiguous interrelationships, presuppositions, and beliefs, we simply listed what we morally ought not to do—such as deceive, cheat, break confidences and promises or deprive a patient of opportunity or freedom. It is extremely limiting (and maybe immoral) to prescribe the infinitely various details of a physician-patient relationship as though that in itself were a moral matter. Why not let many styles flourish? Let patient and physicians establish the kinds of relationships which suit them. Let them find each other and develop together. The constraints, then, would be the constraints that proscribe certain actions and behavior in the society at large, such as deceiving, breaking promises, depriving of self-determination, and so on.

What is the relation between these models and morality? As we have seen, it is by no means clear-cut. It is highly circuitous at best. However, the goal of this delineation of models is relatively clear, by virtue of the article's subtitle: 'What physician-patient roles foster the most ethical relationship?' What is being sought is a format that would most likely maximize morality, a form of relationship that would motivate moral behavior. This assumes a particular view of ethics which is worth exploring. However, since May's arguments boil down (in ethical substance) to this same point, we will look more generally at his article before focussing on it. I see this point as the key link between Veatch and May.

MAY'S CODE AND COVENANT

The reader is referred to the two appropriate paragraphs above [and May's essay] for a quick review of the context and connecting thread of May's in-depth examination of codes and covenants.

May sees codes as very particularized guides to human behavior. That is they are not universal, binding on all, but molded to meet the needs and fancies of myriad sub-groups of human kind. A code dictates style as well as substance of behavior; demeanor as well as deeds; it bespeaks commitments, techniques, aesthetics and world views. These codes are fashioned by and for each particular group as an expression of that group's 'philosophy' of those mentioned items.

May finds the code of the medical profession—through its various expressions down through the centuries—to be typical of the codes just described. As the guiding ideal for dealing with patients, the medical code "has not had altogether favorable consequences for the moral health of the profession" ([2], p. 29). The crippling aspect isn't what one would expect. Rather, it is the ideal of philanthropy, which after all, is a very unusual item to be found in these usually very self-serving, self-aggrandizing codes. Nevertheless,

> This ideal of service, in my judgment, succumbs to what might be called the conceit of philanthropy when it is assumed that the professional's commitment to his fellow man is a gratuitous, rather than a responsive or reciprocal, act ([2], p. 31).

This is a good insight, which May clearly and convincingly elaborates. There is, on the part of physicians, considerable condescension toward patients; a condescension perpetuated by the code which suggests that physicians owe patients absolutely nothing, and that it is only out of the physician's self-generating goodness that the public is so graciously served. Such an attitude is not justified by the facts, and it does not make for a morally healthy relationship between doctor and patient.

The severe misdirection of the code would incline May toward a contractual relationship as preferable. Among other things, the contract would at least involve informed consent, encourage full respect for the dignity of the patient, acknowledge explicitly the 'symmetry and mutuality' of the relationship, and perhaps provide for legal enforcement of its terms.

Nevertheless, the contractual relationship does not capture the spirit, attitude, and commitment that May would find most ideal. Contracts engender a quid pro quo mentality; they lead to a minimalism—a doing of not more than absolutely necessary. Focus ends up on the terms of the contract and not on the well-being of the patient. The very nature of health and illness is such that all their related contingencies and surprises could not possibly be exhaustively detailed in a contract. As May so nicely puts it a contractual relationship produces a professional too grudging, too calculating, too lacking in spontaneity, too quickly exhausted to go the second mile with his patients along the road of their distress ([2], p. 35).

At this point May turns to the notion of covenant as the most adequate model of the physician-patient relationship. The heart of it is that it is a model of the physician-patient relationship. The heart of it is that it is a commitment made (by physicians) in response to gifts and services received (from the public). This is not a tit-for-tat detailing of gifts and responses, but an acknowledgement of overall, undetailable gifts received, so basic and so immense that ledger keeping of reciprocating responses seems inappropriate. Thus neither gratuitous nor contractual mentalities are apt to surface, though, eventually and obviously outdistanced the 'original' gift, even, or circumstances which provoked the covenant, from then on the reciprocating 'responses' could be seen as gratuitous. Furthermore, if one were led to keep score in this fashion, it would begin to resemble a contract of sorts. One way to avoid both of these eventualities would be to ground the covenant in the transcendent. If the gift is boundless and ongoing, then there is no possibility that response can ever make complete repayment. If you are forever beholding to someone, condescension toward him can never be appropriate.

May has many more interesting insights into the covenantal relationship—its provocation, strengths, and limitations—but for our purposes of focusing on the ethics of the physician-patient relationship, we have drawn out all we need.

COMMENTARY ON CODES AND COVENANTS

It is important to raise the question in a very simplistic way: What is it that May is seeking? It certainly is not mainly a search of what in fact is the relationship between physician and patient, though he spends considerable time on that matter. And he certainly is not seeking a list of right and wrong actions which should or should not transpire between physician and patient, though he deals with the like from time to time. He studies the history, context, and connotations of codes, covenants and contracts. To what end? He rejects this or that aspect of codes, covenant, and contracts, and finds others to be acceptable, even ideal. What are the criteria by which he judges? Criteria and ends are clearly at work. What are they? And what is their relationship to ethics, which is, after all, our main interest?

As we found with Veatch, May is searching for a form, format, or structure of relationship which would create, foster, insure, or motivate ethical behavior on the part of the physician. (Very little if any attention is paid to the patient's behavior toward the physician, though very likely the contractual relationship would embrace that aspect.) Of what is this relationship made up? Beliefs? Attitudes? Imagery? Behaviors? May seems to be consciously building a set of beliefs which will create attitudes which will in turn inspire certain kinds of action. Codes are too ego-expressive and protective, too idiosyncratic, and in medicine, they bespeak a condescending philanthropy. Contractual relationships lead to a tit-for-tatness and minimalism. May seems in no doubt as to what results he wants, and all he is looking for is the right set of beliefs to insure those results. May not only wants the physician to do the right thing, but he wants him to do it in the right frame of mind, with the right attitude, and for the right reasons. One gets the impression that May would like to create a wonderful myth which would lead physicians to believe that they were eternally in debt to the people they serve. This would then promote the demeanor and behavior which May finds most acceptable. Again, May apparently already knows how a moral physician acts with patients, and what he is seeking is the right concatenation of truths, beliefs, occurrences, etc. which will ensure that the physician not only acts that way, but does so from the right motives and with the right attitude.

As intriguing as I find all of this with respect to historical, literary, and the physician-patient relationship, I find it bewildering and unhelpful. Models seem to be entities or structures which come between patient and physician, fabricated intermediaries which clog the direct relationship between patient and physician (not unlike the traditional metaphysical/ontological problems with the concept of 'relations').

However much the article purports to be about ethics, I think it really is not. I think it really is about motivation and philosophy of life. The mode—or relationship—does not tell us what actions are moral nor is it an example of morality but rather its role is to mobilize the physician's attitudes, beliefs, perspectives, and emotions so as to produce moral actions. But 'proper' motivation is neither necessary nor sufficient for moral actions to take place. 'Models' thus are more in the category of sermons, commencement addresses, and other exhortations. Hypnosis, brainwashing, and purity pills might also lead to moral actions. Behind the formulation of models for physician-patient relationship, leading to their acceptance or rejection, has been the implicit consideration: Will it force (or lead, or incline, or motivate) the physician to be moral?

But why such concern for motivation? Morality certainly requires that certain actions be done (or more often, not done) but does not require that they be done from this or that motive, or with this or that attitude, or for this or that reason. It seems an inappropriate criticism of a moral theory to say, "But that would never make anyone be moral." The obsession with motivation I think is misleading and dangerous, unless its distinction from ethics is kept clear. This point needs some elaboration, since it gets at the core of the issue of models of physician-patient relationships.

One guesses that the focus on the physician-patient relationship develops something like this: the relationship is so complicated, there are so many variables, so many different concepts and situations, that we could never spell out explicitly all that a physician should or should not do. Therefore, if we could change his inner self—his attitudes, dispositions, and beliefs—so as to motivate him to be moral, then the myriad individual situations would, by and large, be handled morally. The difficulty with this is that the focus ends up on the inner self—the agent's philosophy of life—more than on what actions are morally acceptable. The criteria for moral-making characteristics of an action shifts to the heart from which it flows rather than to objective moral criteria of the action itself. At that point he is in effect suggesting that any action, as long as it proceeds from the proper motivation, is moral. The motivation might be of the purest sort, say, a realization of profound indebtedness, combined with love and concern. But the like has led not infrequently to an act of unjustified paternalism or deception, or to a broken promise. And those actions are immoral by virtue of criteria external of the motivation which inspired them.

That one's actions are in accord with his own philosophy of life does not make them moral. A philosophy of life concerns what goods that person acknowledges, but bringing about those goods for himself of for others might involve downright immoral actions. A philosophy of life is extremely important, and I think that that is primarily what May is helping us with. It is good, for example, to recognize one's indebtedness to others, to give service unbegrudgingly, to find meaning and commitment in events and encounters, and so on. Some philosophies of life might well be such that they help and encourage us to be moral. The important thing to realize is that what is moral is logically independent of and judged by other criteria than our philosophy of life.

Why not allow these external criteria of moral actions determine what actions in a doctor-patient relationship are moral or immoral? What is the point of creating a new entity—'the relationship'—which itself, presumably, can be either moral or immoral. Let any kind of relationship flourish, as long as no immorality is done. Interpersonal styles—including mannerisms, dress, tone of voice, eye contact, sense of humor—should not become susceptible to the straightjacket of 'models' which may be embodying 'philosophies of life' in the name of morality. Rather let relationships develop as creatively and freely as they will, being limited only by the immoralities to be avoided.

MORALITY AND PROFESSIONAL CODES: THEIR CONNECTION

It seems only fair and appropriate that I at least sketch the ethical perspective from which I see these issues. Space considerations rule out supporting arguments, but they can be found elsewhere [3,5]. What follows is grossly oversimplified, but it does give a kind of 'floor plan' to suggest the juxtaposition of some key ideas.

My biggest worry is that ethics has come to mean almost anything. It seems to be an indefinitely malleable concept, stretched to fit everyone's whims, goals, and favorite goods. As such it becomes almost meaningless, and discussion involving it becomes almost pointless. Fudge factors prevail. There is in the center of all this, I believe, a hardcore morality, a basic morality which all rational persons would, in a sense, support. Their very rationality would require them "to publicly advocate" this morality ([3], esp. pp. 86–101) lest, as Hobbes would have it, life be poor, nasty, brutish, and short. This basic morality would comprise rules whose central theme is 'Do not cause evil.' The fact that there is a small number of items all rational persons would agree on as evil makes this possible (unlike goods on which we would get very little agreement). The moral rules proscribe the doing of these evils to each other; they are admonitions that would get the public backing of all rational persons. Following these rules requires no effort; it requires only that one does not cause these evils (unlike promoting goods which require time, effort, risk, and sacrifice). And one can follow these rules universally and impartially, that is, toward everyone, equally, all the time (unlike trying to follow the admonition 'Promote good').

These very basic, 'hardcore,' moral rules of course constitute a minimalist morality. But it is a solid beginning, for at least it can have universal and rational support. The sense of all the moral rules is one of proscribing: for example, 'Do not deceive,' 'Do not break promises,' 'Do not cheat,' 'Do not deprive of freedom or opportunity.' However, one of the rules would be "Do your duty" ([3], esp. pp. 121–125). This rule would be publicly advocated by all rational persons because we all come to count on people—firemen, policemen, pilots, waiters, mothers—to do their jobs. If they fail, evil results. So it is to everyone's best interest to urge that prescribed jobs be done, because the rest of us are counting on it.

It is at this point that 'professional codes' enter the scene. Codes, in effect, are delineations of this basic rule 'Do your duty.' Codes spell out the duty of those involved, the way in which the rest of society can count on them to make efforts, go out of their way, run risks, and make sacrifices. This is not simply the minimalist 'avoid causing evil'; this is more positive and praiseworthy (though it is not the only way to transcend minimal morality).

How these duties get formulated is another matter. Whether it is a self-imposed duty, or one prescribed by the town, council, or one that has a long historical tradition, it is crucial that we realize that there are boundaries and limitations—unlike some of the professional codes described by May. A professional code cannot (morally) be simply the self-expression of some group toward any old 'goods' they see fit to pursue. It must be in accord with all the other basic moral rules. That is, the group may promote any goods that they want to commit themselves to, as long as they are not breaking any other moral rules. Thus, if the physicians' code requires that the physician do whatever is necessary for the health of the patient, the doctor would still not (morally) be justified in deceiving or in taking away the patients' decision-making role.

It is from this sketched perspective that I see the physician-patient relationship. Moral considerations do not specify the details of that relationship nor the frame of the heart and mind the physician must have while doing his job. But it would be important that he not break any of the moral rules with respect to his patients. That of course is no different from our expectations of any person; it is just that, by virtue of the intimate relationship, the physician has so many more opportunities to break moral rules.

What carries the physician beyond the 'mere' of doing no evil is his professional code. Therein is his pledge or his commitment for positive tasks—such as alleviating pain, saving life, comforting the distressed, etc. These then become his duty, people come to depend on these services to be performed, and the physician is morally blameworthy if he defaults on their performance. It is like breaking a promise.

CONCLUSION

Constructing models of doctor-patient relationship seems to be multiplying entities beyond necessity. It gives us a complicated construct which obscures rather than clarifies the relevant moral issues. Models divert our attention from the morality of deeds and duties to the morality of the model itself. Do we need different models for our relation to our accountant, our barber, our grocer, our lawyer, our architect? Model-talk blurs the fact that physicians have the same moral obligation toward their patients that all humans have toward each other. One can get the impression that if the model is 'in place' in a relationship, all moral obligations are being met, as though programmed by insertion of the model. Models obscure the crucial differences between moral issues and style/manner/personality issues.

Furthermore, the attempt to build incentive and motivation into the model cannot work. Reason will not compel one to be moral but only to advocate morality. It is hard enough to be moral without trying to be moral from the 'right' reasons and the 'right' attitudes. Far better it is to see clearly what the morally right actions are. Let the exhortations to be moral be expressed in sermons, commencement addresses, and the preambles of professional codes.

By seeing the physician-patient relationship as having the same basic moral obligations as any other human relationship, we can then more clearly see the role of professional codes as promises to go above and beyond—but not in conflict with—these basic moral rules. And those expressed duties are what we as patients should be particularly alerted to, since those are what makes this professional different from any other. But we have and can have no more assurances that he will live up to those pledges than we have that anyone will live up to their moral obligations. And neither codes, covenants, nor models can make it otherwise.

NOTES

1. Veatch, R. M. "Models for Ethical Medicine in a Revolutionary Age." *Hastings Center Report* 2:5–7, June 1972.
2. May, W. F. "Code, Covenant, Contract, or Philanthropy." *Hastings Center Report* 5:29–38, December 1975 [pages 156–173 in this volume].
3. Gert, B. *The Moral Rules: A New Rational Foundation for Morality.* New York: Harper Torchbook, Harper & Row, 1973.
4. Gert, B. and Culver, C. "Paternalistic Behavior." *Philosophy and Public Affairs* 6:45–57, Fall 1976.
5. Clouser, K. D. "Bioethics." In *Encyclopedia of Bioethics,* Vol. I, edited by W. T. Reich. New York: Macmillan and Free Press, 1978, pp. 115–127.

Thus far all the answers to the question of where ethics is grounded focus on what the profession imposes on itself (Roth), what is contracted or covenanted by hypothetical contractors (May), or some combination of what all rational people would agree to as well as the additional specification of duties by professional groups (Clouser). There is another possibility, however. It could be that there are no norms that all rational people would agree to or that hypothetical contractors would choose, but, still it should not be up to professional groups to invent the norms relative to their relationships with lay people. Especially if professionals are licensed by the broader society and given privileges such as certain monopoly practices, perhaps the norms of the relationship should be defined by agreements involving both actual lay people and actual professionals. The following essay by H. Tristram Engelhardt puts forward the view that ethics is the result of agreements by actual contractors who want to live peaceably, gathering together in sub-communities to agree on different concepts of the good. He concedes that one overarching principle, the principle of liberty or autonomy, is a necessary constraint on all agreements that these sub-groups make, but that, beyond this, there are no preset limits. Ethics is thus invented, not by professionals or by hypothetical contractors, but by communities of actual people including lay persons and professionals.

Ethics and the Resolutions of Controversies: A Closer Look at the Brink

H. TRISTRAM ENGELHARDT

Much can be regained for ethics by remembering what in fact one could hope for from ethics. To ask an ethical question is to seek a rational answer, a ground other than force for resolving a controversy. Ethics is at the very least a means for resolving controversies regarding proper conduct on bases other than direct or indirect appeals to force as the fundamental basis for a resolution. Put in this way, ethics is an enterprise in controversy resolution. Controversies regarding which lines of conduct are proper can be resolved on the basis of (1) force, (2) conversion of one party to the other's viewpoint, (3) sound argument, and (4) agreed-to procedures. The grounds for the resolution of moral controversies are of crucial importance, for they provide the authority for public policy. One must distinguish in this regard between resolutions through what one might term *cloture* (main force) and resolutions that satisfy the intellectual question regarding the correct solution. Using force, even legally authorized force, to close abortion clinics would be by itself simply an act of force. An appeal to force will not answer the ethical question as a rational question regarding why the controversy ought to be resolved in a particular fashion.

Brute force is simply brute force. A goal of ethics is to determine when force can be justified. Force by itself carries no moral authority.

Justification for the resolution of a moral controversy has often been sought in a commonly held moral viewpoint, a viewpoint to which all in a community have in one sense or another been converted. In great proportion, the appeal to "conversion" involves one of the traditional Western hopes for the resolution of moral controversies. The Christian West, especially prior to the Reformation, envisaged a single authoritative viewpoint, available through divine grace, and interpreted by the singular authority of the church, and in particular that of the pope. It completed and fulfilled what reason disclosed regarding the *jus gentium*. The fragmentation of Christendom and the development of a more secular spirit called this ideal into question as a historical possibility. Moreover, the appeal to a transcendent God and His grace cannot resolve controversies in a secular society. Since, by definition, the decisive premises in such a context are available only through divine revelation and grace, they will not be accessible to those not so blessed. Force will need to be employed to coerce those not so favored, and that force will not be justifiable in general rational terms. Religious controversies, which involve other than true believers, will as a result be resolved by force and without the benefit of a generally defensible justification. Such actions will then be against the possibility of a peaceable, generally defensible morality. Indeed, the Christian states of the Middle Ages were without moral authority in much of what they did, as the history of the persecution of Jews and heretics attests. The failure of Christendom's hope is in historical terms a major one.

This failure suggests that it is hopeless to suppose that a general moral consensus will develop regarding any of the major issues in bioethics. There will always be minorities who in a free and open society will take vocal exception to any who claim a consensus. This will be the case from the issue of abortion to that of rights to health care. As a consequence, attempts to force a general consensus will lack the authority of a general endorsement.

The third possibility is that of achieving moral authority through successful rational arguments to establish a particular view of the good moral life. This Enlightenment attempt to provide a rationally justified, concrete view of the good life, and thus a secular surrogate for the moral claims of Christianity, has not succeeded. From the French Revolution to the October Revolution, reason has failed to establish a particular view of the good life as morally authoritative. The problem is outlined earlier. In order rationally to establish a particular concrete understanding of the nature of the good life as morally authoritative, one will need to appeal to a particular moral sense. However, to justify that moral sense one will need to appeal to a yet higher moral sense, *ad indefinitum*. Nor will Marxist claims regarding the inevitability of the triumph of a communist morality secure the normativeness of that viewpoint. Pessimists have long supposed that the morality of the debased and misguided might in the end universally triumph. In short, force, conversion, and sound argument appear to fail as means for resolving moral controversies in a way that stakeholders should rationally hold to be a proper resolution. The only remaining hope is resolution by agreement.

If one cannot clearly establish by sound rational argument a particular concrete moral viewpoint as properly decisive (and one cannot, because the establishment of such a viewpoint itself presupposes a moral viewpoint, and that is exactly what is at stake), then the only mode of resolution is by agreement. Such agreement can be either free or forced. Free agreement can either be on the basis of sharing moral premises for which general justification cannot be given, or on the basis of nonmoral considerations that lead one to agree to a mechanism or procedure for negotiating disputes. Or to rephrase the point, because it does not appear that there will in fact be decisive argument to establish one concrete view of the moral life to be better than its rivals (or at least as we shall show, beyond certain general constraints), and since usually all will not convert to a single moral viewpoint, canons of moral probity will often need to be created by commonly accepted procedures. For this to succeed generally, one will need to discover an inescapable procedural basis for ethics. This basis, if it is to be found at all, will need to be disclosable in the very nature of ethics itself. Such a basis appears to be available in the minimum notion of ethics as an alternative to force in resolving moral controversies. If one is interested in resolving moral controversies without recourse to force as the fundamental basis of agreement, then one will have to accept peaceable negotiation among members of the controversy as the process for attaining the resolution of concrete moral controversies.

This condition is the minimum condition, because it commits one to no particular concrete moral view of the good life (e.g., the importance of health care vis-a-vis other human undertakings). Such a concrete view would require either arguments that do not appear to be successful (i.e., establishing a particular view of the good life by general moral arguments) or special premises available only within special communities endorsing particular religious, metaphysical, or ideological presuppositions. It is a minimal condition in simply underscoring what it is to resolve issues peaceably and with moral authority. Such a defining condition (i.e., ethics as a means for commonly and peaceably discerning or creating canons of moral probity—what I shall refer to as the morality of mutual respect and summarize under the rubric of a negative principle of autonomy) offers ethics as an enterprise that can be accepted by all participants. It establishes an equally acknowledgeable authority for its conclusions: the conclusions to the process of ethical reasoning are those that peaceable negotiators have all agreed to accept. If a participant in a negotiation refuses to participate because of an interest in resolving the dispute by an appeal to force, even if supposedly morally justified (e.g., "God tells me that abortions are wrong, so therefore we will forbid them by law"), others can retort: "When you use force against the innocent on the basis of moral claims that are not generally justifiable, or agreed to by all parties concerned, you cannot rationally protest when we employ force to protect ourselves from you and reject your supposed authority. What is asserted without proof can as easily be rejoined with a counterassertion. Moreover, rational beings anywhere in the cosmos who are interested in resolving moral controversies peaceably, and in not using force as the primary basis for the resolution of disputes, should understand you to be an enemy of the moral community, and therefore blameworthy, and hold us to have acted correctly." On the other hand, when an individual refuses to participate in a particular agreement, as long as that refusal does not involve the use of unconsented-to force against the innocent (e.g., breaking a promise), one has simply discovered a limit to a particular community or area of agreement, and not a warrant to force cooperation. It is here that one also discovers a fundamental equality among all persons. If no hierarchy of values can be established as canonical, then individuals cannot be subordinated one to the other outside of the agreements of particular communities, or the wishes or action of the person subordinated (e.g., as a part of just punishment). Moreover, the right of all persons to refuse to participate in any particular community makes each person equal to any other in the right to be left alone and to seek to fashion community with willing others.

By appealing to the minimum notion of ethics as a means for peaceably negotiating moral disputes, one can disclose as a necessary condition for ethics the requirement to respect the freedom of the participants in a moral controversy. Since moral controversies can in principle encompass all moral agents (and, as we shall see, *only* moral agents), one has a means of characterizing the moral community as the possible intellectual standpoint of persons interested in resolving moral controversies in ways not fundamentally based on force. This view of ethics should not be seen as grounded on a conditional concern for peaceableness. It is not simply based on an interest in establishing the peaceable community. It should, instead, be recognized as a disclosure, to borrow a Kantian metaphor, of a transcendental condition, a necessary condition for the possibility of a general domain of human life and of the life of persons generally. It is a disclosure of the minimum grammar involved in speaking rationally of blame and praise, and in establishing any particular set of moral commitments, other than through force.

Since this is a very radical suggestion, it is worth putting it yet another way. If the expected means for establishing the correctness of a particular moral viewpoint fails, then without some new approach one will not be able (1) to establish *a* particular moral viewpoint as *the* proper moral viewpoint, and therefore (2) one will not be able to establish public policy bodies or individuals as having the moral authority to impose any particular moral points of view by force. Morality would, in fact, lack rational authority, and could at best have authority with a bar sinister, an authority based on force. The foregoing arguments suggest that circumstances are indeed this disparate. The hope of establishing through general secular arguments the moral probity of any particular concrete moral viewpoint appears unfounded. The monotheistic presumption has in short collapsed. However, if authority cannot be acquired through sound arguments, or through the conversion of all to a single moral viewpoint, it can be acquired through mutual agreement. The moral world can be fashioned through free will, even if not on the basis of sound rational arguments with moral content.

Though moral authority does not rest on sound rational arguments establishing the content of the good moral life, the process has a rationality that can lead to the fashioning of a common moral fabric. The general will to have at least a minimum fabric for morality introduces the contexts of mutual respect and peaceable negotiation. If one is to have reasons for actions that all can accept, one must have reasons that all have endorsed. The use of will to fashion a place for reason in moral discourse is a condition for the possibility of a general and inescapable domain of the endeavor of persons: mutual respect. The foundations of the moral point of view are thus best expressed not in the disinterest with respect to personal advantage but rather in terms of mutual respect. Even if one does not attain transcendental rationality, one obtains an immanent, indeed transcendental, rationality for this procedure of will. There is, in short, a remaining means to acquire authority in a straightforward fashion for general secular ethics. If the authority of good arguments and common inspiration fails, the final possibility remains of deriving authority from the consent of those who fashion a community. There is still a generally understandable meaning to acting with moral authority—that is, with the consent of all those involved.

These points concerning of the resolution of moral controversies with authority may benefit from a summary. Resolution by force carries no intellectual authority whether with regard to (a) what viewpoint is correct, or (b) whether the correct viewpoint may be imposed by force. Authority in such cases simply means force to compel. Nor will appeals to conversion by grace suffice for a secular society, though they may for those who form a community of believers who feel the force of the grace of common conversion or who are committed to a particular moral sense or set or moral premises. Others outside the community will not. Moreover, grace of conversion or special commitment has no intellectual authority. Sound arguments would have authority, were they able to justify a particular moral viewpoint. However, it does not appear possible for them to secure a concrete view of the good life, though they may be able to establish certain general, abstract constraints. Differences in the ordering of goods and harms offer numerous competing moral possibilities among which one will not be able to choose on the basis of strong rational arguments.

The only remaining source for authority will be common agreement. That is to say, authority can be derived either from force or from peaceable means. The peaceable means include assent on the basis of rational argument or agreement. Where rational argument fails in principle, one is left with being accepted by all because of all sharing a common moral viewpoint or sense (e.g., through grace of common conversion) or through some form of negotiation. Thus agreement through conversion is a limiting and unlikely (at least for any large society) example of resolution through agreement. The resort to resolution by agreement (hereafter to mean resolution by agreement other than through conversion; resolution by agreement will usually be equivalent to resolution through negotiation) provides authority. One wills rationality and gives authority to the notion of a moral community in asking questions regarding blame and praise, and commits oneself to mutual respect as a means of gaining moral authority, namely, through mutual consent. The use of persuasion, inducements, and market forces is rendered rational as a means of making it worthwhile for individual persons to will to join in particular communal undertakings. Such manipulations, as long as they are peaceable, as long as they do not involve threats of force or unconsented-to interventions that make free choice impossible (this does not foreclose the possibility of peaceably inducing others to agree to make choice impossible—e.g., let's get drunk together, seduce each other, etc.) form a part of the proper fabric of a peaceable community. One encounters a way in which rational agents can will on rational grounds (i.e., an interest in being able with reason to hold persons blameworthy or praiseworthy) a general means (peaceable negotiations) for a general community (the community of all peaceable moral agents), without presupposing rational grounds for directly justifying the concrete moral viewpoint of particular communities.

Mutual peaceable negotiation emerges as the lynchpin of public authority in general and of authority in health care in particular. With the advent of the Reformation (which is the historical metaphor for the unlikelihood of common conversion) and with the collapse of the Enlightenment hope of delivering a secular, rational justification of the authority of a singular concrete understanding of the good life (which is the historical metaphor for the failure of reason to establish a particular concrete view of the good life), one is still left with a process for peaceably creating such a concrete viewpoint.

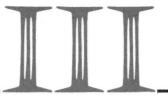

The Principles of Medical Ethics

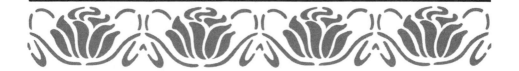

5

Beneficence, Promise-keeping, Veracity, and Autonomy

INTRODUCTION

Once one resolves the question of how an ethic for medicine is to be grounded—whether in the pronouncements of medical professional associations, contracts or covenants under ideal, hypothetical conditions, or in actual agreements involving whole communities of lay people as well as professionals—then one is ready to ask what the actual principles of a medical ethic are. This step will not yet give us actual answers to questions that arise in specific medical ethical cases. It will not even give us concrete rules of conduct to resolve questions in specific medical ethical cases. That will have to wait until later. At this point, however, we can begin to construct a list of principles that will provide the framework for generating rules or guidelines and, eventually, answers to specific case problems.

At this point holders of most medical ethical systems can articulate a single very general, abstract principle or a small number of principles that are seen as morally relevant considerations in moral judgments. These principles provide a general structure for either going directly to specific cases for moral resolution or to articulating more concrete rules that, in turn, provide moral resolution in particular cases.

In medicine, the most commonly accepted general principle is the idea that the physician's duty is to benefit the patient according to the physician's ability and judgment. That is the principle of the Hippocratic Oath and is incorporated into ethical codes in the Hippocratic tradition up until contemporary times. It is a principle that focuses on producing good consequences and avoiding evil consequences, one of the most widely accepted principles of ethics. It differs from the common ethical principle of utilitarianism, however, in several important respects. First, it limits the good to be done to the good of the patient. Whereas classical utilitarianism would calculate the net good for all affected persons resulting from alternative courses of action, the Hippocratic principle limits the good to the patient.

Second, the good is based on the judgment of the clinician. This could be based on the belief that the individual clinician knows the good for the patient better than anyone else, but that is hardly plausible. Individual physicians are known to differ widely over what constitutes the best course for a patient. It is unreasonable that the correct way to produce the most good is to rely on whatever the physician decides who happens to be responsible for the patient's case. Moreover, in order to understand the Hippocratic principle we need to know whether it is the total good of the patient that the physician is to promote or only the medical good. If it is the total good, this requires comparing the medical effects of an action with many other impacts including the financial, social, psychological, familial, legal, and spiritual. It seems unreasonable that the physician would know better how to compare all of these diverse elements than anyone else. On the other hand, if it is only the medical effects, it is hard to see why patients would always want maximum medical benefits if they came at the expense of other kinds of goods. Moreover, it is not even clear whether the individual physician would be the best person to decide what constitutes the maximum medical benefits. Would the individual physician be the best judge of medical benefits for a patient, for instance, when it is known that he differs from the vast majority of his colleagues in dealing with similar cases. Is the physician who believes that aggressive life-prolonging treatment of a patient known to be dying painfully a better judge than his colleagues who would favor simply supportive care? For that matter, is there any reason to believe that the majority view of physicians is the best way to determine what is medically best for a patient faced with such a difficult situation? Some would argue that the patient himself would be a better judge.

There is another element of dispute surrounding the Hippocratic principle. It is commonly said that the duty of the physician can be summarized by the slogan, "First of all, do no harm." In fact, sometimes that is taken to be synonymous with the Hippocratic principle. The meaning and origin of the phrase are, however, in dispute. Some interpret it as giving a special meaning to an ethic of producing good and avoiding evil consequences. In some ethical theories that focus on consequences, it is believed that there is a special, more stringent, or prior duty to avoid evil. That could be what the slogan means. If so, it may be in conflict with the original Hippocratic principle, which appears to give equal weight to producing benefits and avoiding harms.

These are all variations on an ethical principle that focuses exclusively on consequences as judged by physicians. Much of medical ethics, however, does not deal with physician behavior. It has to do with how patients, public policy-makers, or other lay people ought to act in order to do the morally right thing. Moreover, in many ethical systems—liberal political philosophy, Kantianism, and, some would argue, in the mainstream of Judeo-Christian ethics—ethical principles are not simply a matter of producing good consequences and avoiding evil ones (no matter who judges the consequences or which kind have priority). According to this view, there are right-making characteristics of actions other than the fact that they produce good consequences. Some of these characteristics might be that the action involves keeping a promise, being honest, or respecting the autonomy of another. Some hold that the choice of aggressive terminal care is the patient's to make even if the patient would choose some course that all would agree (including the patient) did not produce the most good for the patient. That position could not be explained easily using the classical Hippocratic principle, but is explained easily if one of the principles of right conduct is respect for autonomy.

In some ethical systems there are other right-making characteristics of actions. How does one explain, for example, the widely held intuition that it is wrong to kill someone even if that person is dying, is in terrible pain, and asks to be killed. Some would hold that, in the long run the consequences of killing could be worse (because of errors that could result if people were allowed to kill in such circumstances), but others hold that it is simply wrong to kill even if more good comes from the killing. Holders of this latter position claim that avoiding killing is another right-making characteristic of action.

Still others hold that a right-making characteristic of action is the way goods are distributed as well as how much good is produced. These persons have an independent principle of justice in their ethical systems. Doing right is not simply a matter of producing good; it is a matter of getting the goods to the right people (those who are in need, those who have earned the good, those with the most merit, etc.).

In this chapter we look at the various interpretations of the Hippocratic principle and the principle "First of all, do no harm." These are all special variants on what is sometimes called the principles of beneficence and nonmaleficence (doing good and avoiding evil). Then we look at some critics who believe there is more to right action than simply producing good consequences. In particular, we look at the possibility of principles of promise-keeping, respect for autonomy, and honesty as possible supplements to beneficence and nonmaleficence. In the next two chapters we look at the role of the principles of avoiding killing and justice.

The ethical principle found in the Hippocratic Oath is that the physician should do what will benefit the patient according to his ability and judgment. Sometimes this principle is expressed in other language. One of the most common statements of the core principle of medical ethics is "Do no harm." We shall see in the essay by Albert Jonsen that follows that it is not at all clear exactly what the core principle means or where it comes from. Some people would take it to be simply another wording for the Hippocratic principle. That would be roughly what Jonsen identifies as his third use of the "do no harm" phrase. He argues that others use it in other ways including an exhortation to the proper motivation, to use due care, and to produce special justifications of harms (or detriments) in cases where there are both good and evil effects. Jonsen also makes clear that some people interpret "do no harm" as a special moral injunction to give priority to avoiding harm (even if it means failing to do good). These are all morally different maxims. This leaves us with the question of which, if any, of these maxims are morally appropriate for medicine.

Do No Harm

ALBERT JONSEN

The maxim "do no harm" is often identified as a primary principle of the ethics of the medical profession. A book on malpractice begins "what is needed . . . is a return to basics, to the first principle of medicine, *primum non nocere*; therein lies the answer to the malpractice crisis."[1] Henry Beecher wrote, "if doctors were certain of the benefit of penicillin, for example, yet did not use it, their decision could be construed as running counter to the basic rule of the physician, *primum non nocere.*"[2] A medicolegal expert, writing on "brain death," refers to "the leading axioms of . . . medical ethics, which include . . . *primum non nocere.*"[3] A notable nineteenth-century text on medical ethics, Simon's Deontologie Medicale (1845) insists, "No physician should ever forget the unbending moral precept: do no harm."[4]

Most physicians who quote the venerable text know little of its origin and are unaware of the range of possible meanings it might have in arguing a case in medical ethics. Usually, the maxim is abruptly cited, as if its import is quite obvious. For example, several physicians offer it as a manifest refutation of what they consider unethical informed consent requirements: "Are we needlessly frightening our patients [by the informed consent process] and contributing to the morbidity and mortality of our procedures . . . *primum non nocere.*"[5]

After some remarks about the origin of the maxim and the form in which it is quoted, this paper will suggest four ways in which it might be used in a discussion of medical ethics. These four uses are "ideal types," that is, they are constructed out of occasional allusions to the maxim, which only hint at some fuller argument that might be put together in order to make some ethical point about medical practice. This method of constructing four ideal types of usage is made necessary by the rather surprising dearth of extended arguments based on the maxim. Despite its frequent citation, neither physicians nor philosophers seem to have pressed it very far as a principle of ethical analysis or argument. One such effort, however, has come to my attention and, in the conclusion of this article, I will propose it as an example of the complexity hidden in this apparently obvious phrase.

THE ORIGIN AND FORM OF THE MAXIM

Those who cite *primum non nocere* often attribute it to the Hippocratic Oath. It is not part of the Oath, although the Oath does contain a similar expression: "I will use treatment to help the sick according to my ability and judgment, but I will never use it to injure or wrong them."[6] The actual phrase "do no harm" appears in another work of the Hippocratic literature, The Epidemics. This work, which has been called "the most remarkable product of Greek science,"[7] is a collection of clinical observations made by Greek physicians as they went on their "epidemia," or rounds to various cities and islands. The entire work is devoted to descriptions of signs and symptoms, with occasional remarks about therapeutics. However, in Chapter Eleven of Book I, four peculiar sentences break abruptly into the scientific text. They have a moralistic tone, with something of a copybook naivete. Declare the past, diagnose the present, foretell the future; practice these acts. As to diseases, make a habit of two things—to help, or at least to do no harm. The art has three factors, the disease, the patient, the physician. The physician is servant of the art. The patient must cooperate with the physician in combatting the disease.[8]

In the midst of this brief excursus into medical philosophy appears the aphorism that has won fame as the primary principle of medical ethics. Like the entire passage, it is left unexplained and neither its purpose nor its application is made clear by the text. Its succinctness and directness, however, have endeared it to generations of physicians who recognize it in the ideal and the peril of their labors.

The Latin words *primum non nocere* are translated "above all [or first of all] do no harm." The Greek text is quite stark: "to practice about diseases, two things: to help or not to harm." The origin of the word *primum* is obscure. None of the major modern commentators on the Hippocratic literature mentions it. Professor Oswei Temkin, in a personal communication to the author, states, "I do not know that origin of *primum non nocere,* though I am sure it has its roots in the Hippocratic passage. As with other old medical dicta, it is very difficult, if not impossible to trace the exact origin." In my own search for the source of *primum,* I noted that Gelen, the great commentator on Hippocrates, rephrases the maxim and, in rephrasing it, does insert the Latin expression, *imprimis,* that is, above all. However, he adds it not to the "harm" phrase but to the "help" one: The physician must aim above all at helping the sick; if he cannot, he should not harm them.[9]

The words "at least," often associated with the maxim, pose another exegetical oddity. The standard English translation by W. H. S. Jones reads, "to help or, at least do no harm."[10] The classic French version by E. Littre translates, *avoir dans les maladies, deux choses en vue; etre utile ou du moins ne pas nuire.*[11] Again, the Greek text does not allow for these additional words and, again, I can find no trace of their origin. Its presence in the maxim, although not literal, has seemed to many natural and congenial, as if expressing a resigned acknowledgement of the impotence of medicine: you will probably not do much good, but at least don't make things worse! This reflection brings us directly to the interpretation and use of this first principle of medical ethics.

THE FIRST USE: MEDICINE AS A MORAL ENTERPRISE

Medical skills, in particular the administration of drugs and use of surgery, are designed to effect a change for the better in a physical state or process that distresses, debilitates, or may destroy the life of a person. These same skills, can however, be turned to other purposes: they can create such defective states in a healthy person for purposes of venality, revenge, or torture. They can be directed to benefit, but out of motives of personal profit or aggrandizement rather than the good of the patient. When it is said that the first duty of the physician is to do no harm, it may be intended to assert that practitioners of medicine have the obligation to consider their art as a moral enterprise.

"Medicine as a moral enterprise" might imply that medical skills are, somehow, intrinsically and of themselves, meant to be used for human benefit. "Do no harm" is a warning against their abuse. Although it would be difficult to demonstrate the intrinsically beneficial nature of the medical enterprise, this idea does appear throughout Eastern and Western medicine in the continued insistence that a physician must never refuse to treat a person in need. The inscription on the Asklepieon at the Acropolis reads, "[the physician] should be like a god; savior equally of slaves, or paupers, of rich men, of princes, to all a brother, because we are all brothers."[12] The Hindu Oath states, "You shall assist brahmins, venerable persons, poor people, women, widows and orphans and anyone you meet on your rounds, as if they were your relatives."[13] The Chinese code of Sun Sumiao (seventh century AD) affirms, "aristocrat or commoner, poor or rich, aged or young, beautiful or ugly, friend or enemy, native or foreigner, educated or uneducated, all are to be treated equally."[14]

Indeed, the medical art itself is considered sacred in many traditions, for it is said to come directly from the hand of God and is intended to heal the creatures of God. The prayer of Maimonides ends, "Almighty God, thou has chosen me in thy mercy to watch over the life and death of thy creatures. I now apply myself to my profession. Support me in this great task so that it may benefit mankind."[15] A long tradition, then, supports the view that the physicians are not morally free to dispose of their skills entirely as they see fit, but are bound by the origin, nature, and purpose of their art to use them only for human benefit.

Medicine as a moral enterprise may also mean that, even if the medical skills are indifferent in themselves, they so affect areas of unmistakable human good and evil, such as health and illness, that their use should be guided solely by those needs of others. The physician should be so strongly motivated to secure the good of his or her patient that all other motives will be banished or subordinated. "Do no harm," in this sense, is an injunction to take to heart the motive of acting only for the benefit of the sufferer.

Whether one attends to the nature of the enterprise or to the motives of its practitioners, one cannot fail to notice the ethical importance of "caring." To possess medical skills is to be able to care for the sick. As the origin of the English word "care" reveals, caring means being "troubled by another's trouble." The agreement to care even in a most formal sense, is itself a moral act, for it initiates a series of activities explicitly designed to affect another person as a response to that person's manifest need. Here, as in innumerable other human interactions, the possibility of responsible or irresponsible acts, of praiseworthy or reprehensible behavior, or selfless or selfish motives, in short, of moral action, arises. It is here that "do no harm" in its meaning "do no mischief" applies most fittingly. To assume some power over another so that the other will benefit is to assume care.

In this first usage, then, "do no harm" is an injunction that admonishes medical practitioners that they enter a moral enterprise and exhorts them to have motivations that will focus their skills on the well-being of their patients. The ethical roots of this use are as deep as any ethical roots can go. The maxim, meant in this sense, is equivalent to the first principle or axiom of all morality. As Aquinas wrote, "This is the first precept of the natural law, good is to be done and promoted and evil is to be avoided."[16] John Locke stated the first principle of the natural law as "all being equal and independent, no one ought to harm another in his life, health, liberty or possessions."[17] In this first use, then, the maxim stands for a self-evident first principle of moral discourse. It serves to affirm the moral nature of medical practice as a whole and to enjoin practitioners to hold motives agreeable to that nature.

Stated at a level of such generality, the maxim provides little concrete direction. It would seem only to exclude malicious uses of medical skills. However, common moral opinion would find such acts reprehensible. No principle peculiar to medical ethics seems needed to condemn them. A physician who excises a kidney not because it is diseased, but because it is the kidney of his enemy, is an evil person who only coincidentally has surgical skills. Similarly, a physician who tortures is a moral reprobate who only per accidens has a license to practice medicine. In this first usage, then something most important about medicine in general is announced, but nothing very illuminating about any particular moral problem is provided.

THE SECOND USE: DUE CARE

The second principle of the Principles of Medical Ethics of the American Medical Association requires physicians "to strive continuously to improve their medical knowledge and skill. . . ." Medicine is a practice based on fusion of several sciences, joined to clinical experience. Use of that science and experience in clinical judgment requires accurate information, clear reasoning, sensitive observation, and, occasionally, manual dexterity. Each of these is attained and improved through exercise and through critical reappraisal by oneself and others. They are reappraised in view of certain standards. Attending to these standards and applying them to particular patients is "due care." Benefit should result from applying due care; harm may result from failing to do so. In this use, the maxim could refer both to medical practices in general, calling for their continued improvement by research, and to the skills of particular practitioners, demanding continued study and upgrading.

The admonition to take due care follows reasonably from the maxim in its first use. If medicine is a moral enterprise, under the imperative of benefiting the patient, the specific acts of medicine, diagnosis and therapy, should meet standards which will assure, with some certainty, the beneficial outcome. Just as the maxim in its first use stated the ethical basis of undertaking care, so in this use, it urges the one who has undertaken care to take care. It enjoins careful assessment, careful procedures, careful evaluation, careful follow-up. For example, it is an act of carelessness for a physician to fail to perform a through rectal examination on a patient presenting with rectal bleeding. A casual diagnosis of hemorrhoids may mask the presence of rectal cancer. It is a careless act to treat bronchitis with the antibiotic chloramphenicol which, while very effective, can have fatal complications and is properly indicated only in serious infections, such as typhoid fever. It is careless to ignore, as happened in a leading malpractice case, persistent foul odor from a leg cast which, to the careful practitioner, would suggest the inception of gangrene.

This second use is where questions of morality become issues of legality, for claims of malpractice frequently assert failure to take due care in accord with accepted standards of practice. Several questions arise: Has a physician been negligent? What are accepted standards? What is the boundary between negligence and the fallibility intrinsic to medical knowledge and reasoning? However, there are more objective questions about the very nature of medical knowledge. Contemporary biomedical science makes possible elaborate description of diseases but, because of the plethora of information, may retard identification of the particular illness in a particular patient. Contemporary therapies can have significant theoretical and practical effects in general but may be very difficult to assess in particular patients. The concept of due care, then, not only enjoins carefulness in the practitioner but also reexamination of the methodology of clinical reasoning.

The first use of the maxim has an absolute tone: It declares the morality of medical practice and permits no exceptions. The second use, on the other hand, admits of degrees of carefulness, from the long diagnosis and treatment of neoplasms to the rushed repair of serious trauma. One cannot argue about whether a physician should do harm in the sense of the first use of the maxim: It is obvious that to do so would be unethical. However, in the second sense, there can be interminable arguments about how much care the ethical physician must take.

THE THIRD USE: RISK-BENEFIT RATIO

Any assessment of medical procedures that is carried out in order to establish standards of due care reveals that the outcome of most procedures is only predictable with relative certainty. Some procedures promise an almost certain benefit, which may not, however, come about in a particular application. Other procedures that will certainly benefit entail certain or probable concomitant harm. It has become possible, because of epidemiologic and statistical methods, to determine in quantitative terms some of these possibilities. Thus, the experience of open heart surgery for replacement of multiple valves shows mortality risks of 5% to 20%; use of the anaesthetic halothane carries a risk of causing hepatic dysfunction estimated to be in the range of 1 in 5000 cases. Clinical trials are constantly being designed and carried out to ascertain efficacy and safety of operations and drugs.

Due care requires that these statistics be collected. The careful practitioner will be aware of them as he attempts to match therapy to disease, although one's own experience, one's clinical intuitions, and one's understanding of the nature of statistics should breed caution in their use. "Medical statistics," writes Pappworth, "are like bikinis, concealing what is vital while revealing much that is interesting."[18] Still, the practitioner can use them to steer clear of dangerous or inefficacious treatment. However, any particular patient is a statistic of one. Each patient will respond uniquely; there may be allergic or idiosyncratic reactions. Here, the practitioner, approaching the individual patient, must base a risk-benefit assessment not only on statistics, but also on a focused and full knowledge of the person and the illness. That knowledge will never comprehend the uniqueness of the person but can, by refined experience and sophisticated clinical methodology, draw closer and closer to that uniqueness.

This statistical and clinical risk-benefit equation is not only an element in the diagnostic and therapeutic judgments of the practitioner; it is also an element in the decision of the patient to accept treatment. Physicians may know, statistically and clinically, how much risk of failure or of harm a procedure entails. But patients alone can know how much risk they wish to run and how much they desire the possible benefits. All persons have a "risk budget," as Charles Fried has observed. They calculate in rough ways, out of their experience, emotions, and energy the extent of security and danger they will accept in their lives.[19]

The Oxford English Dictionary defines risk as "exposure to mischance or peril." Although the risk itself is an actuality, as a set of circumstances constituting the exposure, the harm is a possibility. Decisions taken about risks are decisions to place oneself in an exposed position, to dispense with certain securities and protections. When persons do so, they are more uncertain about the consequent situation than they would otherwise be, but only in relation to a certain plan of life. There is, of course, a radical uncertainty about every next situation, given the contingency of existence. But the risks taken within life plans have to do with voluntary steps into more exposed, less protected states of affairs.

In this usage, "do no harm," refers, on the one hand, to the physician's educated assessment of risks. It commands that those procedures be selected that carry the best chance for success with the lowest risk of harm. In this sense, Dr. L. J. Henderson rephrased the maxim as "try to do as little harm as possible."[20] On the other hand, it refers to the patient's own assessment of how those risks and chances fit a lifestyle, with its own personal goals, strengths, and weakness. Here the maxim seems to be assimilated into a familiar form of ethical discourse sometimes called "utilitarian." The objective statement of the equation is translated into a personal "felicific calculus" and choices are made in terms of how the calculation would reveal ways to maximize the goods and minimize the evils of a person's experienced life in its present and future.

In this usage, the word "harm" must be given much more content than in the two previous usages. Although a discussion of harm might begin with an enumeration of possible physical detriments, as is usual in discussions of medical procedures, the scope of meaning quickly expands to wider realms of human experience. Thus, at a first level of meaning, harm might signify an intrusion by physical means upon the physical integrity of oneself or another, leaving an effect of some duration. The intrusion may come from a voluntary or involuntary agent or from an inanimate object or power. One can be harmed by man or beast, by lead weight or lightning, by scalpel or scopolamine. The intrusion comes about because no effort is made, or no effort succeeds, in warding it off. Its effect is more than transient, as a hurt can be, but remains debilitating for a time or permanently. It reduces one's ability to defend oneself, leaving a wounded integrity.

Without distortion, this primitive notion can be expanded from the physical to the psychologic realm, even though psychologic integrity is a more vague concept. Perhaps it can be defined as the ability to respond appropriately and effectively to intellectual and emotional challenges, such as loss or danger. Here the agents of harm move beyond the physical to the psychologic. They include threats, lies, ridicule, shame.

Finally, physical and psychologic integrity imply social integrity, the ability to maintain oneself as a whole person by initiating action and responding to others. This integrity can be harmed by cutting off human contacts, by distorting communication, by rendering ineffectual all efforts at self preservation. At the heart of harming and being harmed is the notion of the ability to respond to challenge. A harmful act is one that cannot be warded off, and its harmful effect is a decreased ability to defend oneself, physically, psychologically, or socially. Response, measured and timely, is the sign of integrity.

"Harming," then, may describe any action or event that results in prolonged diminished ability to respond to physical, psychologic, or social challenge. In this usage, then, the risk to physical integrity of patients. Patients alone are capable of assessing the boundaries of this personal integrity, because it is coterminous with their selfhood. However, it is not uncommon that the patient is incapable of making or expressing an assessment. In such cases, the surrogate, who may or may not be the physician, must attempt to be "in the place of the other." The complexities of this question cannot be discussed here. It should only be noted that if the surrogate is a physician, his duty to do no harm extends not only to controlling the risk of physical harm, but also to adopting the "felicific calculus" of the patient, attempting to imagine in some general way the entire range of possible insults to personal integrity of his patient.

THE FOURTH USE: THE BENEFIT-DETRIMENT EQUATION

Many medical procedures not only carry risk of harm, but necessarily bring about some detriment at the same time as they effect a benefit. Any amputation will, in one and the same act, remove a diseased part in order to save life and always leaves the patient with a physical and, sometimes, a psychologic deficit. Administration of powerful alkylating agents, such as nitrogen mustards, for treatment of lymphomas, produces almost invariably unpleasant and sometimes serious side-effects. Drawing blood for careful monitoring of a tiny premature baby's blood gases significantly reduces the baby's blood volume. Some of these necessarily associated detriments can be remedied; some must be borne.

In situations such as these, the maxim might be rephrased as, "do no harm unless that harm is necessarily associated with a compensating benefit." A certain benefit must be balanced against a certain detriment. Here again, as in the previous risk-benefit usage, a felicific calculus can be employed. How does one sum the benefits and the detriments in terms of a desired life plan? Here also, the physician should know, from science and experience, the ratio, and use it to eliminate disproportionate approaches and inform the patient about the effects of that therapeutic plan that seems most reasonable. Here again, the patient alone is in a position to make the calculation. One person chooses to live even as a quadriplegic; another prefers the limited life on dialysis to the risks of transplantation; a third rejects chemotherapy, which he considers too unpleasant even though it may prolong life.

There are, however, certain problems of benefit-detriment that do not fit easily into the felicific calculus. These are problems in which the benefit accrues to one party and the detriment to another. Four current problems in medical ethics are of this type: abortion, allocation of scarce biomedical resources, nontherapeutic experimentation on subjects incapable of consent, and sterilization of carriers of deleterious genes. In such cases, certain evils are visited upon some in order that others might benefit. Classic utilitarian reasoning, although vaunting its solution to such problems, has generally been considered at its weakest in coming to grips with the distribution of benefits and burdens to different parties.

Another manner of moral reasoning, traditionally called the Principle of Double Effect was designed to deal with problems of this sort. Although much criticized in recent years, from within and without the camp of Roman Catholic moral theologians, who were its creators, it seems at least to ask the right question: Under what circumstances can one be said to act morally when one of the multiple effects of that action is an evil? The death of a fetus, the danger to a nonconsenting subject, refusal of dialysis, the imposed sterility of a dysgenic male are all evils. Is their occurrence or permission justified by some good, presumably "greater," for some other or others?

In its most traditional form, the double-effect argument depends on the distinction between directly intended and indirectly intended (or merely permitted) effects. The object of the direct intention must be a good in itself or, at least, be morally indifferent. An act good in itself could cause a foreseen, but unintended evil result, but no good result, no matter how great, could justify an act vitiated by an intrinsically evil object. Recent attempts by Catholic theologians to untangle this ethical intricacy have turned on the notion of "proportionate reason," which is not merely a "serious reason" but rather an explanation of how the evil effect is an inextricable byproduct of a good that one is obliged to perform.[21] Outside the theologians' camp, philosopher Phillipa Foote argues that it is the concept of positive and negative duties, rather than the intended and the foreseen effects, that determines the justifiability of an evil effect.[22]

We will not enter the debate about the strengths and weaknesses of double-effects reasoning. We simply note that, in arguments about the morality of multiple effects, participants often believe that some of these are undesirable and, perhaps, immoral. They also believe that something other than "greater good of another or of the greater number" must be proposed to justify the commission or permission of an evil effect. They seek for "serious" or "overriding" reasons. The abortion debate, in some of its forms, is the classic example. Abortion is a medical act that has two associated consequences: the mother's well-being and the death of the fetus. Many make an ethical case for abortion by admitting that the fetal death is undesirable and perhaps immoral, but then cite one or several reasons that they consider "to override" or "to justify" that effect. Freedom to control one's own body is considered by some to be such a reason; others refuse to allow this to outrank the right to life of the fetus.

In this use, then, "do no harm" is an imperative that calls for double-effect reasoning in order to reach a conclusion about the morality of an action. It calls for the proposal of serious or proportionate reasons for allowing some detriment that is necessarily concomitant with a desired benefit.

A PARADOXICAL USE

Recently, several authors have invoked the principle "do no harm" to justify involuntary euthanasia. Philosopher-physician H. Tristram Engelhardt writes:

> In the field of medicine, the need is to recognize an ethical category, a concept of wrongful continuance of existence, . . . [which] presupposes that life can be of a negative value such that the medical maxim *primum non nocere* would not require sustaining life.[23]

The proposal is, at first sight, paradoxical. Does not one harm another by allowing him to die? Can sustaining life be properly called harming?

A review of the several uses of the maxim may put Dr. Engelhardt's proposal in perspective. If "do no harm" is intended to bear the meaning of the first usage, always having the motive to care for the other, termination of painful or a seriously debilitated existence might be considered a "caring act." However, this appears to beg the question: Can deprivation of life, of any quality, be a good for the one deprived? The second usage, due care, at first sight, seems irrelevant for it is primarily procedural. However, it may be highly relevant. Due care consists of assessing medical actions in relation to certain goals. It might be argued that sustaining life of low quality is not a goal of medical actions because medicine is concerned only with restoration of health in some functional sense. Medical actions that cannot achieve this are improper and may be ethically discontinued. The physician judges this action to be beyond his or her responsibility. The third usage, risk-benefit equation, bears only on the question, often moot, about whether continued care might possibly bring about restoration. The fourth use, benefit-detriment equation, is most often invoked. If seen as felicific calculus, it is flawed by being always a surrogate judgment and also by the logical peculiarities inherent in the suggestion that someone would be "better off dead." It seems that both benefit and detriment must be experienced in order to be evaluated.

Finally, if the fourth use is seen as a good reasons argument, the good reasons must be scrutinized in terms of some broader ethical theory that gives the criteria whereby a reason is measured as good. For example, Father Richard McCormick proposes such criteria based upon a theological foundation:

> In all of these instances—instances where the life could be saved—the discussion is couched in terms of the means necessary to preserve life. But often enough it is the kind of, the quality of life thus saved (painful, poverty-stricken and deprived, and away from home and friends, oppressive) that established the means as extraordinary. That type of life would be an excessive hardship for the individual. It would distort and jeopardize his grasp on the overall meaning of life. Why? Because, it can be argued, human relationships—which are the very possibility of growth in love of God and neighbor—would be so threatened, strained, or submerged that they would no longer function as the heart and meaning of the individual's life as they should. Something other than the "higher more important good" would occupy first place. Life, the condition of other values and achievements, would usurp the place of these and become itself the ultimate value. When that happens, the value of human life has been distorted out of context.[24]

It seems reasonable to invoke the "do no harm" maxim as a justification for termination of life.[25] The logic of this justification, however, must move through usage two and four, "due care" and "good reasons." The substance of the argument is difficult to make because standards of due care for the dying and the irretrievably comatose are very insufficiently developed by physicians and because theories of good reason for action are very skimpily designed by philosophers. Physicians who do not understand the "end of medicine" and philosophers who do not appreciate the "end of man" are unlikely to succeed in providing the substance of that argument.[26,27]

CONCLUSION

Several generalizations may be drawn about the "do no harm" argument. First, the ancient maxim serves in a variety of ways, each of which represents a somewhat different mode of ethical discourse. We have noted at least four that can be designated as an absolute principle, a counsel of prudence, a calculation of acceptability, a rule of double effect. When the maxim appears, its role as one or another of these should be recognized and the argument analyzed accordingly. Secondly, the maxim as absolute principle and counsel of prudence is directed at the physician as moral agent, urging that he or she have certain motives, intentions, and ways of judging. As calculus of acceptability and as rule of double effect, it is directed primarily at the patient and only indirectly at the physician, for it is the recipient of care who must accept risks and find reasons proportionate. Only occasionally will the physician have to exercise surrogate judgment about these. The "do no harm" maxim, in the third and fourth uses, affirms that physician ethics must be centered on respect for the autonomy of patients. The benefit to others commanded by the absolute principle that initiates that moral enterprise of medicine is seen to be the benefit of fostering the independence of patients. Harming touches not only the body but also the person in his or her personality and community.

In conclusion, it may appear that dwelling on the negative apodosis of the maxim, "do no harm," rather than upon the positive protasis, "be of benefit," creates the impression of a minimalist morality. This may be. But, if we recall the version of the maxim, "at least do no harm," we may see it not so much as a morality of lower limits, but as an admonition to humility. When good persons possess great powers and wield them on behalf of others, they sometimes fail to recognize the harm done as they play their beneficent craft. The medical profession has such power and its practitioners usually intend to use it well. They must become sensitive to its shadow side. A character in a recent novel states the case for humility well: "I was less morally ambitious than you . . . I didn't aspire to do good: that seemed too difficult. I only wanted not to do harm."[28] Only wanting not to do harm, we may conclude, is difficult enough!

NOTES

1. Kramer, C. *The Negligent Doctor.* New York: Crown Publishing, 1968, p. 17.
2. Beecher, H. *Research and the Individual.* Boston: Little, Brown, 1970, p. 94.
3. Van Till, H. A. H. "Diagnosis of Death in Comatose Patients Under Resuscitation Treatment: A Critical Review of the Harvard Report." *American Journal of Law and Medicine* 2:1–40, 1976.

4. Simon, M. "Deontologie Medicale." Paris: J. B. Bailliere, 1845, p. 269.
5. Kaplan, S. R., R. A. Greenwald, and A. I. Rogers. "Neglected Aspects of Informed Consent." *New England Journal of Medicine* 296:1127, 1977.
6. Jones, W. H. S. *Hippocrates I.* Cambridge, Mass.: Harvard University Press, 1923, p. 165.
7. Ibid., p. 141.
8. Ibid., p. 165; cf. A. Jonsen, "Do No Harm." In *Philosophical Medical Ethics: Its Nature and Significance,* edited by S. F. Spicker and H. T. Engelhardt, Jr. Dordrecht, Holland: D. Reidel, 1977, pp. 27–41.
9. Galen. "Commentarium I." In *Hippocratis libri I Epidemiorum,* c. 50, Vol. 17A. Liepzig: C. Cnoblochius, 1828, p. 148.
10. Jones, p. 165.
11. Littre, E. *Oeuvres Comples d'Hippocrate,* Vol. II, Paris: J. B. Bailliere, 1839–1869, p. 635.
12. Etziony, M. B. *The Physicians' Creed.* Springfield, Ill.: Charles C Thomas, Publishing, 1973, p. 21.
13. Ibid., p. 15.
14. Ibid., p. 20.
15. Ibid., p. 30.
16. Aquinas. *Basic Writings,* edited by A. Pegis. New York: Random House, 1945, II, 773 (I–II, 94, 2).
17. Locke, J. *Two Treatises of Government,* edited by T. Cook. New York: Hafner, 1947, p. 73.
18. Pappworth, M. H. *Primer of Medicine.* New York: Appleton-Century-Crofts, 1971, p. 177.
19. Fried, C. *Anatomy of Values.* Cambridge, Mass.: Harvard University Press, 1971, p. 177.
20. Henderson, L. J. "The Physician and the Patient as a Social System." *New England Journal of Medicine* 212:819–823, 1937.
21. Knauer, P. "The Hermaneutic Principle of Double Effect." *Natural Law Forum* 12:132–162, 1962.
22. Foote, P. "The Problem of Abortion and the Doctrine of Double Effect." *Oxford Review* 5:5–15, 1967.
23. Engelhardt, H. T. "Aiding the Death of Young Children." In *Beneficent Euthanasia,* edited by M. Kohl. Buffalo, N.Y.: Prometheus Books, 1975, p. 187.
24. McCormick, R. "To Live or Let Die." *Journal of the American Medical Association* 229:173–175, 1974.
25. Jonsen, A. and M. Garland. *The Ethics of Newborn Intensive Care.* Berkeley, Calif.: Institute of Governmental Studies, 1976.
26. Gustafson, J. *The Contribution of Theology to Medical Ethics.* Milwaukee: Marquette University Press, 1975.
27. Kass, L. "Regarding the End of Medicine and the Pursuit of Health." *Public Interest* 40:11–42, 1970.
28. Lurie, A. *The War Between the Taits.* New York: Random House, 1975, p. 271.

In the previous essay, Jonsen has shown that something as simple as "do no harm" can have many different meanings. Even if we were to agree that the principles of medical ethics should be beneficence and nonmaleficence, it is still not clear exactly what they mean. Matters get more complex when we realize that spokespersons for many ethical systems maintain that production of good and avoidance of evil are not the only right-making characteristics of actions. In the essay that follows, W. D. Ross provides the classical argument that an ethical principle that focuses only on consequences is only one way of thinking about ethics. As an alternative he proposes an ethic with other right-making characteristics (what he calls *prima facie* duties). He suggests such considerations as fidelity to promises, honesty, and justice. Note that he is not arguing that actions are always wrong in the end if they involve breaking a promise or telling a lie, just that these are always elements that tend to make an action wrong—what he calls wrong *prima facie* (other "all other things being equal"). It is thus wrong to conclude that Ross's system of ethics, which includes right-making characteristics other than consequences (sometimes called deontological ethics), is more rigid than consequentialist ethics. Someone could be quite rigid and still be a consequentialist (as, for example, someone who holds that the rule "rape is always wrong because it always produces bad consequences"). On the other hand Ross, though the classical deontologist, can be quite flexible. Sometimes it is right on balance to break a promise, even though it is always *prima facie* wrong to do so.

What Makes Right Acts Right

W. D. Ross

The real point at issue between hedonism and utilitarianism on the one hand and their opponents on the other is not whether 'right' means 'productive of so and so;' for it cannot with any plausibility be maintained that it does. The point at issue is that to which we now pass, viz. whether there is any general character which makes right acts right, and if so, what it is. Among the main historical attempts to state a single characteristic of all right actions which is the foundation of their rightness are those made by egoism and utilitarianism. But I do not propose to discuss these, not because the subject is unimportant, but because it has been dealt with so often and so well already, and because there has come to be so much agreement among moral philosophers that neither of these theories is satisfactory. A much more attractive theory has been put forward by Professor Moore: that what makes action right is that they are productive of more *good* than could have been produced by any other action open to the agent.[1]

This theory is in fact the culmination of all the attempts to base rightness on productivity of some sort of result. The first form this attempt takes is the attempt to base rightness on conduciveness to the advantage or pleasure of the agent. This theory comes to grief over the fact, which stares us in the face, that a great part of duty consists in an observance of the rights and a furtherance of the interests of others, whatever the cost to ourselves may be. Plato and others may be right in holding that a regard for the rights of others never in the long run involves a loss of happiness for the agent, that 'the just life profits a man.' But this, even if true, is irrelevant to the rightness of the act. As soon as a man does an action *because* he thinks he will promote his own interests thereby, he is acting not from a sense of its rightness but from self-interest.

To the egoistic theory hedonistic utilitarianism supplies a much-needed amendment. It points out correctly that the fact that a certain pleasure will be enjoyed by the agent is no reason why he *ought* to bring it into being rather than an equal or greater pleasure to be enjoyed by another, though, human nature being what it is, it makes it not unlikely that he *will* try to bring it into being. But hedonistic utilitarianism in its turn needs a correction. On reflection it seems clear that pleasure is not the only thing in life that we think is good in itself, that for instance we think the possession of a good character, or an intelligent understanding of the world, as food or better. A great advance is made by the substitution of 'productive of the greatest good' for 'productive of the greatest pleasure.'

Not only is this theory more attractive than hedonistic utilitarianism, but its logical relation to that theory is such that the latter could not be true unless *it* were true, which it might be true though hedonistic utilitarianism were not. It is in fact one of the logical bases of hedonistic utilitarianism. For the view that what produces the maximum pleasure is right has for its bases the views (1) that what produces the maximum good is right, and (2) that pleasure is the only thing good in itself. If they were not assuming that what produces the maximum *good* is right, the utilitarians' attempt to show that pleasure is the only good in itself, which is in fact the point they take most pains to establish, would have been quite irrelevant to their attempt to prove that only what produces the maximum *pleasure* is right. If, therefore, it can be shown that productivity of the maximum good is not what makes all right actions right, we shall *a fortiori* have refuted hedonistic utilitarianism.

When a plain man fulfills a promise because he thinks he ought to do so, it seems clear that he does so with no thought of its total consequences, still less with any opinion that these are likely to be the best possible. He thinks in fact much more of the past than of the future. What makes him think it right to act in a certain way is the fact that he has promised to do—that and, usually, nothing more. That his act will produce the best possible consequences is not his reason for calling it right. What lends colour to the theory we are examining, then, is not the actions (which form probably a great majority of our actions) in which some such reflection as 'I have promised' is the only reason we give ourselves for thinking a certain action right, but the exceptional cases in which the consequences of fulfilling a promise (for instance) would be so disastrous to others that we judge it right not to do so. It must of course be admitted that such cases exist. If I have promised to meet a friend at a particular time for some trivial purpose, I should certainly think myself justified in breaking my engagement if by doing so I could prevent a serious accident or bring relief to the victims of one. And the supporters of the view we are examining hold that my thinking so is due to my thinking that I shall bring more good into existence by the one action than by the other. A different account may, however, be given of the matter, an account which will, I believe, show itself to be the true one. It may be said that besides the duty of fulfilling promises I have and recognize a duty of relieving distress,[2] and that when I think it right to do the latter at the cost of not doing the former, it is not because I think I shall produce more good thereby but because I think it the duty which is in the circumstances more of a duty. This account surely corresponds much more closely with what we really think in such a situation. If, so far as I can see, I could bring equal amounts of good into being by fulfilling my promise and by helping some one to whom I had made no promise, I should not hesitate to regard the former as my duty. Yet on the view that what is right is right because it is productive of the most good I should not so regard it.

There are two theories, each in its way simple, that offer a solution of such cases of conscience. One is the view of Kant, that there are certain duties of perfect obligation, such as those of fulfilling promises, of paying debts, of telling the truth, which admit of no exception whatever in favour of duties of imperfect obligation, such as that of relieving distress. The other is the view of, for instance, Professor Moore and Dr. Rashdall, that there is only the duty of producing good, and that 'conflicts of duties' should be resolved by asking 'by which action will most good be produced?' But it is more important that our theory fit the facts than that it be simple, and the account we have given above corresponds (it seems to me) better than either of the simpler theories with what we really think, viz. that normally promise-keeping, for example, should come before benevolence, but that when and only when the good to be produced by the benevolent act is very great and the promise comparatively trivial, the act of benevolence becomes our duty.

In fact the theory of 'ideal utilitarianism,' if I may for brevity refer so to the theory of Professor Moore, seems to simplify unduly our relations to our fellows. It says, in effect, that the only morally significant relation in which my neighbours stand to me is that of being possible beneficiaries by my action.[3] They do stand in this relation to me, and this relation is morally significant. But they may also stand to me in the relation of promisee to promiser, of creditor to debtor, of wife to husband, of child to parent, of friend to friend, of fellow countryman to fellow countryman, and the like; and each of these relation is the foundation of a *prima facie* duty, which is more or less incumbent on me according to the circumstances of the case. When I am in a situation, as perhaps I always am, in which more than one of these *prima facie* duties is incumbent on me, what I have to do is to study the situation as fully as I can until I form the considered opinion (it is never more) that in the circumstances one of them is more incumbent than any other; then I am bound to think that to do this *prima facie* duty is my duty *sans phrase* in the situation.

I suggest '*prima facie* duty' or 'conditional duty' as a brief way of referring to the characteristic (quite distinct from that of being a duty proper) which an act has, in virtue of being of a certain kind (e.g., the keeping of a promise), of being an act which would be a duty proper if it were not at the same time of another kind which is morally significant. Whether an act is a duty proper or actual duty depends on *all* the morally significant kinds it is an instance of. The phrase '*prima facie* duty' must be apologized for, since (1) it suggests that what we are speaking of is a certain kind of duty, whereas it is in fact not a duty, but something related in a special way to duty. Strictly speaking, we want not a phrase in which duty is qualified by an adjective, but a separate noun. (2) '*Prima' facie* suggests that one is speaking only of an appearance which a moral situation presents at first sight, and which may turn out to be illusory; whereas what I am speaking of is an objective fact involved in the nature of the situation, or more strictly in an element of its nature, though not, as duty proper does, arising from its *whole* nature. I can, however, think of no term which fully meets the case. 'Claim' has been suggested by Professor Prichard. The word 'claim' has the advantage of being quite a familiar one in this connection, and it seems to cover much of the ground. It would be quite natural to say, 'a person to whom I have made a promise has a claim on me', and also, 'a person whose distress I could relieve (at the cost of breaking the promise) has a claim on me'. But (1) while 'claim' is appropriate from *their* point of view, we want a word to express the corresponding fact from the agent's point of view—the fact of his being subject to claims that can be made against him; and ordinary language provides us with no such correlative to 'claim'. And (2) (what is more important) 'claim' seems inevitably to suggest two persons, one of whom might make a claim on the other; and while this covers the ground of social duty, it is inappropriate in the case of that important part of duty which is the duty of cultivating a certain kind of character in oneself. It would be artificial, I think, and at any rate metaphorical, to say that one's character has a claim on oneself.

There is nothing arbitrary about these *prima facie* duties. Each rests on a definite circumstance which cannot seriously be held to be without moral significance. Of *prima facie* duties I suggest, without claiming completeness or finality for it, the following division.[4]

(1) Some duties rest on previous acts of my own. These duties seems to include two kinds, (a) those resting on a promise or what may fairly be called an implicit promise, such as the implicit undertaking not to tell lies which seems to be implied in the act of entering into conversation (at any rate by civilized men), or of writing books that purport to be history and not fiction. These may be called the duties of fidelity. (b) Those resting on a previous wrongful act. These may be called the duties of reparation. (2) Some rest on previous acts of other men, i.e., services done by them to me. These may be loosely described as the duties of gratitude.[5] (3) Some rest on the fact or possibility of a distribution of pleasure or happiness (or of the means thereto) which is not in accordance with the merit of the persons concerned; in such cases there arises a duty to upset or prevent such a distribution. These are the duties of justice. (4) Some rest on the mere fact that there are other beings in the world whose condition we can make better in respect of virtue, or of intelligence, or

of pleasure. They are the duties of beneficience. (5) Some rest on the fact that we can improve our own condition in respect of virtue or of intelligence. These are the duties of self-improvement. (6) I think that we should distinguish from (4) the duties that may be summed up under the title of 'not injuring others'. No doubt to injure others is incidentally to fail to do them good; but it seems to me clear that non-maleficence is apprehended as duty distinct from that of beneficience, and as a duty of a more stringent character. It will be noticed that this alone among the types of duty has been stated in a negative way. An attempt might no doubt be made to state this duty, like the others, in a positive way. It might be said that it is really the duty to prevent ourselves from acting either from an inclination to harm others or from an inclination to seek our own pleasure, in doing which we should incidentally harm them. But on reflection it seems clear that the primary duty here is the duty not to harm others, this being a duty whether or not we have an inclination that if followed would lead to unharming them; and that when we have such an inclination the primary duty not to harm others gives rise to a consequential duty to resist the inclination. The recognition of this duty of non-maleficence is the first step on the way to the recognition of their duty of beneficience; and that accounts for the prominence of the commands 'thou shalt not kill,' 'thou shalt not bear false witness,' in so early a code as the Decalogue. But even when we have come to recognize the duty of beneficience, it appears to me that the duty of non-maleficence is recognized as a distinct one, and as *prima facie* more binding. We should not in general consider it justifiable to kill one person in order to keep another alive, or to steal from one in order to give alms to another.

The essential defect of the 'ideal utilitarian' theory is that it ignores, or at least does not do full justice to, the highly personal character of duty. If the only duty is to produce the maximum of good, the question who is to have the good—whether it is myself, or my benefactor, or a person to whom I have made a promise to confer that good on him, or a mere fellow man to whom I stand in no such special relation should make no difference to my having a duty to produce that good. But we are all in fact sure that it makes a vast difference.

NOTES

1. I take the theory that, as I have tried to show, seems to be put forward in *Ethics* rather than the earlier and less plausible theory put forward in *Principia Ethica*. For the difference, cf. Ross, W. D. *The Right and the Good*. Oxford: Oxford University Press, 1939, pp. 8–11.
2. These are not strictly speaking duties, but things that tend to be our duty, or *prima facie* duties. Cf. Ross, pp. 19–20.
3. Some will think it, apart from other considerations, a sufficient refutation of this view to point out that I also stand in that relation to myself, so that for this view that distinction of oneself from others is morally insignificant.
4. I should make it plain at this stage that I am assuming that the correctness of some of our main convictions as to *prima facie* duties, or, more strictly, am claiming that we *know* them to be true. To me it seems as self-evident as anything could be, that to make a promise, for instance, is to create a moral claim on us in someone else. Many readers will

perhaps say that they do not know this to be true. If so, I certainly cannot prove it to them; I can only ask them to reflect again, in the hope that they will ultimately agree that they also know it to be true. The main moral convictions of the plain man seem to me to be, not opinions which it is for philosophy to prove or disprove, but knowledge from the start; and in my own case I seem to find little difficulty in distinguishing these essential convictions from other moral convictions which I also have, which are merely fallible opinions based on an imperfect study of the working for good or evil of certain institutions or types of action.

5.   For needed correction of this statement, cf. Ross, pp. 22–23.

The ethical principles (or *prima facie* duties) that W. D. Ross presents in the previous reading make clear that it is possible to be committed to ethical principles other than beneficence and nonmaleficence (or the production of good on balance). Principles such as fidelity to promises are essential to some moral systems even if they are viewed as not based on consequences. Immanuel Kant offers one of the classic defenses of another possible basic principle of ethics in the following essay in which he argues that telling a lie is inherently a wrong even if it does no harm.

On a Supposed Right to Tell Lies from Benevolent Motives

IMMANUEL KANT

In the work called *France,* for the year 1797, Part VI, No. 1, on "Political Reactions," by Benjamin Constant, the following passage occurs:

> The moral principle that it is one's duty to speak the truth, if it were taken singly and unconditionally, would make all society impossible. We have the proof of this in the very direct consequences which have been drawn from this principle by a German philosopher, who goes so far as to affirm that to tell a falsehood to a murderer who asked us whether our friend, of whom he was in pursuit, had not taken refuge in our house, would be a crime.

The French philosopher opposes this principle in the following manner, "It is a duty to tell the truth. The notion of duty is inseparable from the notion of right. A duty is what in one being corresponds to the right of another. Where there are no rights there are no duties. To tell the truth then is a duty, but only towards him who has a right to the truth. But no man has a right to a truth that injures others." The [primary lie] here lies in the statement that "To tell the truth is a duty, but only towards him who has a right to the truth."

It is to be remarked, first, that the expression "to have a right to the truth" is unmeaning. We should rather say, a man has a right to his own *truthfulness* (*veracitas*), that is, to subjective truth in his own person. For to have a right objectively to truth would mean that, as in *meum* and *tuum* generally, it depends on his *will* whether a given statement shall be true or false, which would produce a singular logic.

Now, the first question is whether a man—in cases where he cannot avoid answering Yes or No—has the *right* to be untruthful. The *second* question is whether, in order to prevent a misdeed that threatens him or some one else, he is not actually bound to be untruthful in a certain statement to which an unjust compulsion forces him.

Truth in utterances that cannot be avoided is the formal duty of a man to everyone, however great the disadvantage that may arise from it to him or any other; and although by making a false statement I do no wrong to him who unjustly compels me to speak, yet I do wrong to men in general in the most essential point of duty, so that it may be called a lie (though not in the jurist's sense), that is, so far as in me lies I cause that declarations in general find no credit, and hence that all rights founded on contract should lose their force; and this is a wrong which is done to mankind.

If, then, we define a lie merely as an intentionally false declaration towards another man, we need not add that it must injure another; as the jurists think proper to put in their definition (*mendacium est falsiioquium in praejudicium alterius*). For it always injures another; if not another individual, yet mankind generally, since it vitiates the source of justice. This benevolent lie *may*, however, by *accident* (*casus*) become punishable even by civil laws; and that which escapes liability to punishment only by accident may be condemned as a wrong even by external laws. For instance, if you have by a lie hindered a man who is even now planning a murder, you are legally responsible for all the consequences. But if you have strictly adhered to the truth, public justice can find no fault with you, be the unforeseen consequence what it may. It is possible that whilst you have honestly answered Yes to the murderer's question, whether his intended victim is in the house, the latter may have gone out unobserved, and so not have come in the way of the murderer, and the deed therefore have not been done; whereas, if you lied and said he was not in the house, and he had really gone out (though unknown to you), so that the murderer met him as he went, and executed his purpose on him, then you might with justice be accused as the cause of his death. For, if you had spoken the truth as well as you knew it, perhaps the murderer while seeking for his enemy in the house might have been caught by neighbours coming up and the deed been prevented. Whoever then *tells a lie*, however good his intentions may be, must answer for the consequences of it, even before the civil tribunal, and must pay the penalty for them, however unforeseen they may have been; because truthfulness is a duty that must be regarded as the basis of all duties founded on contract, the laws of which would be rendered uncertain and useless if even the least exception to them were admitted.

To be *truthful* (honest) in all declarations is therefore a sacred unconditional command of reason, and not to be limited by any expediency.

M. Constant makes a thoughtful and sound remark on the decrying of such strict principles, which it is alleged lose themselves in impracticable ideas, and are therefore to be rejected:—"In every case in which a principle proved to be true seems to be inapplicable, it is because we do not know the *middle principle* which contains the medium of its application." He adduces the doctrine of *equality* as the first link forming the social chain: "namely, that no man can be bound by any laws except those to the formation of which he has contributed. In a very contracted society this principle may be directly applied and become the ordinary rule without requiring any middle principle. But in a very numerous society we must add a new principle to that which we here state. This middle principle is, that the individuals may contribute to the formation of the laws either in their own person or by *representatives*. Whoever would try to apply the first principle to a numerous society without taking in the middle principle would infallibly bring about its destruction. But this circumstance, which would only show the ignorance or incompetence of the lawgiver, would prove nothing against the principle itself." He concludes thus: "A principle recognized as truth must, therefore, never be abandoned, however obviously danger may seem to be involved in it." (And yet the good man himself abandoned the unconditional principle of veracity on account of the danger to society, because he could not discover any middle principle which would serve to prevent this danger; and, in fact, no such principle is to be interpolated here.)

Retaining the names of the persons as they have been here brought forward, "the French philosopher" confounds the action by which one does harm (*nocet*) to another by telling the truth, the admission of which he cannot avoid, with the action by which he does him *wrong* (*laedit*). It was merely an *accident* (*casus*) that the truth of the statement did harm to the inhabitant of the house; it was not a free *deed* (in the juridical sense). For to admit his right to require another to tell a lie for his benefit would be to admit a claim opposed to all law. Every man has not only a right, but the strictest duty to truthfulness in statements which he cannot avoid, whether they do harm to himself or others. He himself, properly speaking, does not *do* harm to him who suffers thereby; but this harm is *caused* by accident. For the man is not free to choose, since (if he must speak at all) veracity is an unconditional duty. The "German philosopher" will therefore not adopt as his principle the proposition: "It is a duty to speak the truth, but only to him who has a right to the truth," first on account of the obscurity of the expression, for truth is not a possession the right to which can be granted to one, and refused to another; and next and chiefly, because the duty of veracity (of which alone we are speaking here) makes no distinction between persons towards whom we have this duty, and towards whom we may be free from it; but is an unconditional duty which holds in all circumstances.

Now, in order to proceed from a *metaphysic* of Right (which abstracts from all conditions of experience) to a principle of *politics* (which applies these notions to cases of experience), and by means of this to the solution of a problem of the latter in accordance with the general principle of right, the philosopher will enunciate:—1. An *Axiom,* that is, an apodictically certain proposition, which follows directly from the definition of external right (harmony of the *freedom* of each with the freedom of all by a universal law). 2. A *Postulate* of external public *law* as the united will of all on the principle of *equality,* without which there could not exist the freedom of all. 3. A *Problem;* how it is to be arranged that harmony may be maintained in a society, however large, on principles of freedom and equality (namely, by means of a representative system); and this will then become a principle of the *political system,* the establishment and arrangement of which will contain enactments which, drawn from practical knowledge of men, have in view only the mechanism of administration of justice, and how this is to be suitably carried out. Justice must never be accommodated in the political system, but always the political system to justice.

"A principle recognized as true (I add, recognized *a priori,* and therefore apodictic) must never be abandoned, however obviously danger may seem to be involved in it," says the author. Only here we must not understand the danger of *doing harm* (accidentally), but of *doing wrong;* and this would happen if the duty of veracity, which is quite unconditional, and constitutes the supreme condition of justice in utterance, were made conditional and subordinate to other considerations; and although by a certain lie I in fact do no wrong to any person, yet I infringe the principle of justice in regard to all indispensably necessary statements *generally* (I do wrong formally, though not materially); and this is much worse than to commit an injustice to any individual, because such a deed does not presuppose any principle leading to it in the subject. The man who, when asked whether in the statement he is about to make he intends to speak truth or not, does not receive the question with indignation at the suspicion thus expressed towards him that he might be a liar, but who asks permission first to consider possible exceptions, is already a liar (*in potentia*), since he shows that he does not recognize veracity as a duty in itself, but reserves exceptions from a rule which in its nature does not admit of exceptions, since to do so would be self-contradictory.

All practical principles of justice must contain strict truths, and the principles here called middle principles can only contain the closer definition of their application to actual cases (according to the rules of politics), and never exceptions from them, since exceptions destroy the universality, on account of which alone they bear the name of principles.

The Kantian view that veracity or honesty is an independent moral principle not conditional on considerations of consequences is not the only justification of the intuition that it is generally morally right to be honest. The famous utilitarian, Henry Sidgwick, has a very different account of why it is generally considered right to speak the truth. He grounds it in the observation that generally good comes from being honest. In special cases, however, where more good might come from a deception or a dishonest statement, a consistent consequentialist will admit to the appropriateness of the less than honest communication in the special situation.

The Methods of Ethics

Henry Sidgwick

THE CLASSIFICATION OF DUTIES—VERACITY

It may easily seem that when we have discussed Benevolence, Justice, and the observance of Law and Contract, we have included in our view the whole sphere of social duty, and that whatever other maxims we find accepted by Common Sense must be subordinate to the principles which we have been trying to define.

For whatever we owe definitely to our fellow-men, besides the observance of special contracts, and of positive laws, seems—at least by a slight extension of common usage—to be naturally included under Justice: while the more indefinite obligations which we recognize seem to correspond to the goodwill which we think ought to exist among all members of the human family, together with the stronger affections appropriate to special relations and circumstances. And hence it may be thought that the best way of treating the subject would have been to divide Duty generally into Social and Self-regarding, and again to subdivide the former branch into the heads which I have discussed one by one; afterwards adding such minor details of duty as have obtained special names and distinct recognition. And this is perhaps the proper place to explain why I did not adopt this course. The division of duties into Social and Self-regarding, though obvious, and acceptable enough as a rough *prima facie* classification, does not on closer examination seem exactly appropriate to the Intuitional Method. For these titles naturally suggest that the happiness or well-being, of the agent or of others, is always the end and final determinant of right action: whereas the Intuitional doctrine is, that at least certain kinds of conduct are prescribed absolutely, without reference to their ulterior consequences. And if a more general meaning be given to the terms, and by Social duties we understand those which consist in the production of certain effects upon others, while in the Self-regarding we aim at producing certain effects upon ourselves, the division is still an unsuitable one. For these consequences are not clearly recognized in the enunciation of common rules of morality: and in many cases we produce marked effects both on ourselves and on others, and it is not easy to say which (in the view of Common Sense) are most important: and again, this principle of division would sometimes make it necessary to cut in two the class of duties prescribed under some common notion; as the same rule may govern both our social and our solitary conduct. Take, for example, the acts morally prescribed under the head of Courage. It seems clear that the prominence given to this Virtue in historic systems of morality has been due to the great social importance that must always attach to it, so long as communities of men are continually called upon to fight for their existence and well-being: but still the quality of bravery is the same essentially, whether it be exhibited for selfish or social ends.

It is no doubt true that when we examine with a view to definition the kinds of conduct commended or prescribed in any list of Virtues commonly recognized, we find, to a great extent, that the maxims we obtain are clearly not absolute and independent: that the quality denoted by our term is admittedly only praiseworthy in so far as it promotes individual or general welfare, and becomes blameworthy— though remaining in other respects the same—when it operates adversely to these ends. We have already noticed this result in one or two instances, and it will be illustrated at length in the following chapters. But though this is the case to a great extent, it is, for our present purpose, of special importance to note the—real or apparent—exceptions to the rule; because they are specially characteristic of the method that we call Intuitionism.

One of the most important of these exceptions is Veracity: and the affinity in certain respects of this duty—in spite of fundamental difference—to the duty of Good Faith or Fidelity to Promises renders it convenient to examine the two in immediate succession. Under either head a certain correspondence between words and facts is prescribed: and hence the questions that arise when we try to make the maxims precise are somewhat similar in both cases. For example, just as the duty of Good Faith did not lie in conforming our acts to the *admissible* meaning of certain words,[1] but to the meaning which we knew to be put on them by the promise; so the duty of Truthspeaking is not to utter words which *might*, according to common usage, produce in other minds beliefs corresponding to our own, but words which we believe will have this effect on the persons whom we address. And this is usually a very simple matter, as the natural effect of language is to convey our beliefs to other men, and we commonly know quite well whether we are doing this or not. A certain difficulty arises, as in the case of promises, from the use of set forms imposed either by law or by custom; to which most of the discussion of the similar difficulty in the preceding chapter applies with obvious modifications. In the case of formulae imposed by law—such (e.g.) as declarations of religious belief—it is doubtful whether we may understand the terms in any sense which they commonly bear, or are to take them in the sense intended by the Legislature that imposed them; and again, a difficulty is created by the gradual degradation or perversion of their meaning, which results from the strong inducements offered for their general acceptance; for thus they are continually strained and stretched until a new general understanding seems gradually to grow up as to the meaning of certain phrases; and it is continually disputed whether we may veraciously use the phrases in this new signification. A similar process continually alters the meaning of conventional expressions current in polite society. When a man declares that he 'has great pleasure in accepting' a vexatious invitation, or is 'the obedient servant' of one whom he regards as a inferior, he uses phrases which were probably once deceptive. If they are so no longer, Common Sense condemns as over-scrupulous the refusal to use them where it is customary to do so. But Common Sense seems doubtful and perplexed where the process of degradation is incomplete, and there are still persons who may be deceived: as in the use of the reply that one is 'not at home' to an inconvenient visitor from the country.

However, apart from the use of conventional phrases the rule 'to speak the truth' is not generally difficulty of application in conduct. And many moralists have regarded this, from its simplicity and definiteness, as a quite unexceptionable instance of an ethical axiom. I think, however, that patient reflection will show that this view is not really confirmed by the Common Sense of mankind.

In the first place, it does not seem clearly agreed whether Veracity is an absolute and independent duty, or a special application of some higher principle. We find (e.g.) that Kant regards it as a duty owed to oneself to speak the truth, because 'a lie is an abandonment or, as it were, annihilation of the dignity of man.' And this seems to be the view in which lying is prohibited by the code of honour, except that it is not thought (by men of honour as such) that the dignity of man is impaired by *any* lying: but only that lying for selfish ends, especially under the influence of fear, is mean and base. In fact there seems to be circumstances under which the code of honour prescribes lying. Here, however, it may be said to be plainly divergent from the morality of Common Sense. Still, the latter does not seem to decide clearly whether truth-speaking is absolutely a duty, needing no further justification: or whether it is merely a general right of each man to have truth spoken to him by his fellows, which right however may be forfeited or suspended under certain circumstances. Just as each man is thought to have a natural right to personal security generally, but not if he is himself attempting to injure others in life and property: so if we may even kill in defense of ourselves and others, it seems strange if we may not lie, if lying will defend us better against a palable invasion of our rights: and Common Sense does not seem to prohibit this decisively. And again, just as the orderly and systematic slaughter which we call war is thought perfectly right under certain circumstances, though painful and revolting: so in the word-contests of the law-courts, the lawyer is commonly held to be justified in un-truthfulness within strict rules and limits: for an advocate is thought to be over-scrupulous who refuses to say what he knows to be false, if he is instructed to say it.[2] Again, where deception is designed to benefit the person deceived, Common Sense seems to concede that it may sometimes be right: for example, most persons would not hesitate to speak falsely to an invalid, if this seemed the only way of concealing facts that might produce a dangerous shock: nor do I perceive that any one shrinks from telling fictions to children, on matters upon which it is thought well that they should not know the truth. But if the lawfulness of benevolent deception in any case be admitted, I do not see how we can decide when and how far it is admissible, except by considerations of expediency; that is, by weighing the gain of any particular deception against the imperilment of mutual confidence involved in all violation of truth.

The much argued question of religious deception ('pious fraud') naturally suggests itself here. It seems clear, however, that Common Sense now pronounces against the broad rule, that falsehoods may rightly be told in the interests of religion. But there is a subtler form in which the same principle is still maintained by moral persons. It is sometimes said that the most important truths of religion cannot be conveyed into the minds of ordinary men, except by being enclosed, as it were, in a shell of fiction; so that by relating such fictions as if they were facts, we are really performing an act of substantial veracity.[3] Reflecting upon this argument, we see that it is not after all so clear wherein Veracity consists. For from the beliefs immediately communicated by any set of affirmations inferences are naturally drawn, and we may clearly foresee that they will be drawn. And though commonly we intend that both the beliefs immediately communicated and the inferences drawn from them should be true, and a person who always aims at this is praised as candid and sincere: still we find relaxation of the rule prescribing this intention claimed in two different ways by at least respectable sections of opinion. For first, as was just now observed, it is sometimes held that if a conclusion is true and important, and cannot be satisfactorily communicated otherwise, we may lead the mind of the hearer to it by means of fictitious premises. But the exact reverse of this is perhaps a commoner view: viz. that it is only an absolute duty to make our actual affirmations true: for it is said that though the ideal condition of human converse involves perfect sincerity and candour, and we ought to rejoice in exhibiting these virtues where we can, still in our actual world concealment is frequently necessary to the well-being of society, and may be legitimately effected by any means short of actual falsehood. Thus it is not uncommonly said that in defense of a secret we may not indeed lie,[4] i.e., produce directly beliefs contrary to fact; but we may "turn a question aside," i.e., produce indirectly, by natural inference from our answer, a negatively false belief; or "throw the inquirer on a wrong scent," i.e., produce similarly a positively false belief. These two methods of concealment are known respectively as *suppressio veri* and *suggestio falsi,* and many think them legitimate under certain circumstances: while others say that if deception is to be practiced at all, it is mere formalism to object to any one mode of effecting it more than another.

On the whole, then, reflection seems to show that the rule of Veracity, as commonly accepted, cannot be elevated into a definite moral axiom: for there is no real agreement as to how far we are bound to impart true beliefs to others: and while it is contrary to Common Sense to exact absolute candour under all circumstances, we yet find no self-evident secondary principle, clearly defining when it is not to be exacted.

There is, however, one method of exhibiting *a priori* the absolute duty of Truth, which we must not overlook; as, if it be valid, it would seem that the exceptions and qualifications above mentioned have been only admitted by Common Sense from inadvertence and shallowness of thought.

It is said that if it were once generally understood that lies were justifiable under certain circumstances, it would immediately become quite useless to tell the lies, because no one would believe them; and that the moralist cannot lay down a rule which, if generally accepted, would be suicidal. To this there seem to be three answers. In the first place it is not necessarily an evil that men's confidence in each other's assertions should, *under certain peculiar circumstances,* be impaired or destroyed: it may even be the very result which we should most desire to produce: e.g., it is obviously a most effective protection for legitimate secrets that it should be universally understood and expected that those who ask questions which they have no right to ask will have lies told them: nor, again, should we be restrained from pronouncing it lawful to meet deceit with deceit, merely by the fear of impairing the security which rogues now derive from the veracity of honest men. No doubt the ultimate result of general unveracity under the circumstances would be a state of things in which such falsehoods would no longer be told: but unless this ultimate result is undesirable, the prospect of it does not constitute a reason why the falsehoods should not be told as long as they are useful. But, secondly, since the beliefs of men in general are not formed purely on rational grounds, experience shows that unveracity may long remain partially effective under circumstances where it is generally understood to be legitimate. We see this in the case of the law-courts. For though jurymen are perfectly aware that it is considered the duty of an advocate to state as plausibly as possible whatever he has been instructed to say on behalf of any criminal he may defend, still a skillful pleader may often produce an impression that he sincerely believes his client to be innocent: and it remains a question of casuistry how far this kind of hypocrisy is justifiable. But, finally, it cannot be assumed as certain that it is never right to act upon a maxim of which the universal application would be an undoubted evil. This assumption may seem to be involved in what was previously admitted as an ethical axiom, that what is right for me must be right for 'all persons under similar conditions.'[5] But reflection will show that there is a special case within the range of the axiom in which its application is necessarily self-limiting, and excludes the practical universality which the axiom appears to suggest: i.e., where the agent's conditions include (1) the knowledge that his maxim is not universally accepted, and (2) a reasoned conviction that his act will not tend to make it so, to any important extent. For in this case the axiom will practically only mean that it will be right for all persons to do as the agent does, if they are sincerely convinced that the act will not be widely imitated; and this conviction must vanish if it is widely imitated. It can hardly be said that these conditions are impossible: and if they are possible, the axiom that we are discussing can only serve, in its present application, to direct our attention to an important danger of unveracity, which constitutes a strong—but not formally conclusive utilitarian ground for speaking the truth.[6]

NOTES

1. The case where set forms are used being the *exceptio probans regulam.*
2. It can hardly be said that the advocate merely reports the false affirmations of others: since the whole force of his pleading depends upon his adopting them and working them up into a view of the case which, for the time at least, he appears to hold.
3. *E.g.,* certain religious persons hold—or held in 1873—that it is right solemnly to affirm a belief that God created the world in six days and rested on the seventh, meaning that 1:6 is the divinely ordered proportion between rest and labor.
4. Cf. Whewell, *Elements of Morality,* Book II, Chapter XV, p. 299.
5. Cf. Sidgwick, *The Methods of Ethics,* Chap. I, para. 3.
6. See Sidgwick, Book IV, Chapter V, para. 3 for further discussion of this axiom.

The dispute between Kant and Sidgwick over whether honesty is an inherent principle of ethics or only a matter of determining what will produce the best consequences is manifest dramatically in the beliefs of physicians about whether they ought to disclose traumatic diagnoses to patients, such as the discovery of a malignancy. It has long been the practice of physicians to approach the issue Hippocratically; that is, they ask themselves what they could do to benefit the patient as much as possible and protect the patient from harm. Often the answer has been that, in order to protect the patient from harm, the diagnosis of cancer or similar findings that would be very upsetting to the patient should be kept from the patient. In 1961 Donald Oken studied physicians' practices regarding disclosure of a terminal malignancy. He found that, based apparently on concern about consequences, the vast majority of physicians would not disclose the diagnosis.

During the 1970s the pattern changed. Dennis Novack and his colleagues repeated Oken's study and found almost all physicians willing to disclose such a diagnosis. Was this because they had reassessed the consequences and now believed that, because of psychological, medical, and other factors, patients are really better off knowing or do those who have changed their positions now hold that people simply have a right to know based on the inherent rightness of being honest, of giving patients the right to autonomous choice about their care?

Changes in Physicians' Attitudes Toward Telling the Cancer Patient

DENNIS H. NOVAK, ROBIN PLUMER, RAYMOND L. SMITH, HERBERT OCHITIL, GARY R. MORROW, AND JOHN M. BENNETT

In answer to a questionnaire administered in 1961, 90% of responding physicians indicated a preference for not telling a cancer patient his diagnosis. To assess attitudinal changes, the same questionnaire was submitted to 699 university-hospital medical staff. Of 264 respondents, 97% indicated a preference for telling a cancer patient his diagnosis—a complete reversal of attitude. As in 1961, clinical experience was the major policy determinant, but the 1977 population emphasized the influence of medical school and hospital training. Our respondents indicated less likelihood that they would change their present policy or be swayed by research. Clinical experience was the determining factor in shaping two opposite policies. Physicians are still basing their policies on emotion-laden personal conviction rather than the outcome of properly designed scientific studies.

A number of surveys since 1953 have investigated the physician's approach to the cancer patient regarding the issue of disclosing the diagnosis.

Of 442 physicians surveyed through the mail in 1953, 31% said they always or usually tell the patient, while 69% said they usually do not or never tell the patient. Of those who generally did not make the diagnosis known, exception occurred when the patient refused treatment or needed to plan. Of those inclined to share the diagnosis, reluctance arose when they were discouraged by the family or afraid of the patient's response.[1] In 1960, of 5,000 physicians, 16% said that they always told the patient, and 22% responded that they never told the patient. Their decisions were influenced by such factors as the stability of the patient, the insistence by the patient or family, the necessity for the patient to put affairs in order, and the unavailability of anyone else who could be told.[2]

In Oken's[3] survey of 219 physicians at Michael Reese Hospital, based on questionnaires and personal interviews, 90% generally did not inform the patient. Although more than three fourths of the group cited clinical experience as the major determinant of their policies, the data bore no relationship to length of experience or age. Many showed inconsistencies in attitudes, personal bias, and resistance to change and to further research, suggesting that emotion-laden a priori personal judgments were the real determinants of policy. Underlying were feelings of pessimism and futility about cancer.

By 1970 a questionnaire survey responded to by 178 physicians showed that 66% sometimes inform the patient, 25% always tell the patient, and only 9% never tell the patient.[4] This suggests a modification of previous practice. To assess whether this represents a genuine change, the present survey was undertaken.

METHODS

Two hundred seventy-eight, or 40% usable responses, were returned from a single mailing. Nine specialties were represented: internal medicine represented 35% of total returns; pediatrics, 7.5%; obstetrics and gynecology, 2.5%; surgery and neurosurgery, 10%; oncology, 11.7%; family practice, 2.1%; radiology, 2.1%; subspecialty, 18.7%; others, 7.9%; and specialty not indicated, 2.5%. The sample appeared to represent a cross section of specialties within the hospital's physician population, with the exceptions that oncology was slightly overrepresented, and surgery and obstetrics and gynecology were slightly underrepresented.

In comparing the 1977 and 1961 populations, the present sample had a mean age of 37 years and was 91% men, while the 1961 sample had a mean age of 50 years and was 97% men. Oken reported that the great bulk of physicians in the sample were in active private practice in addition to taking a regular part in the teaching program. Two thirds of our respondents were older than 31 years and were involved in the practice of their specialties. Many took an active role in the hospital's teaching program.

Table 1.—Physicians' Policies About Telling Cancer Patients

Exceptions	Do Not Tell, No. (%)		Tell, No. (%)	
	1977	1961	1977	1961
Never	1(0.4)	18(9)	17(7)	0(0)
Very rarely	2(0.8)	90(47)	152(61)	6(3)
Occasionally	1(0.4)	56(29)	71(28)	10(5)
Often	2(0.8)	5(3)	5(2)	8(4)
Usual policy	6(2)	169(88)	245(98)	24(12)

*1961 data from Oken.[3]

As shown in Table 1, 98% reported that their general policy is to tell the patient. Two thirds of this group say that they never or very rarely make exceptions to this rule. This stands in sharp contrast with Oken's 1961 data, which showed that 88% generally did not tell the patient, with 56% saying that they never or very rarely made exceptions to this rule.

No differences between specialties were found, with the exception that the pediatricians, while reporting that their usual policy is to tell the patient, make exceptions to this rule more frequently than other physicians. With minor exceptions this lack of specialty difference was a consistent finding for all questionnaire items.

The results seem to indicate that the many factors that went into the decision to tell the patient influenced not only whether a physician would tell the patient but also the manner in which he made the diagnosis known, perhaps influencing the timing or wording of the communication.

The four most frequent factors considered in the decision to tell the patient were age (56%), intelligence (44%), relative's wish about telling the patient (51%), and emotional stability (47%).

Four factors most frequently believed to be of special importance were the patient's expressed wish to be told (52%), emotional stability (21%), age (11%), and intelligence (10%).

Eighteen percent of the sample reported they were less likely to tell a child, while approximately 10% were inclined to tell a patient who was old or who had poor comprehension. Fourteen percent said that they would tell the patient less frequently or might delay telling if they thought the patient was prone to depression or suicide. Approximately 12% would tell the patient somewhat more frequently if personal affairs needed to be put in order.

The bases for policies in 1977 and 1961 are tabulated in Table 2.

The topic of communication with the cancer patient seems to be more frequently discussed now in medical schools and hospital training programs. Twenty-four percent of the 1977 sample vs 7% in the 1961 sample mention hospital training as sources from which policies are acquired.

Table 2.—Sources From Which Policies Were Acquired

Source	Every Source, No. (%) 1977	Every Source, No. (%) 1961	Major Source, No. (%) 1977	Major Source, No. (%) 1961
Medical school teaching	59(24)	14(7)	7(3)	0(0)
Hospital training	128(53)	72(35)	33(15)	10(5)
Clinical experience	222(92)	191(94)	153(70)	146(77)
Illness in friends or family	89(37)	61(30)	15(7)	15(8)
Other	22(9)	24(12)	10(5)	17(9)
Total	520*	362*	218(100)†	188(100)†

*More than one answer can be given by respondent.
†Figures rounded to nearest percent.

As before, clinical experience was given the major credit in both studies, with more than 90% citing it as a source and more than 70% citing it as a major source. As in Oken's data, analysis of the age of respondents citing clinical experience as a major policy determinant showed that younger physicians were just as likely to cite clinical experience as their seniors. Seventy-four percent of our group (and 86% of Oken's group) said that their policy had not changed in the past.

Thus, as in 1961, it appears that personal and emotional factors are of major importance in shaping policy, perhaps even more so in the present study. Subsequent to the general inquiry, "How did you acquire your policy?" it was specifically asked if personal issues were determinants. Seventy-one percent of the 1961 survey and 92% of the current survey reported that personal elements were involved. Again, as in 1961, these respondents were about equally divided as to whether these factors were most important. The physicians specializing in oncology (12% of total respondents) indicated that personal factors were less important in shaping their policies, suggesting that they believed there was some objective policy to be followed that was independent of personal considerations.

There is further evidence of the continuing importance of personal and emotional factors in shaping policy. Our sample evidences an even greater resistance to change and opposition to further research. Questioned about the likelihood of policy change in the future, our respondents show significantly less likelihood that they would change their policy in the future (P less than .01). Five percent said that there was no possibility of change, 48% said that change was very unlikely, although they were not sure. Only 9% said that change was probable, and 4% said that it was certain.

This resistance to change was also evident with 28% responding that their policy would not be swayed by research as opposed to 16% on Oken's sampling. Only 15% of our sample said that perhaps their policy would be changed; 29% responded this way in 1961. One of the comments seemed to sum up the general feeling: "I would not be swayed by research (but I think my opinion is correct)."

Responses to the last two survey questions are perhaps indicative of the conviction with which the present policies are held. One hundred percent (vs 60% of the 1961 sample) indicated a preference for being told if they themselves had cancer. One hundred percent thought that the patient has the right to know.

COMMENT

There appears to have been a major change in physicians' attitudes concerning telling patients their diagnosis of cancer. Even if only those physicians who believed strongly about telling the patient responded to our survey, there has still been a significant change since Oken's study. Indeed, there is some evidence that our results may be representative of more widely held views. In a recent study in which 50 patients undergoing radiotherapy were interviewed, 94% used the word "cancer" or "malignant tumor" to describe the reason for being treated. All patients were told their diagnosis by the physician who referred them for therapy.[5] How might we account for this change in attitude? Our respondents' written replies and additional comments suggest several explanations.

Therapy for many forms of cancer has notably improved in recent years. Oken's data suggested that the great majority of physicians believed that cancer connoted certain death. As many patients shared this pessimism, this common belief was often an effective deterrent to free communication. Today advances in therapy have brought longer survival, improved quality of life, and, in many cases, permanent cure. Physicians believe they can offer their cancer patients more hope.

There has been an increase in public awareness of cancer at many levels. The media are constantly presenting evidence of the ubiquity of carcinogens. Public figures such as Betty Ford and Happy Rockefeller spoke openly about their malignant neoplasms. The American Cancer Society publicizes the "Seven Danger Signals of Cancer." Perhaps all of this has led to a lesser stigmatization of cancer, a greater ease in talking about its reality, and a greater awareness of its signs and symptoms.

Oken suggested that most physicians thought that the diagnosis of cancer, with its expectation of death, deprived the patient of hope, and hence they were reluctant to tell cancer patients the diagnosis. Our data suggest that this attitude has also changed. Even when death is expected from the disease, physicians are nevertheless telling their patients the diagnosis. Perhaps improved therapy allows physicians to be overly optimistic with their patients. Perhaps some physicians feel more comfortable in relating to dying patients. At least, many understand better the dying process. This is certainly due, in part, to the recent upsurge of interest in death and dying. Good empirical studies have been done, and many authors have made important contributions to our knowledge in this field.[6–12] This knowledge may have led to more effective communication with dying patients, a reduction in the fear that the dying process necessarily engenders loss of hope, and a greater understanding of the concerns and needs of dying patients. Our data show that these issues are more frequently discussed in medical schools and hospital training programs.

Perhaps more patients are being told because more need to know. Many university hospitals are major clinical research centers, and patients who agree to participate in research protocols must be told their diagnosis to satisfy the legal requirements of informed consent. At the University of Rochester, in 1975, 15% of patients with all newly diagnosed cancer participated in national protocols.

It is impossible to know to what extent the literature on telling the cancer patient has shaped attitudes. If it has had any effect, however, it would be in the direction of encouraging frankness. Koenig[13] systematically reviewed 51 articles appearing in the professional journals between 1946 and 1966 that discussed the treatment of fatally ill patients. He concluded that the tendency of authors appears to be strongly in favor of informing fatally ill patients of their conditions. This has been more recently reaffirmed by Cassem and Stewart,[14] who, in suggesting a general policy of frankness, cite two sets of empirical studies. The first set includes those studies in which patients were asked whether or not they should be told. These indicate overwhelming positive favor for telling. The second set looks at the effects of telling on patients and their families. These studies dispelled the myth of the harm that telling the patient might engender.

The comments of some of our respondents indicate that the reason for the present reversal in attitude is due, in part, to more sweeping social changes. The rise in the consumerism movement and increasing public scrutiny of the medical profession have altered the physician-patient relationship. In this era of "patient's rights," an attitude of frankness feels right and, indeed, given the current disputatious atmosphere of medical practice, may be the safest one to adopt.

Many questions remain. Do physicians tell patients they have "cancer," or are euphemisms such as "tumor" or "growth" still widely used, and if so what does that mean for the communication process? Are changing attitudes on telling the patient accompanied by the emotional support that a patient's knowledge of his diagnosis may demand of a physician? Saunders[15] wrote, "The real question is not 'What do you tell your patients?' but rather, "What do you let your patients tell you?'" Now that we tell our patients more, are we also listening more? Unfortunately one survey cannot answer these questions.

Is the present policy of telling the patient the best policy? The majority of our respondents cite clinical experience as shaping their present policy, even though most of them have never had experience with another policy. The majority of Oken's respondents also cited clinical experience in shaping the exact opposite policy. While not discounting the value of clinical experience, its use as a determinant of policy must be called into question.

Our data suggest that, as in Oken's study, the present policy is supported by strong belief and emotional investment in its being right. One hundred percent of our respondents stated that patients have a right to know. Yet in asserting this in a blanket manner, are physicians sometimes abdicating a responsibility to make subtle judgments in individual cases? Do patients also have a right not to know?

Is it possible to determine who should be told what, when, and how? What are the criterions by which we judge if telling is right? Patient evaluation in future studies on telling might include assessments of compliance with the medical regimen, quality of communication with physician and family members, ratings of adjustment to illness, or psychological tests of depression and anxiety.

Our respondents' written comments seem to indicate that the current policy of telling the patient is accompanied by increased sensitivity to patients' emotional needs. There is some evidence that telling is the best policy.[16] Yet how rational is the process of deciding what to tell the patient with cancer? Even though the policies have reversed, many physicians are still basing their communication with cancer patients on emotion-laden personal convictions. They are relying on honesty, sensitivity, and patients' rights rather than focusing on the following relevant scientific psychological question: Does telling the diagnosis of cancer help or harm (which) patients and how? Only further systematic research can answer these question.

NOTES

1. Fitts, W. T., Jr., Ravdin IS. "What Philadelphia Physicians Tell Patients with Cancer." *Journal of the American Medical Association* 153:901–904, 1953.
2. Rennick, D. (ed). "What Should Physicians Tell Cancer Patients?" *N Med Material* 2:51–53, 1960.
3. Oken, D. "What to Tell Cancer Patients: A Study of Medical Attitudes." *Journal of the American Medical Association* 175:1120–1128, 1961.
4. Friedman, H. S. "Physician Management of Dying Patients: An Exploration." *Psychiatry Med* 1:295–305, 1970.
5. Mitchell, G. W., and A. S. Glicksman. "Cancer Patients: Knowledge and Attitudes." *Cancer* 40:61–66, 1977.
6. Feifel, H. (ed). *The Meaning of Death.* New York: McGraw-Hill, 1959.
7. Saunders, C. "Care of the Dying." *Nursing Times* 55:960–995, ff. 1031, 1959.
8. Hinton, J. M. *Dying.* Baltimore: Penguin Books, 1967.
9. Glaser, B. G., and A. C. Strauss. *Awareness of Dying.* Chicago: Aldine Publishing, 1965.
10. Kubler-Ross, E. *On Death and Dying.* New York: Macmillan, 1969.
11. Engel, G. L. "Psychological Responses to Major Environmental Stress." In *Psychological Development in Health and Disease.* Philadelphia: Saunders, 1962, pp. 272–305.
12. Greene, W. A. "The Physician and His Dying Patient." In *The Patient, Death and the Family,* edited by S. B. Troupe and W. C. Greene. New York: Scribner's, 1974, pp. 85–99.
13. Koenig, R. R. "Anticipating Death from Cancer—Physician and Patient Attitudes." *Michigan Medicine* 68:899–905, 1969.
14. Cassem, N. H., and R. S. Stewart. "Management and Care of the Dying Patient." *International Journal of Psychiatry in Medicine* 6:293–304, 1975.
15. Saunders, C. "The Moment of Truth: Care of the Dying Person." In *Death and Dying,* edited by L. Pearson. Cleveland: Case Western Reserve University Press, 1969, pp. 49–78.
16. Gerle, B., G. Landen, and P. Sandblom. "The Patient with Inoperable Cancer from the Psychiatric and Social Standpoint." *Cancer* 13:1206–1217, 1960.

Thus far the principles of promise-keeping and honesty or veracity have been considered as principles of actions that make them right. Both were proposed by W. D. Ross. One characteristic of action that many now consider to be inherently right-making is respect for another person's autonomy. According to this view, even if one is certain that interfering with another's autonomous choices will do more good for that person than respecting them, there is still some moral reason to forego intervening. Some people consider respect for autonomy along with fidelity to promises and honesty to be aspects of a broader principle of respect for persons while others see them as more independent. The following excerpt from James Childress's volume on paternalism spells out what is meant by autonomy.

Autonomy

JAMES CHILDRESS

One aspect of respecting persons is respecting their *autonomy;* this is an implication of respecting persons as independent ends in themselves. Etymologically, "autonomy" is compounded of *autos* (self) and *nomos* (law or rule). *Autonomia* originally was used to indicate the independence of Greek city-states from outside control, perhaps from a conqueror, and their determination of their own laws. The notions of independence, self-rule, and self-determination recur in explications of "autonomy," and their analysis is essential if we are to understand "what is essentially a metaphor."

It is customary to contrast "autonomy" and "heteronomy," "autonomy" referring to self-rule and "heteronomy" referring to rule by other objects or persons. Heteronomous persons, for example, might have surrendered their judgment-making and decision-making to the state or to the church; their actions would be heteronomous because they would be determined by what the state or the church dictates. But although such persons may fall short of the ideal of autonomy (which will be discussed later), they may have exercised and even continued to exercise autonomy in the choice of the state or the church as the source of their judgments and decisions. Thus, there is an important distinction between *first-order* and *second-order* autonomy.[1] Persons who are subservient to state or church would lack first-order autonomy, i.e., self-determination regarding the content of decisions and choices, because of their exercise of second-order autonomy, i.e., selection of the institution to which they are subordinate. In other situations, first-order choices and actions such as the use of some drugs may appear to be under inner compulsion or addiction. But these agents retain some *second-order* autonomy: when they are made aware of their condition, they may choose to seek help or to remain under compulsion or addiction because they want to. As Gerald Dworkin contends, a person who is a drug addict and cannot break his physiological dependence on the drug, and yet who wants to be under this compulsion, is autonomous at least in this second-order sense, for he identifies with *his* addiction.[2]

Autonomy does not imply that an individual's life plan is his or her own creation and that it excludes interest in others. The first implication focuses on the *source,* the second on the *object* of autonomy.[3] Neither implication holds. Autonomy simply means that a person chooses and acts freely and rationally out of her own life plan, however ill-defined. That this life plan is her own does not imply that she created it de novo or that it was not decisively influenced by various factors such as family and friends. Some existentialists who use the language of autonomy suggest that if an individual does not create his own life plan, or at least an independent series of choices, he is guilty of "bad faith." Recall Jean-Paul Sartre's advice to the young man who was trying to decide whether to join the Free French Forces or to remain to help his mother: "You're free, choose, that is, invent."[4] More satisfactory interpretations of autonomy recognize that it may be rooted in both society and history. The source of an individual's life plan may well be, for example, a religious tradition with which he identifies and which he appropriates. An example is a Jehovah's Witness' life plan which gives everlasting life priority over earthly life if the latter can be maintained only by blood transfusions. Thus, personal autonomy does not imply on asocial or ahistorical approach to life plans. It only means that whatever the life plan, and whatever its source, an individual takes it as his own.

Likewise, the object of autonomous life plans and choices is not limited to the individual himself or herself but may include various principles and values such as altruistic beneficence. Autonomy does not presuppose that the individual is uninterested in the positive or negative impact on others. For example, some discussions of autonomous suicide seem to suppose that the agent is acting autonomously only if she is uninterested in an impact on others. But the agent may view the act of suicide primarily as expression and communication. This was certainly true of Jo Roman, who committed suicide in order to create "on [her] own terms the final stroke of [her] life's canvas". A 62-year-old artist, she had originally planned to commit suicide on her seventy-fifth birthday but acted earlier because of her breast cancer. In addition, she carefully staged her suicide in order to have a public impact, particularly to convince others that "life can be transformed into art."[5] Her desire for expression and communication did not, however, make her act less autonomous. It is a distortion of autonomy to limit the object to the agent's own self. Both points can be summarized: in terms of input and output, autonomy is not asocial or ahistorical. Both communication and influence occur both ways.

Does this analysis of autonomy imply the "separateness of persons," a conception that undergirds several recent critiques of utilitarianism? According to these criticisms, utilitarianism tends to view separate individuals as having only instrumental, not intrinsic, value as either depositors or depositories of good. Against utilitarianism, they emphasize either the separateness of agents or the separateness of recipients or patients (i.e., those acted upon). In the former, the emphasis will be on the patient's rights.[6] But because the separateness of persons tends to suggest an atomistic individualism, it is better to focus on the distinctiveness of persons, while recognizing that both their sources and their objects may be social.

Respect for persons who are autonomous may differ from respect for persons who are not autonomous. Formal equality, sometimes referred to as the formal principle of justice, demands that similar cases be treated similarly and that equals be treated equally. But because it does not specify relevant similarities or dissimilarities, it is formal and thus empty until it receives material content from other sources. My interpretation of the principle of respect for persons identifies autonomy as one relevant similarity. When persons are autonomous, respect for them requires (or prohibits) certain actions that may not be required (or prohibited) in relation to nonautonomous persons. Several principles, particularly nonmaleficence, may establish minimum standards of conduct, such as noninfliction of harm in relation to all persons whatever their degree of autonomy. But what the principle of respect requires (and prohibits) in relation to autonomous persons will differ. Thus Kant excluded children and the insane from his discussion of the principle of respect of persons and Mill applied his discussion of liberty only to those who are in "The maturity of their faculties."[7] I will examine some aspects or criteria of autonomy before considering some specific requirements of respect for autonomous persons.

Two essential features of autonomy are (1) acting freely and (2) deliberating rationally. I will provide only a brief statement of these features which will be discussed in more detail in subsequent chapters. First, what is the relationship between competence and these two features of autonomy? Logically competence might be viewed as a precondition of deliberating rationally and acting freely or as a summary term for these two (and perhaps other) conditions. A person suffering from mental defects, for example, that would preclude either acting freely or deliberating rationally would be incompetent to make decisions. Competence is not an all or nothing matter. It may vary over time and from situation to situation. A person may be competent part of the time but incompetent the rest of the time; this will be called intermittent competence. And a person may be competent to act in X (e.g., to drive a car) but not in Y (e.g., to make decisions in a large family-operated business); this will be called limited competence.[8] One difficult question that will occupy out attention in later chapters is which way to err in borderline cases of competence.

ACTING FREELY

To act freely is, in part, to be outside the control of others. This point is implied by independence, and it excludes coercion, duress, undue influence, and manipulation. If a person is coerced—"your money or your life"—she is not acting freely even though she is deliberating rationally and acting intentionally. But, as we have seen, a person may exercise second-order autonomy by freely choosing to become dependent on a religious community for moral guidance. For example, a woman may decide not to have an abortion to save her life because she freely accepts the authority of the Catholic Church. To act freely also involves the absence of certain internal constraints such as compulsion and drug addiction. A person's action can be seriously encumbered or limited by either internal or external constraints that he or she cannot be said to be autonomous.

Indeed, internal constraints, for example, may be so severe that we do not hold the agent responsible for what he does. In some cases although the agent was causally responsible for what occurred, we do not hold him morally or legally responsible because he lacked the capacity for responsibility. Nonetheless a general use of the language of disease to discount responsibility for wrongful conduct is a sign of disrespect for persons:

> A *total* reinterpretation of wrong doing in terms of disease amounts to a denial of personal responsibility altogether. It *insults* the wrongdoer under the guise of *safeguarding* his interests. It treats him as though he were *not* a person, and falls foul accordingly of the very principle of respect to which it appeals. This is the element of vital truth in the doctrine which to many has seemed merely a bad joke, that a man has a *right* to be punished.[9]

DELIBERATING RATIONALLY

Deliberation is "an imaginative rehearsal of various courses of action."[10] It can be encumbered or limited in various ways, particularly by a person's inability to reason because of mental illness or to reason fully because of inadequate or incomplete information about various courses of action and their consequences. It is possible in some cases to judge that a person's deliberation is irrational without calling into question the life plans, values, and ends on which the deliberation is based and without calling into question the weighting of the alternatives and their consequences. For example, a person may seek incompatible ends (such as preservation of a gangrenous leg) or choose ineffective means to his ends.[11] Suppose two patients refuse amputations of gangrenous feet, one because she wants to die and the other because she does not believe that the condition is fatal. In the latter case there may be grounds for holding that the patient is not deliberating rationally and thus is not autonomous. Nevertheless, as Bruce Miller reminds us, it is not always possible to separate factual and valuative errors in nonrational deliberation.

> A patient may refuse treatment because of its pain and inconvenience, e.g. Kidney dialysis, and choose to run the risk of serious illness and death. To say that such a patient has the relevant knowledge, if all other alternatives and their likely consequences have been explained, but that non-rational assignment of priorities has been made is much too simple. A good accurate characterization may be that the patient misappreciates certain as-

pects of the alternatives. The patient may be cognitively aware of the pain and inconvenience of the treatment, but because he or she has not experienced them, the assessment of their severity may be too great. If the patient has begun dialysis, assessment of the pain and inconvenience may not take into account the possibilities that the patient will adapt to them or that they may be reduced by adjustments in the treatment. Misappreciating the consequences of treatment in this way is not a lack of knowledge, nor is it simply a non-rational weighting; it involves matters of fact and value.[12]

In addition, even when it is possible to identify errors in factual beliefs, it may be difficult to determine that the person is not autonomous.

Several philosophers have used the notion of authenticity to explicate autonomy. For example, Gerald Dworkin views autonomy as authenticity plus independence, while Bruce Miller identifies four aspects of autonomy as free action, authenticity, effective deliberation, and moral reflection. For Dworkin, authenticity is a person's identification with the determinants of his behavior so that they become *his* own. For Miller, it means that "an action is consistent with the attitudes, values, dispositions and life plans of the person."[13] The intuitive idea of authenticity is "acting in character." We wonder whether actions are autonomous if they are not consistent with what we know about a person (e.g., a sudden and unexpected decision to discontinue dialysis by a man who had displayed considerable courage and zest for life despite his years of disability). If they are in character (e.g., a Jehovah's Witness' refusal of a blood transfusion), we are less likely to suspect that they do not represent genuine autonomy. In addition, the notion of authenticity captures our sense that selves develop over time with persistent and enduring patterns; they are not simply collections of choices and acts. And yet it would be a mistake to make authenticity a criterion of autonomy. At most authenticity alerts us to relevant questions. If it is not satisfied, if the choice or action (such as refusal of treatment) is inconsistent with what we know of the person and his character, then we should seek justifications or explanations, some of which may indicate that the action is not autonomous (perhaps because it was under inner compulsion). We should also consider whether the person has experienced a change or even conversion in basic values and life plan and even whether we really knew the person as well as we previously thought. Actions apparently out of character and inauthentic can be caution flags that alert others to press for justifications and explanations in order to determine whether the actions are autonomous. By contrast, actions that are not free cannot count as autonomous.

An important distinction, drawn from Robert Nozick, may help to clarify the meaning of the principle of respect for persons: (1) autonomy as an end state or goal and (2) autonomy as a side constraint.[14] Frequently debates about paternalism are confused because all parties appeal to autonomy to justify their proposals without attending to differences that result from viewing autonomy as an end state as opposed to a side constraint. If autonomy is a *side constraint*, it limits the pursuit of goals such as health and survival; it even limits the pursuit of the goal of the preservation and restoration of autonomy itself. In pursuing goals for ourselves or for others we are not permitted to violate others' autonomy. Because what we do, not merely what happens is morally important, or nonviolation of autonomy is required. Whether autonomy is an absolute limit would depend on the moral theory; perhaps it could be violated in order to prevent a catastrophe. In contrast, when autonomy is viewed as an end state to be realized, its function in moral argument is very different. Autonomy is a condition, not a constraint, and the goal might be to minimize damage to autonomy whether that damage results from nature, disease, or other persons. In this view, some violations of autonomy (such as some decisions to reject patients' refusals of treatment) might be justified because overall more autonomy would result, and that is the desirable end state.

Eric Cassell, a strong proponent of autonomy, views it mainly as an end state rather that as a side constraint. He contends that autonomy (for which he uses Gerald Dworkin's formula, autonomy = authenticity + independence) is seriously compromised by illness, "the most important thief of autonomy," and that the primary function of medicine is to preserve, to repair, and to restore the patient's autonomy. When we are sick, our autonomy is greatly diminished because we are not "ourselves," our freedom of choice is limited, our knowledge is incomplete, and our reason is impaired. Although Cassell emphasizes the importance of relationships with family, friends, and physicians, he affirms that the best way to restore autonomy is "to cure the patient of the disease that impairs autonomy and return him to his normal life."[15]

To be sure, autonomy is an important end state of health care that professionals should pursue for their patients in order to benefit them. But it is an end state that individuals may autonomously choose not to pursue. By expanding the notion of autonomy to include freedom from the effects of disease,[16] and by conceiving it as a goal rather that as a right, Cassell fails to address the most important and difficult question: Can autonomy as a goal override autonomy as a right? Or does autonomy as a side constraint preclude its violation even to achieve the end state of restored or increased autonomy? The principle of respect for persons requires that autonomy be conceived as a side constraint and as a right, rather that as an end state, even if it does not establish an absolute limit (an issue that I will consider later). Pursuit of another's autonomy as an end state may be an important goal of altruistic beneficence, but the patient, rather that the agent, should determine how important it is.

The *ideal* of autonomy, especially moral autonomy, is neither a presupposition nor an implication of the principle of respect for persons, however much we admire persons who realize or approximate this ideal, so widely praised in the tradition of Western individualism. Recognition of this ideal and praise for the "autonomous person" would require additional premises that are not required for a defense of autonomy as a side constraint without denying the burden of autonomy for individuals and the importance of community and tradition. Gerald Dworkin argues that the ideal of moral autonomy

> represents a particular conception of morality—one that, among other features, places a heavy emphasis on rules and principles rather that

virtues and practices. Considered purely internally there are conceptual, moral, and empirical difficulties in defining and elaborating a conception of autonomy which is coherent and provides us with an ideal worthy of pursuit. It is only through a more adequate understanding of notions such as tradition, authority, commitment, and loyalty, and of the forms of human community in which these have their roots, that we shall be able to develop a conception of autonomy free from paradox and worthy of admiration.[17]

My argument is that the principle of respect for persons requires that we construe autonomy as a constraint upon our pursuit of goals for ourselves or for others' wishes, choices, and actions in that they constrain and limit our pursuit of goals, whether these goals are for them, for others, or for ourselves, without committing ourselves to the goal of promoting autonomy or to the ideal of autonomous existence.

NOTES

1. Dworkin, Gerald. "Autonomy and Behavior Control," *Hastings Center Report* 6:23, February 1976; for an important discussion, see Harry G. Frankfurt. "Freedom of the Will and the Concept of a Person." *Journal of Philosophy* 58:5–20, 14 January 1971. Frankfurt argues that "it is having second-order volitions [when one wants a certain desire to be his will], and not having second-order desires generally that I regard as essential to being a person" (p. 10). Yet reason is presupposed because it is "only in virtue of his rational capacities that a person is capable of becoming critically aware of his own will and of forming volitions of the second order" (p. 12).
2. Dworkin, "Autonomy and Behavior Control," p. 25.
3. For use of this distinction between *source* and *object* in relation to ethical individualism, see Lukes, Steven. *Individualism.* New York: Harper & Row, 1973, Chap. 15.
4. Sartre, Jean-Paul. "Existentialism." In *Existentialism and Human Emotions.* New York: Philosophical Library, 1957, pp. 24f.
5. See " 'Rational Suicide'?" *Newsweek,* 2 July 1979, 87; Laurie Johnston, "Artist Ends Her Life. . . ." *The New York Times,* 17 June 1979; and *Choosing Suicide,* a Documentary on PBS, 16 June 1980.
6. As a matter of emphasis, Bernard Williams represents the former, while Robert Nozick represents the latter. Also, see the illuminating discussion of the debate about the separateness of persons by Hart, H. L. A. "Between Utility and Rights." in *The Idea of Freedom: Essays in Honour of Isaiah Berlin,* edited by Alan Ryan, 77–98. Oxford: Oxford University Press, 1979.
7. See Kant, *The Doctrine of Virtue,* p. 122; and Mill, *On Liberty,* edited by Gertrude Himmelfarb. Harmondsworth, Eng.: Penguin, 1976. For an argument that paternalistic treatment is not necessarily incompatible with a concern to respect moral autonomy, see Husak, Douglas N. "Paternalism and Autonomy." *Philosophy and Public Affairs* 10:27–46, Winter 1981.
8. For a fuller discussion of competence, including these terms, see Beauchamp, Tom L. and James F. Childress. *Principles of Biomedical Ethics.* New York: Oxford University Press, 1979, Chapter 3. I do not treat competence as merely or primarily a legal matter, although the law has much to say about it.
9. Maclagan. "Respect for Persons as a Moral Principle," p. 301.

10. Dewey, John. *Theory of the Moral Life.* New York: Holt, Rinehart & Winston, 1960, p. 135.

11. Mabbott, J. B. "Reason and Desire." *Philosophy* 28:113–123, 1953.

12. Miller. "Autonomy and the Refusal of Life-Saving Treatment." *Hastings Center Report* 11:22–28, August 1981.

13. Dworkin, G. "Autonomy and Behavior Control"; and Miller. "Autonomy and the Refusal of Life-Saving Treatment."

14. This distinction is developed by Nozick, Robert. *Anarchy, State, and Utopia.* New York: Basic Books, 1974, pp. 28–35. I use it for analytical purposes without accepting his normative theory.

15. I have drawn this statement of Cassell's postion from his article "The Function of Medicine." *Hastings Center Report* 7:16–19, December 1977. See also his *The Healer's Art: A New Approach to the Doctor-Patient Relationship.* Philadelphia: Lippincott, 1976. Elsewhere he also considers cases of chronic care: "Naturally, autonomy is best served by a return to health. Increasingly, however, success in medicine does not mean a return to normalcy as it did with the infectious diseases. Rather, we are successful when patients requiring continuing care are able to function and live their lives with the least possible interference from their diseases or their medical care." Cassell. "Autonomy and Ethics in Action." *New England Journal of Medicine* 297:333–334, 11 August 1977. His discussion of cases sometimes expresses appreciation of autonomy as a side constraint, which is usually absent from his more theoretical statements.

16. This sort of expansion shifts the argument away from human interactions to conditions and goals: people are less autonomous when they are sick. While it is true that people are affected in various ways when they are sick, including having their options more severely limited, they can still be self-determining within these conditions. That is the important point, sometimes obscured by Cassell's contention that a sick person is not simply a person with a disease added on but a "sick person." See *The Healer's Art.*

17. Dworkin, Gerald. "Moral Autonomy." In *Morals, Science and Sociality, Vol. III of The Foundations of Ethics and Its Relationship to Science,* edited by H. Tristram Engelhardt, Jr., and Daniel Callahan, 170. Hastings-on-Hudson, N.Y.: The Hastings Center, 1978. p. 170.

The principle of autonomy has gained increasing importance in contemporary medical ethics as the philosophical system of secular liberalism begins to replace more paternalistic Hippocratic assumptions. It is manifest most conspicuously in the moral defense of the requirement that patients consent to any treatment and that they have a moral right to refuse treatment by withholding or withdrawing their consent.

The following essay shows how the notion of informed consent can be grounded in various ethical principles including Hippocratic beneficence (patient welfare), more general beneficence (total net good considering the effects on everyone), and autonomy. The differences in the principles are manifest in cases where respecting autonomy may do harm to the individual patient or to society.

Why Get Consent?

Robert M. Veatch

Members of the Human Experimentation Committee in a large inner-city hospital debated hotly over whether it was necessary to obtain consent when researchers took placentas for their research from clinic patients in the course of normal childbirth. Some felt strongly that consent should be obtained from the women. Others objected, saying they felt this was another example of over-protectionist ethics obstructing scientific progress. It was not necessary, they said, to inform the patients that the placentas were to be used in research rather than being discarded.

The use of the placentas, or other experiments with body wastes such as tissue removed during routine surgery, raises the question of why we get consent in the first place. Is consent required only to protect the human subjects of medical research from possible harm, or does it serve some other purpose?

The fact that this issue is so controversial implies that something fundamental is at stake. Let us concede at the outset that at least some of this research has potential value to humans, and that risks to those from whom the wastes are taken are negligible. Some institutions routinely make use of human blood, urine, and feces as well as skin, organs, and internal tissues in their scientific investigations. The increasing use of waste body tissues has been justified by one of the fundamental principles of the ethics of experimentation with humans—that the potential benefits to the subject and/or the value of the knowledge to be gained must outweigh the risks to the subject and cannot be carried out in another way that involves less risk to the subject.

The issue has been complicated, however, by the growing influence of the principle of informed consent. Since the mid-1940s, when the Nuremburg Code was formulated following the Nazi war crimes trial, researchers have been expected to obtain consent from subjects of medical research. In the late 1960s the Department of Health, Education, and Welfare developed regulations regarding human subjects. Consent was required for most kinds of research on human subjects carried out with HEW funds. Although these regulations helped the notion of informed consent, they did not resolve the question of consent for the use of waste body tissues.

If the object of consent is to protect the subject, then it appears foolish—and even an obstruction of scientific progress—to demand that researchers get consent to use body wastes. In this case, consent must have an object that goes beyond protecting the human subject. I am convinced what is at issue is a disagreement about the basic principles of medical research itself.

Those who feel it is not necessary to obtain consent for the use of a placenta appear to base their justification on the central principle of the Hippocratic Oath—that the physician's duty is to do what he thinks will benefit the patient. If patient protection is the physician's duty, they reason, and the purpose of consent is to avoid harm, then consent is not necessary, since no harm is envisioned.

It is not that simple however. Even when the researcher actually believes there is no risk, consent may protect the subject. It is inevitable that errors will sometimes occur, either because the researcher incorrectly evaluates the risks or fails to concede they exist. To provide protection in such cases, the rule, "Get consent even when you think the subject is not at risk," may protect the subject. Some risks may actually be involved in contributing wastes such as placentas and urine—the risk of going to another part of the hospital, or the risk that illegal drugs might be found in the urine, for example.

There is also a more fundamental problem associated with the classical principle of benefitting the patient. While it might justify waiving consent, it will rule out the experiment as well, except in cases where the subject stands to benefit from the research. That is why the Nuremburg Code and HEW have had to abandon the old, individualistic patient-benefit principle in favor of a more socially-oriented concern. Even if the individual subject does not stand to benefit directly, the research could be justified by the classic "utilitarian" principle of the greatest good for the greatest number. By itself, however, this principle would justify conducting very risky research without subject consent—provided the potential benefits to society are great enough. Accordingly, the Nuremburg Code adopted the principle of social benefit, recognizing that the human is a social animal with responsibilities to the human community. It did, however, subordinate it to a very strongly worded principle of consent. The key point is that legally, such contributions to society are permitted, but they are not required even if there is great potential benefit.

Why is consent required if the goal is to benefit society? It simply may be that consent itself would benefit society in the long run. Consent not only minimizes gross risks, it reassures the public that subjects are reasonably safe because they will at least be informed of potential risks. This is important—especially in an urban hospital where the medical community in general, and the research community in particular, are already under suspicion. Consent, even for experiments using waste body tissues, may in the long run actually serve the interests of the research enterprise by assuring a supply of volunteers. It may even avoid community pressures to stop using the hospital as a research facility.

But this does not seem to be the primary reason for the heavy emphasis on consent in the Nuremburg Code. At least in the modern West, human freedom is valued independently of social utility. It seems reasonable that the consent requirement has its roots in this belief, although the principle of self-determination is not equally central to all cultural or social groups. More authoritarian societies seem not to uphold its importance. The medical profession, at least in its classical codes, gives the principle very little attention. And research committees may tend to put more emphasis on "protecting human subjects" from physical or mental harm, and less emphasis on their subjects' right to self-determination. That, however does not imply that subjects or society in general do not consider subject self-determination crucial.

While the principle of autonomy requires consent independent of whether there is risk to the subject, it cannot, by itself, justify research. Benefitting society is a legitimate consideration. Potential gain to society is essential for research to be ethical. But that gain must be subordinated to, or at least filtered through the principle of individual autonomy. Research is justified when it will benefit the patient and/or society, only when an autonomous subject or guardian for that subject permits the research. The mere fact that the subject will not be harmed physically cannot justify abandoning this principle of autonomy.

Informed consent requires informing the patient of the nature and purpose of the experiments. While this knowledge may not be relevant to subject risk, it is necessary in order for the subject to exercise self-determination. The fact that a woman from whom a placenta has been taken is not at risk should not mean she should be deprived of the right to determine whether she wants to cooperate in achieving an objective. It is quite conceivable that a patient might object to experiments in genetic testing or hypothetically, to the development of techniques for blood or urine screening for IQ.

Social benefits from medical research are potentially great, and reasonable people should not normally refuse to participate if there are no costs to themselves. But the principle of self-determination is also fundamental. Getting consent to use a patient's body wastes preserves this principle. If it is feared that requesting consent will produce many refusals, then the information is indeed important to the subjects and consent is all the more imperative. It does seem reasonable that at least some people would want to know whether their tissues are being used in research. Those who want to preserve autonomy will support consent whether or not there is thought to be a risk.

As can be seen from the above discussion, three principles can be applied to the decision about whether to require consent for the use of body wastes. Each is plausible, and each leads to a unique solution of the problem. The three principles can be summarized as: consent should benefit the patient and/or protect him from harm; consent should benefit society; consent should protect the subject's right to self-determination.

Killing and Prolonging Life

INTRODUCTION

The principles of medical ethics that we have examined thus far (beneficence, fidelity to promises, veracity, and autonomy), do not complete the list of possible principles for a medical ethic. It is often said that a central principle of medical ethics has something to do with prolonging life, the notion that life is sacred, that killing is morally wrong. The question addressed in the two essays in this chapter is whether there is some additional principle in medical ethics that reflects this perception.

The first question is whether physicians have actually held historically that they have a duty to prolong life, and, if so, under what circumstances. Of course, we have already seen that Hippocratic ethics holds that the physician's duty is to do what the physician believes is beneficial to the patient. That is a form of the principle of beneficence. Often preserving the life of the patient will be beneficial; avoiding killing the patient is a good thing for the patient. The morally interesting case, however, is the special situation where the physician perceives that the patient has been so afflicted with illness that prolonging the patient's life will actually do him no good and may, in fact, do him harm. Some physicians may go even further to maintain that some patients are suffering intractably so that they are better off, all things considered, if they are mercifully killed. The first question, then, is whether physicians have held that in such cases they have a duty to prolong life or avoid killing even when such interventions cannot be justified on the grounds that it is doing the patient good.

Determining what physicians have traditionally held about preserving life and killing is only the first step in understanding the ethics of these morally vital issues in medicine. Regardless of what traditional physician ethics has held, it is necessary to establish whether preserving life or avoiding killing is morally an independent right-making characteristic of action. Some scholars have insisted that this is a question that ought to be answered by examining the consequences—to see whether avoiding killing or preserving life does good. A pure consequentialist would hold that in order to decide whether it is right to kill someone or to preserve someone's life, one needs to examine the results. Since normally preserving life has good results and killing has bad ones, the answer usually is that life should be preserved. When preserving life leaves the patient unconscious or, worse, in severe pain, some would hold that life should then not be preserved while others would hold that, even then that morally it is right to preserve life.

Many people hold that in such circumstances life need not be preserved, especially against the wishes of the patient, but that it is still wrong to kill even if doing so would relieve the individual of severe pain. These people make a distinction between killing and letting die. One of the great arguments in medical ethics today is over whether there is any moral difference between killing and letting die. People who hold that acts are judged solely on their consequences usually hold there is no difference, while those who accept other right-making characteristics sometimes hold on to the difference between the two. This might be, as in the essay presented here, on the grounds that the consequences of acting on the rule that distinguishes killing and letting die are different from the rule that makes no distinction (even if there are no discernable differences in individual cases). Others—including many working in Jewish and Catholic traditions as well as many secular thinkers—hold that killing is simply a wrong-making characteristic of action independent of consideration of consequences. Those who take the latter view would add avoiding killing (but not life preservation) to their list of principles of ethics.

The first issue needing attention is whether physicians have believed historically in the Hippocratic tradition that they have a duty to preserve life. Historian and classicist Darrel Amundsen argues that there was no such duty in Hippocratic medicine; that the duty, as it is perceived in modern medicine, comes from other more recent sources.

The Physician's Obligation to Prolong Life: A Medical Duty without Classical Roots

DARREL W. AMUNDSEN

Is the physician's duty to prolong life a modern phenomenon, or does it have its roots in Hippocratic or other strains of classical medicine? First, we must ask, what is meant by the phrase "the physician's duty to prolong life"? If this question were put to a physician in classical antiquity, he might reasonably ask whether, by prolonging life, we mean increasing longevity generally; preserving health by prophylaxis; combating curable diseases and injuries; temporarily prolonging the unhealthy life of a terminally ill patient; or refusing to assist in terminating the life of any man with or without his consent, whether healthy or ill, and if ill, whether a painful but curable or an incurable ailment.

He might also ask what we mean by life. Would we limit the term to useful, productive, happy, and healthy life; to that of the citizen, the foreigner, the freeman, the slave? And of the word "duty" he might quite rightly ask: "Duty to whom? to the patient, even against the patient's wishes? to the medical art or profession? to the public opinion, to the state, to religion? to his own conscience, simply as a man, or as a physician?"

This list of hypothetical questions is by no means exhaustive, and of course most of them are still being asked. But there are a few that may seem slightly alien to modern considerations. We should first, at least indirectly, address our attention to these questions for they will provide us with a heightened awareness of some important differences between the ethos of the classical world and that of modern Western cultures.

PHYSICIANS IN CLASSICAL ANTIQUITY

The practice of medicine was a right, not a privilege, in classical antiquity. It remained so in the Western world until some geographically limited licensure requirements were instituted beginning in the twelfth century. There was no system of medical licensure and anyone who wished to could set himself up as practitioner of the healing arts. Therefore, one can speak of a "medical profession" in classical Greece and Rome only in the sense that the phrase designates the aggregate of those who called themselves physicians. This designation does not exclude those medical practitioners or schools of medical theory and practice that seem to us, and may have seemed to some contemporary practitioners, to typify charlatanism rather than medical professionalism.Given this qualification, it should come as no surprise that the phrase "ethics of the profession" can be very misleading. There were no professional standards that were enforceable by law or by inclusive medical organizations. Although certain exclusive medical societies set standards of conduct for their members, at no time was the swearing of any oath or the acceptance of any informal or formal code of ethics required of anyone calling himself a physician and undertaking to treat patients.

This is not to say there were no ethical standards; diverse examples are evident in both medical and lay classical literature. But those that seem consonant with modern medical ethics or appear as "timeless ideals" of medicine may have been held by only an unrepresentative minority of medical practitioners at any given time during the classical period.

What was the physician, the *iatros* of the Greek, the *medicus* of the Roman? By the most basic definition, he was one who practiced the art of preserving or restoring health. If the primary function of the classical physician was preserving or restoring health, ideally he should be a compassionate man. When I say "ideally," I am thinking in terms of the "ideal" physician as he appears, at least in simile and metaphor, especially in philosophical or political literature. When thus used, the word "physician" was not a neutral term, but denoted a "compassionate, objective, unselfish man, dedicated to his responsibilities." In this manner the good ruler, legislator or statesman was sometimes called the physician of the state; essentially, "the statesman should be to the state what the physician is to his patient."[1]

Although some of the medical literature deals with etiquette, little is said about the "ideal" physician or the moral basis for medical practice. In the Hippocratic Corpus appears the statement, "Where there is love of man, there is also love of the art,"[2] which is often cited as if ancient medical ethics were founded upon this lofty principle. Yet it rests in the context of a discussion about fees introduced by the admonition, "I urge you not to be too unkind." Attempts to find any assertions in the Hippocratic Corpus that would set up philanthropy as an indispensable motivation for practicing medicine are fruitless.[3] Occasional medical sources strongly emphasize that the physician should be moved by love of humanity.[4] But as Galen laments, philanthropy is the inspiration of only a minority of physicians; the majority pursue money, honor, or glory. Proficiency in the art, not one's motivation for practicing determines whether or not one is a physician.[5] "The motive . . . is a matter of personal choice," as Ludwig Edelstein summarizes Galen's opinion; "it has not intrinsic connection with the pursuit of medicine."[6]

Regardless of the motivation behind engaging in medical practice, an apparently constant ideal was that the physician was "to help, or at least to do no harm," a familiar aphorism found in the Hippocratic Corpus.[7] This famous adage appears in a variety of forms in other classical medical literature and seems to be axiomatic.[8] Although the literature of many cultures, not excluding Greece and Rome, is rife with accusations of physicians using their art to evil ends, it is reasonable to assume that physicians thus accused were viewed as having acted in violation of an inherent principle undergirding their calling. Thus rhetoricians, when giving examples of contradictions or opposites, were wont to cite the adulterous philosopher, the temple-robbing priest, and the murderous physician.[9] When a physician used the opportunities provided by his relationship with a patient to kill him for political, financial, or other selfish or malicious reasons, not only would he as a physician have been viewed as having acting evilly, but he as a legal *persona* would have been culpable as an agent of homicide.[10]

Aside from such obvious examples of using the art of medicine to cause harm, were there other activities that would commonly have been so classified? Here we come to the crux of the problem of understanding the ancient physician's conception of his duty to his patients and to the art of medicine. Let us exclude from our discussion the small number of physicians who might have admitted to disagreeing with the proposition that as physicians they should render help, or at least not cause harm. How then would the ancient physician have defined or delimited the terms "helping" and "harming"? Would he have thought it helping or harming (1) to refuse to treat a terminally ill patient if medical intervention would temporarily prolong the patient's life; or (2) to agree to assist a man who, for any reason wished to end his life? Now it can be objected that such questions are meaningless. They can only be addressed if fleshed out by specific sets of circumstances of definite cases, real or hypothetical. But if forced to put these two questions under the rubric of helping or harming, a probably strong, if not overwhelming, majority of ancient physicians would have classified these actions as "helping, or at least not harming."

Plutarch preserves a favorite saying of Pausanias, King of Sparta from 408–394 BC, to the effect that the best physician was the man who did not cause his patients to linger on, but buried them quickly.[11] Although Pausanias was well known as an excoriator of physicians, his remark represents a quite commonly held attitude. The medical art's two functions were preserving and restoring health. Preserving or restoring health was the emphasis, not prolonging life *per se.*

Plato is perhaps better known than any other classical source for ardently opposing any effort on the part of physicians to prolong the lives of patients who had no chance of regaining their health.[12] Plato, at least within the context of the *Republic,* may be an extreme case, for there his concern was much more with eugenics than with the personal worth of the individual. But aside from utopian literature, there is abundant evidence that, at least among the Greeks of the fifth century BC and later, health was considered both a virtue and an indicator of virtue.[13] Health was an ideal, indeed the highest good, set above beauty, wealth, and inner nobility. Health was a goal in itself, for without health all else was without value. The statement in the Hippocratic Corpus that without health nothing avails, neither money, nor any other thing,[14] expresses a strong popular, philosophical, and medical statement.

REFUSING TO TREAT THE TERMINALLY ILL

Let us now directly address the first ethical question posed: would ancient physicians have thought it helping or harming to refuse to treat a terminally ill patient if medical intervention would temporarily prolong the patient's life? The treatise entitled *The Art* in the Hippocratic Corpus defines medicine as having three roles: doing away with the sufferings of the sick, lessening the violence of their diseases, and refusing to treat those who are overmastered by their diseases, realizing in such cases medicine is powerless.[15]

Again I emphasize that in classical Greece and Rome there was no system of medical licensure. Bound by no duty to a licensing authority or professional organizations, the physician exercised his art at his own pleasure. He sold his services at his own discretion to those who asked and paid for treatment. Lucian emphasizes that the physician should be completely free to treat or to refuse to treat. In one of his treatises he has a physician state that "in the case of the medical profession, the more distinguished it is and the more serviceable to the world, the more unrestricted it should be for those who practice it. It is only just . . . that no compulsion and no commands should be put upon a holy calling, taught by the gods and exercised by men of learning; moreover, it should not be subject to enslavement by the law. . . . The physician ought to be persuaded, not ordered; he ought to be willing, not fearful; he ought not to be hailed to the bedside, but to take pleasure in coming of his own accord."[16] To such a physician, any whim or reason not to treat a particular patient would be a justification not to give treatment. It could be merely a matter of personal sentiment. If, however, the physician were basing his decision whether or not to undertake a case only on the consideration that the treatment he gave would simply prolong the life of a patient for whom there was no hope of recovery, he of course would still be completely free to refuse. No legal or, even in the broadest sense of the word, ethical pressures could compel him to undertake treatment. It was entirely his decision and, regardless of what he decided, he would receive approbation from some medical or lay persons and condemnation from others.

I have already mentioned that in a treatise in the Hippocratic Corpus one role of medicine was to refuse to treat those who are overmastered by their diseases, realizing that in such cases medicine is powerless. This represents a very strong and, in my opinion, prevailing sentiment among ancient physicians. It is one for which precedent could easily have been found in Egyptian and Assyro-Babylonian medicine.[17] And it was a medical sentiment that remained strong throughout most, if not all, of the Middle Ages.[18]

In Greco-Roman medicine, the decision to refuse to treat such a patient was motivated by a variety of factors. If treatment would simply prolong life, the patient's interests would not have been served. Indeed the physician would have been considered by many physicians and lay persons as having harmed rather than helped the patient. While the patient's interests may have been a partial motivation behind the decision not to treat, the most frequently articulated concern in the medical sources was the possible damage that such a case might cause to a physician's reputation. Many, if not most, of the ethical principles expressed in the medical literature were motivated by the physician's concern for his reputation. Although from a modern vantage point this seems reprehensible, we must remember that the physician's only credential was his reputation.[19] Earning and preserving a good reputation was a precarious enterprise. Charlatans were criticized for avoiding dangerous cases and exaggerating the severity of ailments that yielded easily to treatment.[20] Thus the conscientious physician, although he might shy away from hopeless cases, was urged in the medical literature not to refuse dangerous or uncertain ones.[21] But the decision of whether to take on a dangerous case was entirely the individual physician's. Some cases in the therapeutic treatises in the Hippocratic Corpus are introduced with the advice that certain procedures should be allowed *if the physician chooses to attempt treatment.*[22] Indeed it appears that physicians might have based their decisions on whether they were liable to earn less reprobation from refusing to treat than from agreeing to treat such cases.

If the physician did elect to take on a dangerous case, the importance of the art of prognosis or forecasting became evident. The physician who declared before beginning treatment that the prospects of a cure were only slight thereby avoided responsibility for an unfavorable outcome.[23] The medical literature is divided on the question of whether a physician should withdraw from a case once it became clear that he would be no meaningful help. Some urged that the physician ought not to withdraw, even if by so doing he might avoid blame.[24] Others felt that he should withdraw if he had a respectable excuse, particularly if continuing treatment might hasten the patient's death.[25]

There is no denying, however, that physicians did sometimes attend cases considered incurable. In the Hippocratic Corpus many diseases that ended in death are described with no mention of prognosis and with no recommendation to the physician that such cases be undertaken or rejected. In most of these, medications to be employed are named. It was recognized that it was necessary to deal with incurable complaints in order to learn how to prevent curable states from advancing to incurability, particularly in the case of wounds. Even a cursory look at the *Epidemics* in the Hippocratic Corpus should convince the reader that the author's intention was not to show how to cure. Nearly 60 percent of the cases end in death and treatment is very seldom mentioned. Such a physician's medical attendance was perhaps less designed for the individual patient's good than for the advancement of medical knowledge.

Opinions certainly varied on the physician's responsibility to undertake treatment of hopeless or dangerous cases. But the following quotation from Celsus represents what appears to have been the mainstream of medical thought: "For it is the part of a prudent man first not to touch a case he cannot save, and not to risk the appearance of having killed one whose lot is but to die; next when there is grave fear without, however, absolute despair, to point out to the patient's relatives that hope is surrounded by difficulty, for then if the art is overcome by the malady, he may not seem to have been ignorant or mistaken."[26] Taking on a hopeless or, under some circumstances, an extremely dangerous case is perhaps the closest issue in ancient medicine to the modern question of employing "extraordinary measures."

Danielle Gourevitch writes of the Greco-Roman physician: "Far from feeling any liability for abandoning his patient, he would feel guilty if he undertook a cure he could not successfully carry out."[27] This is perhaps somewhat overstated. While it is true that if the physician were motivated by greed to continue inefficacious treatment, he would be viewed as acting reprehensibly; nevertheless, if he were attempting a novel treatment in an effort to effect a cure, the ethical implications would not be as clear-cut.[28] Markwart Michler views the "Hippocratic" admonition to refuse to treat patients overwhelmed by their diseases ("an inhuman attitude") as a taboo finally broken by authors on the treatises *On Fractures* and *On Joints* in the Hippocratic Corpus. In these works the authors are said to be motivated by a desire to advance knowledge so as to be able ultimately to render more effective treatment to the suffering.[29] The objective even here was not an ethically based imperative to prolong the life of the incurable patient, but rather a very pragmatic desire to increase the boundaries of the art.

Lain Entralgo bases much of his understanding of Greek medical ethics on the idea that the Greek physician's sense of responsibility both to his art and to his patient rested on his *physiophilia,* that is, love of nature. Since, in Lain Entralgo's view, physis (nature) "was 'divinity' to the Hippocratic doctor, he was deeply and spontaneously conscious of the religious and ethical imperative to respect the limits of his art. . . . The frequency and sternness with which [the] injunction to abstain from therapy is formulated in the *Corpus Hippocraticum* . . . clearly shows that it was not a mere piece of technical advice, but a religious and ethical injunction. Under the influence of his belief about nature, man and his own art, the Greek physician understood that it was his duty to abstain from treating the incurably and mortally ill. . . ."[30]

The diverse opinions of many more scholars could be quoted, but to little profit. The issues were usually not wrestled with in the primary sources that have survived, and modern appraisals of ancient attitudes often are not tempered by the consideration that divergent opinions existed side by side in antiquity and that society was not static. There are significant differences between, for example, fifth-century BC Athens, third-century BC Rome, and the Roman Empire of the first century AD. The attitudes toward old age and death held by the Athenian gentleman of the fifth century BC were, in certain respects, significantly different from those of a Roman aristocrat of a later period. "Generally speaking, the Greeks judged old age unfavorably. The Romans, however, cherished and respected it."[31]

It is noteworthy that an increased interest in the investigation of chronic diseases and the development of geriatric medicine were probably due in great part to the influence of Roman ideals. I cannot here deal adequately with the sundry issues that impinge upon the ancient physician's willingness to take on dangerous or hopeless cases. I am, however, confident that, although attitudes varied, generally a physician who prolonged, or attempted to prolong, the life of a man who could not ultimately recover his health was viewed as acting unethically.

ASSISTING IN SUICIDE

We turn now to the second ethical question: would the ancient physician have thought it helpful or harmful to agree to assist a man who, for any reason, wished to end his life? To this question *probably* a majority of ancient physicians would also have given the reply: "Helping, or at least not harming." It is absolutely essential that we consider the ancient physician as a functioning member of a highly complex and diverse society whose moral responses arose from ethical foundations sometimes strikingly different from what may seem typical of the Western world today. Except among some groups on the periphery of classical thought, the "sanctity of human life" was an idea partially obfuscated by, or at least subservient to, the belief in the inherent right of the free man to dispose of his life as he saw fit, if not always in its living, at least in its termination.

In neither Greek nor Roman law was suicide a concern of the state, except the suicide of a slave or of a soldier. Indeed even murder, at least in Greek law, was not a crime against the state (a public offense); it was considered solely a matter between the victim (and his family) and the killer. Although murder was classified as a public offense in Roman law, it did not follow that suicide was viewed as self-murder but instead was outside the purview and interest of law. Should a person who wished to commit suicide enlist the aid of a second party, the latter, in rendering such assistance, was not culpable. Turning to extralegal sources, we find few objections in classical literature to suicide in general, fewer still to the suicide of the hopelessly ill.[32] Granted, a few cults or philosophical schools condemned all suicide, regardless of the circumstances. But these were both comparatively small in number and quite insignificant in long-range influence. Christianity is of course an exception, but the rise of its influence corresponds roughly with the decline of classical culture.

Platonists, Cynics, and Stoics considered suicide an honorable alternative to hopeless illness;[33] some philosophers regarded it as the greatest triumph of man over fate.[34] The Aristotelean and Epicurean schools did not censure suicide, but condoned it under any circumstances.[35] Porphyry wrote a treatise entitled "On Sensible Removal," and some authors went so far as to compose lists of conditions justifying suicide.[36] Pliny, for example, considered pain due to bladder stones, stomach disorders, and headache valid reasons for suicide.[37] Whether or not to commit suicide was completely up to the individual; whether or not to assist in the act was up to the physician, if asked. The literature contains references to physicians cutting the veins of patients, both ill and well, who asked for such a procedure.[38] Poison was even more common than sustained phlebotomy, and various poisons were developed by physicians who were praised for employing their toxicological knowledge in the production of drugs for inducing a pleasant and painless death.[39] Assisting in suicide was a relatively common practice for Greco-Roman physicians; the very infrequent criticism of such physicians was made *primarily* by sources that would have to be considered as atypical of classical thought. The so-called Hippocratic Oath must be placed into such a category.

THE HIPPOCRATIC OATH: AN ESOTERIC DOCUMENT

Although scholarly opinion varies considerably as to how many (if any) of the treatises in the Hippocratic Corpus were written by Hippocrates,[40] few (if any) scholars today hold that the Oath that bears his name was written by the historically elusive "father of medicine."[41] Even the date of the composition of the Oath is unknown; some scholars place it as early as the sixth century BC and others as late as the first century AD.[42] It apparently did not excite a great deal of attention on the part of physicians or others earlier than the beginning of the Christian era; the first known reference to it was made by Scribonius Largus in the first century AD.[43]

Some of the stipulations in the Oath are not consonant either with ethical precepts prevalent elsewhere in the Hippocratic Corpus and in other classical literature or with the realities of medical practice as revealed in the sources. This has inspired a number of attempts either to explain away those inconsistencies or to attribute the Oath to an author or school whose views were, in other respects as well, discordant with those characteristic of classical society.[44] Most significant is Edelstein's theory that the Oath was a product of the Pythagorean school. Edelstein's thesis is tempting and, in my opinion, the most convincing so far advanced.[45] The Pythagorean origin of the Oath, however, should not be considered proved. It is reasonable to say with absolute certainty that the Oath, taken as a whole, is an esoteric document that is often inconsonant with the larger picture of Greco-Roman medical ethics.

Among other stipulations in the so-called Hippocratic Oath are the prohibitions of performing abortions and of practicing surgery, both of which were common practices of Greco-Roman physicians. Immediately before these two injunctions is the famous passage that reads "I will neither give a deadly drug to anybody, not even if asked for it, nor will I make a suggestion to this effect."[46] These three prohibitions have at least this much in common: they are inconsistent with values expressed by the majority of sources and atypical of the realities of ancient medical practice.

I do not want to debate the various possible origins of an oath that must be considered esoteric in many of its essentials. But it is known that, while these three prohibitions remained atypical of medical ethics for the entirety of the classical period, during the first and second centuries AD a greater sensitivity to two of them began to be evidenced. During the early Christian era some pagan physicians, influenced by the Oath, refused to perform abortions under any circumstances, others would perform them only to preserve the health of the mother, and others would perform them on request for any reason.[47] Some physicians began emphasizing philanthropy as their essential motive and extended philanthropy to include what we may generally term "respect for life."[48] Stressing, on the basis of the Oath, that medicine is the science of healing, not of harming, Scribonius Largus credits "Hippocrates," in condemning abortion, with going "a long way toward preparing the mind of the learners for the love of humanity. For he who considers it a crime to injure future life still in doubt, how much more criminal must he judge it to hurt a full grown human being."[49] He then asserts that unless medicine "strives fully in each of its parts to help those in need, it is not better than promising sympathy to men." Later he writes that the medical art should never be injurious to anyone. But Scribonius' insistence that the physician not harm or be injurious to anyone is just as neutral in respect to the issue of active or passive euthanasia as the Hippocratic aphorism "to help, or at least to do no harm."

Some physicians may have preferred not to assist in a suicide for it could prove to be a messy business, at least from a legal point of view. Physicians were frequently charged with, or at least suspected of, poisoning their patients. Other physicians, however, who may have refused to aid a person in committing suicide, perhaps condemned suicide under all circumstances for philosophical or religious reasons, but these seem to have left few records of their sentiments, much less professional justification.

Aretaeus, who lived in either the first or the second century AD, can perhaps be placed in this last category of physicians. He writes that some patients suffering from a particularly painful disease still shrink from death, while others beg for it. In these cases, he writes it still *is not proper for the responsible physician*[50] to cause the patients' death but it *is proper* to drug such patients in order to relieve their anguish.[51] On the basis of the paucity of such statements as Aretaeus' and the plethora of evidence of opposite sentiments, it is safe to conclude that the author of the Oath and perhaps Aretaeus represented a minority opinion on the question of active euthanasia.[52]

PROLONGING LIFE: A SEARCH FOR THE ORIGINS

Does the modern physician's duty to prolong life have its roots in Hippocratic or other strains of classical medicine? The answer to this question must be a qualified "no." The only duty common to probably all Greco-Roman physicians was "to help, or at least to do no harm." Taking on a hopeless case was entirely the prerogative of the individual physician and few voices would condemn a refusal, particularly if such a decision were based on the conviction that the patient's unhealthy life would only be temporarily extended. Prolonging the life of a patient who did not want to live would probably have been considered as harming the patient and therefore as unethical by all, or nearly all, classical physicians, even by those constituting that minority that would not assist actively in terminating a patient's life.

While the physician's duty to prolong life does not have its roots in any strains of classical medicine, the idea of "respect for life" is quite a different matter. Owsei Temkin writes, concerning the so-called Hippocratic Oath and sources expressing compatible attitudes, that "sufficient material has now been gathered to prove the existence of a tradition which, in its uncompromising form, did not sanction any limit to the respect for life, not even therapeutic abortion. . . ."[53] This tradition that would sanction no limit to the respect for life appears, in its emphasis, to have been entirely negative: the physician would not actively terminate life by abortion or euthanasia. But it laid no stress, apparently, on the positive correlate that would require the physician actively to prolong life. This negative tradition did indeed become stronger with the rise of Christianity: abortion, suicide, and euthanasia became sins. As Temkin says, "God has given life, and man must not interfere with His purposes."[54] Many early Christians and Church Fathers, however, insisted that God also either inflicts or permits disease and the practitioner of the secular healing arts thus works against divine purposes.[55] Wide acceptance by Christians of the medical art as consonant with the sanctified life of faith took centuries. While abortion, suicide, and euthanasia became sins, the prolonging of life did not become either a virtue or a duty.

If the duty to prolong life is not found in classical medicine, where might we begin to look for it? Francis Bacon (late sixteenth, early seventeenth centuries), in his *De augmentis scientiarum*, divides medicine into three offices (the preservation of health, the cure of diseases, and the prolongation of life). He then writes that "the third part of medicine which I have set down is that which relates to the prolongation of life, which is new, and deficient; and the most noble of all."[56] He protests that physicians have not recognized the significance of the "new" branch of medicine, but have confused it with the other two. He urges physicians to investigate means of developing a regimen designed to contribute to longevity.

Coming closer to our subject, in the same work Bacon writes that physicians "in their inquiry concerning diseases . . . find many which they pronounce incurable, some at their commencement, and others after a certain period."[57] At first sight he may seem to be castigating physicians for refusing to treat patients with incurable diseases. But this is not his concern here. Rather, his criticism is directed against the lack of concern with finding cures for conditions regarded as incurable. He exhorts "some physicians of eminence and magnanimity" to produce "a work on the cure of diseases which are held incurable . . . since the pronouncing of these diseases incurable gives a legal sanction as it were to neglect and inattention, and exempts ignorance from discredit."[58]

Expanding his discussion of the deficiencies of the medical art and profession of his day, Bacon writes that he considers it "to be clearly the office of a physician, not only to restore health, but also to mitigate the pains and torments of diseases; and not only when such mitigation of pain, as of a dangerous symptom, helps and conduces to recovery; but also when, all hope of recovery being gone, it serves only to make a fair and easy passage from life. For it is no small felicity which Augustus Caesar was wont so earnestly to pray for, that same *Euthanasia* [Bacon's emphasis]; which likewise was observed in the death of Antoninus Pius, which was not so much like death as like falling into a deep and pleasant sleep."[59]

Bacon then levels another criticism against the profession: "But in our times, the physicians make a kind of scruple and religion to stay with the patient after he is given up, whereas in my judgment if they would not be wanting to their office, and indeed to humanity, they ought both to acquire the skill and to bestow the attention whereby the dying may pass more easily and quietly out of life. This part I call the inquiry concerning *outward Euthanasia* [Bacon's emphasis], or the easy dying of the body (to distinguish it from that Euthanasia which regards the preparation of the soul); and set it down among the desiderata."[60] So, at least in the estimation of Bacon, the medical profession of his day was deficient owing, among other things, to its lack of concern with finding cures for supposedly incurable conditions and with finding and applying means for making death less unpleasant. He uses the term "euthanasia" in its etymological meaning, that is, an easy death, probably devoid of any implication of expediting death.

Most germane is Bacon's assertion that, in his time, "the physicians make a kind of scruple and religion to stay with the patient after he is given up." What is Bacon saying? What, if his statement is taken at face value, are these physicians, who feel obliged to stay with their patients after they are given up, doing? It is difficult to say how fair and objective Bacon is being here. He might very likely be saying that, on the one hand, physicians declare patients terminally ill who are suffering from diseases that the medical art has declared incurable without giving adequate attention to attempting to find a cure. But, on the other hand, physicians feel obligated to continue treating such patients for whom medical science holds out no hope, although they do not feel any compulsion to provide the means of an easy and felicitous death.

Now the statement that "the physicians make a kind of scruple and religion to stay with the patient after he is given up" can be taken to imply a sense of duty on the part of physicians to make an attempt, however inept or futile, to prolong the lives of terminally ill patients or simply not to desert them. Even if it means only the latter (and I do not so limit it), it is still a significant step toward the former. Bacon claims no recent origin for this scruple. But such a statement as his most certainly would not have been made, at least not commonly, in classical antiquity nor during the greater part of the Middle Ages. It is my opinion that there were significant changes in the ethical bases for medical practice during the late Middle Ages, roughly from the twelfth through the fifteenth centuries. Many converging factors played roles in the formation of medical professionalism in a relatively "modern" sense of the word: the development of guilds which, in exchange for the right to hold a monopoly in service or commodity, were bound to adopt and enforce ethical codes; the creation of universities (which were themselves guilds); the institution of medical licensure requirements in some areas; and very importantly, the increasing importance of the Catholic Church as a factor in moral and ethical definition. Canon lawyers and moral theologians, including casuists and authors of *Summae Confessorum* and confessional manuals, directed considerable attention to defining and classifying the sins, both of omission and commission, as well as the moral obligations of various professions. Needless to say, the medical profession excited a great deal of their interest.

I have only begun to scratch the surface of the vast quantity of relevant primary sources, but I have found some tantalizing hints in certain authors. For example, the fifteenth-century moral theologian and casuist, Saint Antonius of Florence, in his *Summa Theologica*, devotes a lengthy section to the medical profession. In it are such statements as these: ". . . even if the sick man forbids any medicines to be given to him, a physician called by him or by his relatives, can treat the patient against the patient's will, just as a man ought to be dragged against his will from a house that is about to collapse"[61] and "succor must be given, following the rule of charity, to those who are in danger, however stubborn they may be."[62]

I must stress that these two quotations by themselves prove nothing, but are merely a sliver from a vast beam of primary evidence begging to be investigated by the historian of medical ethics. For it is there that I am reasonably certain that solutions can be found for, or at least significant light shed upon, many problems in the development of medical ethics. One of these problems is of course the question of the origin of the physician's duty to prolong life, a duty that does not, except in its negative side, have direct roots in classical medicine, but was, in my opinion, probably well established by the seventeenth century.

NOTES

1. For example, Thucydides, *The Peloponnesian War* VI, 14; Euripides, *The Phoenician Women* 893; Plato, *The Statesman* 293 A–C; *Laws* 862 B, 720 D–E (cf. *Gorgias* 464 B); *Republic* 342 D; Aristotle, *Nicomachaen Ethics* 1180 b: *Politics* 1287 a; pseudo-Demosthenes, *Against Aristogeiton* II, 26; Aeschines, *Against Ctesiphon* 225 f., cf. Cicero, *Republic* I, 62; V, 5; *De oratore* II, 186; *Disputations* III, 82. Even epigraphy yields an example: *Supplementum Epigraphicum Graecum* X, 98, 14.
2. *Precepts* 6.
3. P. Lain Entralgo (*Doctor and Patient*, F. Partridge, trans; New York: McGraw-Hill, 1969) argues that the Greek physician's relationship with his patients was based on a combination of *philanthropia* and *philotechnia* (pp. 17 ff.). Later he maintains that "a careful study of the Hippocratic writings leads to the conclusion that Hippocrates and his direct and indirect followers were 'philanthropists' *avant la lettre*" (p. 243, n. 1). His thesis, unfortunately rests upon his belief that "there is an 'instinct to help' at work in human moving a man to succour the sick. . . ." (p. 45).
4. *E.g.,* Scribonius Largus (in Karl Deichgraber, *Professio Medici. Zum Vorwort des Scribonius Largus.* Abhandlungen der Akademie der Wissenschaften und der Literatur Nr. 9, Mainz, 1950) and Oliver, James H. and Maas, Paul Lazarus. "An Ancient Poem on the Duties of a Physician." *Bulletin of the History of Medicine* 7:315–323, 1939. For a discussion of the changing attitudes in classical antiquity toward philanthropy as the basis for medical practice, see Kudlien, Fridolf, "Medical Ethics and Popular Ethics in Greece and Rome." *Clio Medica* 5:91–121, 1970, especially pp. 91–97.
5. Galen, *De Placitis* 9, 5.

6. Edelstein, Ludwig. "The Professional Ethics of the Greek Physician." In *Ancient Medicine: Selected Papers of Ludwig Edelstein*, edited by Owsei and C. Lilian Temkin. Baltimore: Johns Hopkins Press, 1967, p. 336.

7. *Epidemics* 1, 11.

8. See the discussion by Sandulescu, C. "Primum non Nocere: Philological Commentaries on Medical Aphorism." *Acta Aniqua Hungarica* 13:359–368, 1965.

9. For the motif of the physician as a poisoner, see Quintilian, *Institutio oratoria* 7, 2, 17, f.; 2, 16, 5; Calpurnius Flaccus, *Declamationes* 13; pseudo-Quintilian, *Declamationes minores* 321; Libanius Progymnasmata 7, 3.

10. See Amundsen, Darrel W. "The Liability of the Physician in Classical Greek Legal Theory and Practice." *Journal of the History of Medicine and Allied Science* 32:172–203, 1977; and "The Liability of the Physician in Roman Law." In *International Symposium on Society, Medicine and Law*, edited by H. Karplus. Amsterdam: Elsevier, 1973, pp. 17–31.

11. Plutarch, *Moralia* 231 A.

12. Plato, *Republic* 406 C, 407 D, 408 B; cf., Euripides, *The Suppliant Women* 1109 ff. (quoted by Plutarch in his "Consolation to Appollonius," *Moralia* 110 C); Aristotle, *Rhetoric* 1361 b; Demosthenes, *Third Olynthiac* 33.

13. See, e.g., Edelstein, Ludwig. "The Distinctive Hellenism of Greek Medicine." in *Ancient Medicine* (supra, n. 6), pp. 386 ff.; Jaeger, Werner. *Paideia: The Ideals of Greek Culture*, G. Highet, trans. New York: Oxford University Press, 1944, III, 44 f. For a discussion of health as the greatest good by a late classical source, see Sextus Empiricus, *Against the Ethicist*, 48 ff.

14. *Regimen*, 3, 69; cp. Herophilis in Sextus Empiricus, *Adversus Mathematicos* 11, 50.

15. *The Art* 3; cf. *Diseases* 2, 48.

16. Lucian, *The Disinherited* 23.

17. See Amundsen, Darrel W. "History of Medical Ethics: Ancient Near East." In the *Encyclopedia of Bioethics*.

18. See Amundsen, Darrel W. "History of Medical Ethics: Medieval Europe." *Ibid.*; and "Medical Deontology and Pestilential Disease in the Late Middle Ages." *Journal of the History of Medicine and Allied Sciences* 32:403–421, 1977, especially pp. 414 ff.

19. See Edelstein, Ludwig. "Hippocratic Prognosis." In *Ancient Medicine* (supra, n. 6), pp. 76 f., and "The Hippocratic Physician," *Ibid.*, pp. 88 ff; Sigerist, Henry. *A History of Medicine*, Vol. II. New York: Oxford University Press, 1961, p. 305.

20. E.g., in the Hippocratic Corpus, *Precepts* 7; Celsus, *De Medicina* 5, 26 1 C (quoted below), Menander, *Phanium* 497, K. See also Barbrius (*Fables* 75) and Ausonius (*Epigrams* 4) for the motif of the deserted patient who recovers and encounters his physician. There is a slightly variant rendition attributed to Aesop: *Fables of Aesop*, S. A. Handford, trans. Baltimore: Penguin Books, 1954, nr. 189.

21. E.g., in the Hippocratic Corpus, *Precepts* 7; *Ancient Medicine* 9; *On Joints* 69; cf. *The Art* 8; Paulus Aegineta 6, 88; Ctesias in Oribasius, *Collect. Medic. Reliquiane* 8, 8.

22. E.g., *De Morbis* 3, 7; *De Intern. Affect.* 12.

23. What responsibility a physician may have felt is open to discussion. There are many passages in the Hippocratic Corpus where the concern with incurring blame is expressed. (See e.g., *On Joints* 67; *Decorum* 14; *Ancient Medicine* 9.) Gert Preiser ("Uber die Sorgfaltspflicht der Artze von Kos," *Medical History Journal* 5:1–9, 1970, maintains that there seems to have been no liability for the physician in Greek law. Thus, although the concern with the use of prognosis as a means to protect the physician from accusations suggests legal liability, Preiser holds that this concern was motivated by a professional responsibility based upon the "Hippocratic physician's" broad conception of his duty to his *techne*. I have attempted elsewhere to demonstrate that Greek, or at least Attic, law allowed for the prosecution of the dolose, incompetent or negligent physician, as did Roman law. See Amundsen (supra, n. 10, both articles cited).

24. See Edelstein, Ludwig. "The Professional Ethics of the Greek Physician" and "The Hippocratic Physician" in *Ancient Medicine* (supra n. 6), pp. 323 and 90 ff.

25. E.g., in the Hippocratic Corpus, *On Fractures* 36; cp., *Aphorisms* 6, 38; *Prorrhetic* 2, 9.

26. Celsus, *De Medicina* 5, 26, 1, C.

27. Gourevitch, Danielle. "Suicide Among the Sick in Classical Antiquity." *Bulletin of the History of Medicine* 43:503, 1969.

28. See pseudo-Quintilian, *Declamationes Maiores* 8, where both sides of the question are argued.

29. Michler, Markwart. "Medical Ethics in Hippocratic Bone Surgery." *Bulletin of the History of Medicine* 42:297–311, 1968.

30. Entralgo, P. Lain (supra, n. 3), p. 48.

31. Edelstein, Ludwig. "The Distinctive Hellenism of Greek Medicine." in *Ancient Medicine* (supra, n. 6), p. 381. Edelstein's statement is generally true; but it would be an easy task to cull from Greek literature sentiments of reverence for old age and from Roman souces statements of the opposite opinion.

32. There is extensive literature on the history of suicide. A classical study is Rudolf Hirzel's "Der Selbstmord," *Archiv für Religionswissenschaft* (1908), 75–104, 243–84, 417–76. David Daube's "The Linguistics of Suicide" (*Philosophy and Public Affairs* [1972], 387–437) is well worth consulting for its historical perspective. Danielle Gourevitch's article, already cited (supra, n. 27), is of the most immediate relevance for the subject under discussion.

33. See especially Rudolf Hirzel (ibid.), pp. 279 ff. A very cogent expression of the Stoic attitude toward suicide is Seneca's *Letters to Lucillus* 77. See also Diogenes Laertius, *Lives of the Eminent Philosophers* 4, 3 and 6, 18, where criticism is directed against those who would cling to life when suffering from disability or extreme pain.

34. Hirzel, Rudolph. *ibid.*, p. 279, n. 1. It should be noted that Plato, for example, condemned suicide as opprobrious if one is "not compelled to it by the occurrence of some intolerable and inevitable misfortune" (*Laws* 873 C). On the origin of the famous prohibition in the *Phaedo*, see Strachan, J. C. C. "Who Did Forbid Suicide at *Phaedo* 62 B?" *Classical Quarterly* 20:216–220, 1970.

35. See Edelstein, "The Hippocratic Oath." In *Ancient Medicine* (supra, n. 6), p. 17. Aristotle argues in *Nicomachean Ethics* (1138 a) that since law does not expressly permit suicide, it forbids the act. Aristotle is concerned here with a citizen acting unjustly toward the state by thus depriving his city of a useful citizen. Elsewhere he unequivocally condemns the cowardice of one who kills himself simply to escape from poverty or love or pain (*Nicomachean Ethics* 1116 a). It is very doubtful, in my opinion, that Aristotle would extend this castigation to the terminally ill suicide.

36. For some examples, see Danielle Gourevitch (supra, n. 27), pp. 509 ff.

37. Pliny the Elder, *Historia naturalis* 25, 7, 23.

38. See, e.g., Tacitus, *Annals* 15, 69. Cf., Suetonius, *Life of Lucan.*

39. See Danielle Gourevitch (supra, n. 27), p. 508.

40. For a discussion of the problem, see Edelstein, Ludwig. "The Genuine Work of Hippocrates." in *Ancient Medicine* (supra, n. 6), pp. 133–144; and Lloyd, G. E. R. "The Hippocratic Question" *Classical Quarterly* 25:171–192, 1975.

41. Savas Nittis' thesis that Hippocrates himself composed the Oath in Athens between March and October of 421 BC is unconvincing; "The Authorship and Probable Date of the Hippocratic Oath." *Bulletin of the History of Medicine* 8:1012–1021, 1940.

42. Ludwig Edelstein dates the composition of the Oath to the mid-to-late fourth century BC; "Hippocratic Oath," in *Ancient Medicine* (supra, n. 8), pp. 55ff.

43. Scribonius Largus, *Professio Medici*, p. 24 in Deichgraber's edition (supra, n. 4).

44. Edelstein's discussion of the Oath (originally published in 1943) includes a summary of previous scholarly treatment.

45. There has been much written on the oath since Edelstein's monograph, and several

leading scholars have questioned the validity of his central thesis of the Pythagorean origin of the Oath. See, for example, Fridolf Kudlien (supra, n. 4), and Karl Deichgraber, *Der Hippokratische Eid* (Stuttgart: Hippokrates-Verlag, 1955), especially p. 40.

46. I have followed Fridolf Kudlien's translation (supra, n. 4), p. 118, n. 47.

47. So writes Soranus, *Gynaecia* 1, 60.

48. For a discussion, see Temkin, Owsei. "The Idea of Respect for Life in the History of Medicine." In *Respect for Life in Medicine, Philosophy, and the Law*, edited by Owsei Temkin, William K. Frankena, and Sanford H. Kadish. Baltimore: The Johns Hopkins Press, 1977, pp. 1–23.

49. Scribonius Largus, *Professio Medici*, p. 24 in Deichgraber's edition (supra, n. 4).

50. The subject under discussion here is intestinal obstruction.

51. *Corpus Medicorum Graecorum* II, p. 133, lines 10 ff. In another passage Aretaeus, when discussing the treatment of inflammation of the lungs, writes that "if you give a drug to a patient at the height of choking and at the point of death, you would be responsible for his death in the opinion of the common people" (ibid., p. 120 line 8 f.). Aretaeus' concern here seems to be less with the ethical issue than with reputation and possible legal implications.

52. There are three other sources sometimes cited as evidence for opposition to active euthanasia in classical antiquity. (1) There is a passage in the Oxyrhynchus Papyri (#437, third century AD) where the oath is quoted as the basis for the rejection of giving poison, (2) a metrical oath of unknown date. A possible translation is "nor would anyone bribe me to alleviate a painful condition by giving baneful drugs (*i.e.*, poison) to a man (sc., a patient)" (*Corpus Medicorum Graecorum* I, 1, pp. 5 f., lines 15 ff.), and (3) A physician in *The Golden Ass*, a novel written by Apuleius in the second century AD, makes a statement that can be interpreted as a condemnation of medical assistance in effecting euthanasia or as simply an assertion that the medical art should not supply the means for murder. On this passage see Owsei Temkin (supra, n. 48, p. 4); Darrell W. Amundsen, "Romanticizing the Ancient Medical Profession: The Characterization of the Physician in the Graeco-Roman Novel." *Bulletin of the History of Medicine* 48:325, 1974; Danielle Gourevitch (supra, n. 27, pp. 506 f.), and Ludwig Edelstein, "Hippocratic Oath," in *Ancient Medicine* (supra, n. 6, pp. 13 f. and nn. 23 and 24).

53. Owsei Temkin (supra, n. 48), p. 5.

54. Ibid., p. 16.

55. E.g., Arnobius, *Adversus gentes* I, 48, and Tatian, *Oratio ad Graecos* 18. See Dawe Victor G. *The Attitude of the Ancient Church Toward Sickness and Healing*. Unpublished doctoral dissertation, Boston University School of Theology, 1955, especially pp. 153 ff.

56. *The Philosophical Works of Francis Bacon* (Ellis and Spedding's translation), edited by J. M. Robertson, 1905. Reprinted, Freeport, N.Y.: Books for Libraries Press, 1970 pp. 485 and 489.

57. Ibid.

58. Ibid.

59. Ibid.

60. Ibid.

61. Antoninus of Florence, *Summa Theologica* 3, 7, 2, 3. The context is the physician's obligation to treat the miser who, because of the expense, refuses to allow himself to be treated.

62. Ibid., 3, 7, 2, 4. Some interpreters of canon law had rigidly maintained that a physician sins mortally who treats a patient who has not first confessed. Antoninus here maintains that such an opinion is too harsh, and justifies his position by the statement quoted in the text.

The historical problem of whether physicians have traditionally perceived a duty to prolong life raises the related ethical question of whether physicians ought always to strive to prolong life. This would require using all means possible to preserve all lives. This is a position held by some Orthodox Jews and apparently by a minority of physicians. Virtually no other groups hold such a rigorous position. Instead, many contemporary thinkers make use of what is called the distinction between passive and active euthanasia or the omission/commission distinction. According to this view it is not acceptable to kill a patient even if that patient is terminally ill and suffering and the killing is done for reasons of mercy. On the other hand, holders of the more moderate position claim that there is not always a duty to do everything possible to preserve life. For example, if a patient refuses a treatment, that treatment may morally be omitted according to this view. One interpretation is that active killing is an inherently wrong-making characteristic of action, just as is breaking a promise, or violating autonomy.

The American Medical Association has adopted the position that physicians may not actively kill but may, under certain circumstances, withhold treatment even though it may lead to the death of the patient. James Rachels has questioned the validity of this distinction. He has argued that it might make moral sense to oppose both omissions and commissions that lead to a death or to accept both kinds of behavior, but that the bare difference between omission and commission cannot be decisive. In the following essay Tom L. Beauchamp responds to this argument of Rachels. Beauchamp examines ways in which the distinction might be morally relevant. He does not argue that there is an independent principle that makes active killing wrong. Rather, he examines the utility of the rule that permits omissions, but not commissions.

A Reply to Rachels on Active and Passive Euthanasia

Tom L. Beauchamp

James Rachels has recently argued that the distinction between active and passive euthanasia is neither appropriately used by the American Medical Association nor generally useful for the resolution of moral problems of euthanasia.[1] Indeed he believes this distinction—which he equates with the killing/letting die distinction—does not in itself have any moral importance. The chief object of his attack is the following statement adopted by the House of Delegates of the American Medical Association in 1973:

The intentional termination of the life of one human being by another—
mercy killing—is contrary to that for which the medical profession stands

and is contrary to the policy of the American Medical Association. The cessation of the employment of extraordinary means to prolong the life of the body when there is irrefutable evidence that biological death is imminent is the decision of the patient and/or his immediate family. The advice and judgment of the physician should be freely available to the patient and/or his immediate family (78).

Rachels constructs a powerful and interesting set of arguments against this statement. In this paper I attempt the following: (1) to challenge his views on the grounds that he does not appreciate the moral reasons which give weight to the active/passive distinction; (2) to provide a constructive account of the moral relevance of the active/passive distinction; and (3) to offer reasons showing that Rachels may nonetheless be correct in urging that we ought to abandon the active/passive distinction for purposes of moral reasoning.

I

I would concede that the active/passive distinction is sometimes morally irrelevant. Of this Rachels convinces me. But it does not follow that it is always morally irrelevant. What we need, then, is a case where the distinction is a morally relevant one and an explanation why it is so. Rachels himself uses the method of examining two cases which are exactly alike except that "one involves killing whereas the other involves letting die" (79). We may profitably begin by comparing the kinds of cases governed by the AMA's doctrine with the kinds of cases adduced by Rachels in order to assess the adequacy and fairness of his cases.

The second paragraph of the AMA statement is confined to a narrowly restricted range of passive euthanasia cases, viz., those (a) where the patients are on extraordinary means, (b) where irrefutable evidence of imminent death is available, and (c) where patient or family consent is available. Rachels' two cases involve conditions notably different from these:

> In the first, Smith stands to gain a large inheritance if anything should happen to his six-year-old cousin. One evening while the child is taking his bath, Smith sneaks into the bathroom and drowns the child, and then arranges things so that it will look like an accident.
>
> In the second, Jones also stands to gain if anything should happen to his six-year-old cousin. Like Smith, Jones sneaks in planning to drown the child in his bath. However, just as he enters the bathroom Jones sees the child slip and hit his head, and fall face down in the water. Jones is delighted; he stands by, ready to push the child's head back under if it is necessary, but it is not necessary. With only a little thrashing about, the child drowns all by himself, "accidently," as Jones watches and does nothing.
>
> Now Smith killed the child, whereas Jones "merely" let the child die. That is the only difference between them (79).

Rachels says there is no moral difference between the cases in terms of our moral assessments of Smith's and Jones' behavior. This assessment seems fair enough, but what can Rachels' cases be said to prove, as they are so markedly disanalogous to the sorts of cases envisioned by the AMA proposal? Rachels concedes important disanalogies, but thinks them irrelevant:

> The point is the same in these cases: the bare difference between killing and letting die does not, in itself, make a moral difference. If a doctor lets a patient die, for humane reasons, he is in the same moral position as if he had given the patient a lethal injection for humane reasons (79).

Three observations are immediately in order. First, Rachels seems to infer that from such cases we can conclude that the distinction between killing and letting die is always morally irrelevant. This conclusion is fallaciously derived. What the argument in fact shows, being an analogical argument, is only that in all relevantly similar cases the distinction does not in itself make a moral difference. Since Rachels concedes that other cases are disanalogous, he seems thereby to concede that his argument is as weak as the analogy itself. Second, Rachels' cases involve two unjustified actions, one of killing and the other of letting die. The AMA statement distinguishes one set of cases of unjustified killing and another of justified cases of allowing to die. Nowhere is it claimed by the AMA that what makes the difference in these cases is the active/passive distinction itself. It is only implied that one set of cases, the justified set, involves (passive) letting die while the unjustified set involves (active) killing. While it is said that justified euthanasia cases are passive ones and unjustified ones active, it is not said either that what makes some acts justified is the fact of their being passive or that what makes others unjustified is the fact of their being active. This fact will prove to be of vital importance.

The third point is that in both of Rachels' cases the respective moral agents—Smith and Jones—are morally responsible for the death of the child and are morally blameworthy—even though Jones is presumably not causally responsible. In the first case death is caused by the agent, while in the second it is not; yet the second agent is no less morally responsible. While the law might find only the first homicidal, morality condemns the motives in each case as equally wrong, and it holds that the duty to save life in such cases is as compelling as the duty not to take life. I suggest that it is largely because of this equal degree of moral responsibility that there is no morally relevant difference in Rachels' cases. In the cases envisioned by the AMA, however, an agent is held to be responsible for taking life by actively killing but is not held to be morally required to preserve life, and so not responsible for death, when removing the patient from extraordinary means (under conditions a–c above). I shall elaborate this latter point momentarily. My only conclusion thus far is the negative one that Rachels' arguments rest on weak foundations. His cases are not relevantly similar to euthanasia cases and do not support his apparent conclusion that the active/passive distinction is always morally irrelevant.

II

I wish first to consider an argument that I believe has powerful intuitive appeal and probably is widely accepted as stating the main reason for rejecting Rachels' views. I will maintain that this argument fails, and so leaves Rachels' contentions untouched.

I begin with an actual case, the celebrated Quinlan case.[2] Karen Quinlan was in a coma, and was on a mechanical respirator which artificially sustained her vital processes and which her parents wished to cease. At least some physicians believed there was irrefutable evidence that biological death was imminent and the coma irreversible. This case, under this description, closely conforms to the passive cases envisioned by the AMA. During an interview the father, Mr. Quinlan, asserted that he did not wish to kill his daughter, but only to remove her from the machines in order to see whether she would live or would die a natural death.[3] Suppose he had said—to envision now a second and hypothetical, but parallel case—that he wished only to see her die painlessly and therefore wished that the doctor could induce death by an overdose of morphine. Most of us would think the second act, which involves active killing, morally unjustified in these circumstances, while many of us would think the first act morally justified. (This is not the place to consider whether in fact it is justified, and if so under what conditions.) What accounts for the apparent morally relevant difference?

I have considered these two cases together in order to follow Rachels' method of entertaining parallel cases where the only difference is that the one case involves killing and the other letting die. However, there is a further difference, which crops up in the euthanasia context. The difference rests in our judgments of medical fallibility and moral responsibility. Mr. Quinlan seems to think that, after all, the doctors might be wrong. There is a remote possibility that she might live without the aid of a machine. But whether or not the medical prediction of death turns out to be accurate, if she dies then no one is morally responsible for directly bringing about or causing her death, as they would be if they caused her death by killing her. Rachels finds explanations which appeal to causal conditions unsatisfactory; but perhaps this is only because he fails to see the nature of the causal link. To bring about her death is by that act to preempt the possibility of life. To "allow her to die" by removing artificial equipment is to allow for the possibility of wrong diagnosis or incorrect prediction and hence to absolve oneself of moral responsibility for the taking of life under false assumptions. There may, of course, be utterly no empirical possibility of recovery in some cases since recovery would violate a law of nature. However, judgments of empirical impossibility in medicine are notoriously problematic—the reason for emphasizing medical fallibility. And in all the hard cases we do not know that recovery is empirically impossible, even if good evidence is available.

The above reason for invoking the active/passive distinction can now be generalized: Active termination of life removes all possibility of life for the patient, while passively ceasing extraordinary means may not. This is not trivial since patients have survived in several celebrated cases where, in knowledgeable physicians' judgments, there was "irrefutable" evidence that death was imminent.[4]

One may, of course, be entirely responsible and culpable for another's death either by killing him or by letting him die. In such cases, of which Rachels' are examples, there is no morally significant difference between killing and letting die precisely because whatever one does, omits, or refrains from doing does not absolve one of responsibility. Either active or passive involvement renders one responsible for the death of another, and both involvements are equally wrong for the same principled moral reason: it is (*prima facie*) morally wrong to bring about the death of an innocent person capable of living whenever the causal intervention or negligence is intentional. (I use causal terms here because causal involvement need not be active, as when by one's negligence one is nonetheless causally responsible.) But not all cases of killing and letting die fall under this same moral principle. One is sometimes culpable for killing, because morally responsible as the agent for death, as when one pulls the plug on a respirator sustaining a recovering patient (a murder). But one is sometimes not culpable for letting die because not morally responsible as agent, as when one pulls the plug on a respirator sustaining an irreversibly comatose and unrecoverable patient (a routine procedure, where one is *merely* causally responsible.)[5] Different degrees and means of involvement assess different degrees of responsibility, and our assessments of culpability can become intricately complex. The only point which now concerns us, however, is that because different moral principles may govern very similar circumstances, we are sometimes morally culpable for killing but not for letting die. And to many people it will seem that in passive cases we are not morally responsible for causing death, though we are responsible in active cases.

This argument is powerfully attractive. Although I was once inclined to accept it in virtually the identical form just developed,[6] I now think that, despite its intuitive appeal, it cannot be correct. It is true that different degrees and means of involvement entail different degrees of responsibility, but it does not follow that we are not responsible and therefore are absolved of possible culpability in any case of intentionally allowing to die. We are responsible and perhaps culpable in either active or passive cases. Here Rachels' argument is entirely to the point: It is not primarily a question of greater or lesser responsibility by an active or a passive means that should determine culpability. Rather, the question of culpability is decided by the moral justification for choosing either a passive or an active means. What the argument in the previous paragraph overlooks is that one might be unjustified in using an active means or unjustified in using a passive means, and hence not be culpable in using either. Fallibility might just as well be present in a judgment to use one means as in a judgment to use another. (A judgment to allow to die is just as subject to being based on knowledge which is fallible as a judgment to kill.) Moreover, in either case, it is a matter of what one knows and believes, and not a matter of a particular kind of causal connection or causal chain. If we kill the patient, then we are certainly causally responsible for his death. But similarly, if we cease treatment, and the patient dies, the patient might have recovered if treatment had been continued. The patient might have been saved in either case, and hence there is no morally relevant difference between the two cases. It is, therefore, simply beside the point that "one is sometimes culpable for killing . . . but one is sometimes not culpable for letting die"—as the above argument concludes.

Accordingly, despite its great intuitive appeal and frequent mention, this argument from responsibility fails.

III

There may, however, be more compelling arguments against Rachels, and I wish now to provide what I believe is the most significant argument that can be adduced in defense of the active/passive distinctions. I shall develop this argument by combining (1) so-called wedge or slippery slope arguments with (2) recent arguments in defense of rule utilitarianism. I shall explain each in turn and show how in combination they may be used to defend the active/passive distinction.

(1) *Wedge arguments* proceed as follows: if killing were allowed, even under the guise of a merciful extinction of life, a dangerous wedge would be introduced which places all "undesirable" or "unworthy" human life in a precarious condition. Proponents of wedge arguments believe the initial wedge places us on a slippery slope for at least one of two reasons: (i) It is said that our justifying principles leave us with no principled way to avoid the slide into saying that all sorts of killings would be justified under similar conditions. Here it is thought that once killing is allowed, a firm line between justified and unjustified killings cannot be securely drawn. It is thought best not to redraw the line in the first place, for redrawing it will inevitably lead to a downhill slide. It is then often pointed out that as a matter of historical record this is precisely what has occurred in the darker regions of human history, including the Nazi era, where euthanasia began with the best intentions for horribly ill, non-Jewish Germans and gradually spread to anyone deemed an enemy of the people. (ii) Second, it is said that our basic principles against killing will be gradually eroded once some form of killing is legitimated. For example, it is said that permitting voluntary euthanasia will lead to permitting involuntary euthanasia, which will in turn lead to permitting euthanasia for those who are a nuisance to society (idiots, recidivist criminals, defective newborns, and the insane, e.g.). Gradually other principles which instill respect for human life will be eroded or abandoned in the process.

I am not inclined to accept the reason (i).[7] If our justifying principles are themselves justified, then any action they warrant would be justified. Accordingly, I shall only be concerned with the second approach (ii).

(2) *Rule utilitarianism* is the position that a society ought to adopt a rule if its acceptance would have better consequences for the common good (greater social utility) than any comparable rule could have in that society. Any action is right if it conforms to a valid rule and wrong if it violates the rule. Sometimes it is said that alternative rules would be measured against one another, while it has also been

suggested that whole moral codes (complete sets of rules) rather than individual rules should be compared. While I prefer the latter formulation (Brandt's), this internal dispute need not detain us here. The important point is that a particular rule or a particular code of rules is morally justified if and only if there is no other competing rule or moral code whose acceptance would have a higher utility value for society, and where a rule's acceptability is contingent upon the consequences which would result if the rule were made current.

Wedge arguments, when conjoined with rule utilitarian arguments, may be applied to euthanasia issues in the following way. We presently subscribe to a no-active-euthanasia rule (which the AMA suggests we retain). Imagine now that in our society we make current a restricted-active-euthanasia rule (as Rachels seems to urge). Which of these two moral rules would, if enacted, have the consequence of maximizing social utility? Clearly a restricted-active-euthanasia rule would have some utility value, as Rachels notes, since some intense and uncontrollable suffering would be eliminated. However, it may not have the highest utility value in the structure of our present code or in any imaginable code which could be made current, and therefore may not be a component in the ideal code for our society. If wedge arguments raise any serious questions at all, as I think they do, they rest in this area of whether a code would be weakened or strengthened by the addition of active euthanasia principles. For the disutility of introducing legitimate killing into one's moral code (in the form of active euthanasia rules) may, in the long run, outweigh the utility of doing so, as a result of the eroding effect such a relaxation would have on rules in the code which demand respect for human life. If, for example, rules permitting active killing were introduced, it is not implausible to suppose that destroying defective newborns (a form of involuntary euthanasia) would become an accepted and common practice, that as population increases occur the aged will be even more neglectable and neglected than they now are, that capital punishment for a wide variety of crimes could be increasingly tempting, that some doctors would have appreciably reduced fears of actively injecting fatal doses whenever it seemed to them propitious to do so, and that laws of war against killing would erode in efficacy even beyond their already abysmal level.

A hundred such possible consequences might easily be imagined. But these few are sufficient to make the larger point that such rules permitting killing could lead to a general reduction of respect for human life. Rules against killing in a moral code are not isolated moral principles; they are pieces of a web of rules against killing which forms the code. The more threads one removes, the weaker the fabric becomes. And if, as I believe, moral principles against active killing have the deep and continuously civilizing effect of promoting respect for life, and if principles which allow passively letting die (as envisioned in the AMA statement) do not themselves cut against this effect, then this seems an important reason for the maintenance of the active/passive distinctions. (By the logic of the above argument passively letting die would also have to be prohibited if a rule permitting it had the serious adverse consequence of eroding acceptance of rules protective of respect of life. While this prospect seems to me improbable, I can hardly claim to have refuted those conservatives who would claim that even rules which sanction letting die place us on a precarious slippery slope.)

A troublesome problem, however, confronts my use of utilitarian and wedge arguments. Most all of us would agree that both killing and letting die are justified under some conditions. Killing in self-defense and in "just" wars are widely accepted as justified because the conditions excuse the killing. If society can withstand these exceptions to moral rules prohibiting killing, then why is it not plausible to suppose society can accept another excusing exception in the form of justified active euthanasia? This is an important and worthy objection, but not a decisive one. The defenseless and the dying are significantly different classes of persons from aggressors who attack individuals and/or nations. In the case of aggressors, one does not confront the question whether their lives are no longer worth living. Rather, we reach the judgment that the aggressors' morally blameworthy actions justify counteractions. But in the case of the dying and the otherwise ill, there is no morally blameworthy action to justify our own. Here we are required to accept the judgment that their lives are no longer worth living in order to believe that the termination of their lives is justified. It is the latter sort of judgment which is feared by those who take the wedge argument seriously. We do not now permit and never have permitted the taking of morally blameless lives. I think this is the key to understanding why recent cases of intentionally allowing the death of defective newborns (as in the now famous case at the Johns Hopkins Hospital) have generated such protracted controversy. Even if such newborns could not have led meaningful lives (a matter of some controversy), it is the wedged foot in the door which creates the most intense worries. For if we once take a decision to allow a restricted infanticide justification or any justification at all on grounds that a life is not meaningful or not worth living, we have qualified our moral rules against killing. That this qualification is a matter of the utmost seriousness needs no argument. I mention it here only to show why the wedge argument may have moral force even though we already allow some very different conditions to justify intentional killing.

There is one final utilitarian reason favoring the preservation of the active/passive distinction.[8] Suppose we distinguish the following two types of cases of wrongly diagnosed patients:

1. Patients wrongly diagnosed as hopeless, and who will survive even if a treatment is ceased (in order to allow a natural death).
2. Patients wrongly diagnosed as hopeless, and who will survive only if the treatment is not ceased (in order to allow a natural death.)

If a social rule permitting only passive euthanasia were in effect, then doctors and families who "allowed death" would lose only patients in class 2, not those in class 1; whereas if active euthanasia were permitted, at least some patients in class 1 would be needlessly lost. Thus, the consequence of a no-active-euthanasia rule would be to save some lives which could not be saved if both forms of euthanasia were allowed. This reason is not a decisive reason for favoring a policy of passive euthanasia, since these classes (1 and 2) are likely to be very small and since there might be counterbalancing reasons (extreme pain, autonomous expression of the patient, etc.) in favor of active euthanasia. But certainly it is a reason favoring only passive euthanasia and one which is morally relevant and ought to be considered along with other moral reasons.

IV

It may still be insisted that my case has not touched Rachels' leading claim, for I have not shown, as Rachels puts it, that it is "the bare difference between killing and letting die that makes the difference in these cases" (80). True, I have not shown this, and in my judgment it cannot be shown. But this concession does not require capitulation to Rachels' argument. I adduced a case which is at the center of our moral intuition that killing is morally different (in at least some cases) from letting die; and I then attempted to account for at least part of the grounds for this belief. The grounds turn out to be other than the bare difference, but nevertheless make the distinction morally relevant. The identical point can be made regarding the voluntary/involuntary distinction, as it is commonly applied to euthanasia. It is not the bare difference between voluntary euthanasia (i.e., euthanasia with patient consent) and involuntary euthanasia (i.e., without patient consent) that makes one justifiable and one not. Independent moral grounds based on, for example, respect for autonomy or beneficence, or perhaps justice will alone make the moral difference.

In order to illustrate this general claim, let us presume that it is sometimes justified to kill another person and sometimes justified to allow another to die. Suppose, for example, that one may kill in self-defense and may allow to die when a promise has been made to someone that he would be allowed to die. Here conditions of self-defense and promising justify action. But suppose now that someone A promises in exactly similar circumstances to kill someone B at B's request, and also that someone C allows someone D to die in an act of self-defense. Surely A is obliged equally to kill or to let die if he promised; and surely C is permitted to let D die if it is a matter of defending C's life. If this analysis is correct, then it follows that killing is sometimes right, sometimes wrong, depending on the circumstances, and the same is true of letting die. It is the justifying reasons which make the difference whether an action is right, not merely the kind of action it is.

Now, if letting die led to disastrous conclusions but killing did not, then letting die but not killing would be wrong. Consider, for example, a possible world in which dying would be indefinitely prolongable even if all extraordinary therapy were removed and the patient were allowed to die. Suppose that it costs over one million dollars to let each patient die, that nurses consistently commit suicide from caring for those being "allowed to die," that physicians are constantly being successfully sued for malpractice for allowing death by cruel and wrongful means, and that hospitals are uncontrollably overcrowded and their wards filled with communicable diseases which afflict only the dying. Now suppose further that killing in this possible world is quick, painless, and easily monitored. I submit that in this world we would believe that killing is morally acceptable but that allowing to die is morally unacceptable. The point of this example is again that it is the circumstances that make the difference, not the bare difference between killing and letting die.

It is, however, worth noticing that there is nothing in the AMA statement which says that the bare difference between killing and letting die itself and alone makes the difference in our differing moral assessment of rightness and wrongness. Rachels forces this interpretation on the statement. Some philosophers may have thought bare differences makes the difference, but there is scant evidence that the AMA or any thoughtful ethicist must believe it in order to defend the relevance and importance of the active/passive distinction. When this conclusion is coupled with my earlier argument that from Rachels' paradigm cases it follows only that the active/passive distinction is sometimes, but not always, morally irrelevant, it would seem that his case against the AMA is rendered highly questionable.

V

There remains, however, the important question as to whether we ought to accept the distinction between active and passive euthanasia, now that we are clear about (at least one way of drawing) the moral grounds for its invocation. That is, should we employ the distinction in order to judge some acts of euthanasia justified and others not justified? Here, as the hesitant previous paragraph indicates, I am uncertain. This problem is a substantive moral issue—not merely a conceptual one—and would require at a minimum a lengthy assessment of wedge arguments and related utilitarian considerations. In important respects empirical questions are involved in this assessment. We should like to know, and yet have hardly any evidence to indicate, what the consequences would be for our society if we were to allow the use of active means to produce death. The best hope for making such an assessment has seemed to some to rest in analogies to suicide and capital punishment statutes. Here it may reasonably be asked whether recent liberalization of laws limiting these forms of killing have served as the thin end of a wedge leading to a breakdown of principles protecting life or to widespread violation of moral principles. Nonetheless, such analogies do not seem to me promising, since they are still fairly remote from the pertinent issue of the consequences of allowing active humanitarian killing of one person by another.

It is interesting to notice the outcome of the Kamisar-Williams debate on euthanasia—which is almost exclusively cast by both writers in a consequential, utilitarian framework.[9] At one crucial point in the debate, where possible consequences of laws permitting euthanasia are under discussion, they exchange "perhaps" judgments:

> I [Williams] will return Kamisar the compliment and say: "Perhaps." We are certainly in an area where no solution is going to make things quite easy and happy for everybody, and all sorts of embarrassments may be

conjectured. But these embarrassments are not avoided by keeping to the present law: we suffer from them already.[10]

Because of the grave difficulties which stand in the way of making accurate predictions about the impact of liberalized euthanasia laws—especially those that would permit active killing—it is not surprising that those who debate the subject would reach a point of exchanging such "perhaps" judgments. And that is why, so it seems to me, we are uncertain whether to perpetuate or to abandon the active/passive distinction in our moral thinking about euthanasia. I think we do perpetuate it in medicine, law, and ethics because we are still somewhat uncertain about the conditions under which passive euthanasia should be permitted by law (which is one form of social rule). We are unsure about what the consequences will be of the California "Natural Death Act" and all those similar acts passed by other states which have followed in its path. If untoward results occur (on a widespread scale), then we would be most reluctant to accept further liberalizations and might even abolish natural death acts.

In short, I have argued in this section that euthanasia in its active and its passive forms presents us with a dilemma which can be developed by using powerful consequentialist arguments on each side, yet there is little clarity concerning the proper resolution of the dilemma precisely because of our uncertainty regarding proclaimed consequences.

VI

I reach two conclusions at the end of these several arguments. First, I think Rachels is incorrect in arguing that the distinction between active and passive is (always) morally irrelevant. It may well be relevant, and for moral reasons—the reasons adduced in section III above. Second, I think nonetheless that Rachels may ultimately be shown correct in his contention that we ought to dispense with the active/passive distinction—for reasons adduced in sections IV–V. But if he is ultimately judged correct, it will be because we have come to see that some forms of active killing have generally acceptable social consequences, and not primarily because of the arguments he adduces in his paper—even though something may be said for each of these arguments. Of course, in one respect I have conceded a great deal to Rachels. The bare difference argument is vital to his position, and I have fully agreed to it. On the other hand, I do not see that the bare difference argument does play or need play a major role in our moral thinking—or in that of the AMA.

NOTES

1. "Active and Passive Euthanasia." *New England Journal of Medicine* 292:78–80, 9 January 1975. (All page references in parentheses refer to Rachels' article.)

2. As recorded in the Opinion of Judge Robert Muir, Jr., Dockett No. C-201-75 of the Superior Court of New Jersey, Chancery Division, Morris County (10 November 1975).

3. See Judge Muir's Opinion, p. 18—a slightly different statement but on the subject.

4. This problem of the strength of evidence also emerged in the Quinlan trial, as physicians disagreed whether the evidence was "irrefutable." Such disagreement, when added to the problems of medical fallibility and causal responsibility just outlined, provides in the eyes of some one important argument against the legalization of active euthanasia, as perhaps the AMA would agree.

5. Among the moral reasons why one is held to be responsible in the first sort of case and not responsible in the second sort are, I believe, the moral grounds for the active/passive distinction under discussion in this section.

6. In *Social Ethics,* as cited in the permission note to this article. *This paper is a heavily revised version of an article by the same title first published in *Social Ethics,* edited by T. Mappes and J. Zembaty. New York: McGraw-Hill, 1976. Copyright 1975, 1977 by Tom L. Beauchamp.

7. An argument of this form, which I find unacceptable for reasons given below, is Dyck, Arthur. "Beneficent Euthanasia and Benemortasia: Alternative Views of Mercy." In *Beneficent Euthanasia,* edited by M. Kohl. Buffalo, N.Y.: Prometheus Books, 1975, pp. 120f.

8. I owe most of this argument to James Rachels, whose comments on an earlier draft of this paper led to several significant alterations.

9. Williams bases his pro-euthanasia argument on the prevention of two consequences: (1) loss of liberty and (2) cruelty. Kamisar bases his anti-euthanasia position on three projected consequences of euthanasia laws: (1) mistaken diagnosis, (2) pressured decisions by seriously ill patients, and (3) the wedge of the laws will lead to legalized involuntary euthanasia. Kamisar admits that individual acts of euthanasia are sometimes justified. It is the rule that he opposes. He is thus clearly a rule-utilitarian, and I believe Williams is as well (cf. his views on children and the senile). Their assessments of wedge arguments are, however, radically different.

10. Williams, Glanville. "Mercy-Killing Legislation—A Rejoinder." *Minnesota Law Review* 43 (No. 1):5, 1985.

Z

The Principle of Justice

INTRODUCTION

The principles that might appear in a system of biomedical ethics examined thus far all are relevant to the care of the individual patient. An individual patient's care can be assessed based on the Hippocratic principle of benefiting the patient and protecting him or her from harm according to the clinician's judgment. The principles of fidelity or contract-keeping, autonomy, and veracity or honesty all indicate additional right-making characteristics of actions as they may be applied to individual patients. These may often present considerations that will incline a clinician to abandon the mere focus on good consequences for the patient. In the name of fidelity the promise to keep confidences may be perceived as binding even in cases where the clinician believes the patient would be better off if information about her were disclosed. In the name of autonomy patients may be recognized as having the right to refuse treatment even in cases where the clinician believes the patient would be better off if he were forced to undergo treatment against his will. In the name of veracity some patients claim that they have a right to terminal diagnoses even in cases where the clinician believes the patient would be better off not knowing. All of these have ethical implications at the personal level of health care.

Many contemporary medical ethical dilemmas, however, necessarily involve more than single isolated patients. Clinicians may be asked to choose among several patients all needing care. Hospitals may be forced to limit access to care in order to conserve scarce resources. The society as a whole may have to decide whether to fund expensive high technology, life-sustaining interventions, such as heart transplants, or to spend scarce resources on immunizations, maternal-child health programs, or campaigns to promote healthy life-styles.

In these cases ethical principles such as the Hippocratic formula that focuses on the patient in the singular will not be sufficient. In any full medical ethical system there needs to be some principle for resolving matters of distribution whenever there is competition for scarce resources, whether they be money, rare pharmaceuticals, or the time of health professionals.

One response is that if only waste and inefficiency were eliminated, there would be enough to go around so that everyone could receive all the health care that was medically necessary. Certainly, that ought to be eliminated. The ethical principle of doing what produces the most good requires that waste be eliminated. But that is not as easy as it sounds. People have vested interests in the systems that supply wasteful care. More importantly there are legitimate ethical disputes about what counts as a useless intervention. Maintenance of a patient in a permanent coma can require a terribly expensive, labor intensive effort. Some people will say that such efforts are utterly useless, that they would actually prefer that such efforts not be made. Others, however, will disagree claiming that they stand in philosophical or religious traditions that hold that life is valuable even if it is a life in a permanent coma. Determining what counts as useless care is morally very controversial.

Moreover, even if we could eliminate all useless, wasteful care there would still be an enormous amount of care that would be somewhat beneficial. Some of that care is terribly expensive in relation to the amount of benefit projected. Aggressive treatment of the cancer patient may produce a one in a thousand chance of cure. However, it may be judged by the patient to be worth the try. The expected benefit may be small, but considering the alternative, it may be worth the try. Frequent physical exams, blood tests, drug therapies with low probability of success, and even experimental surgical procedures are all more appropriately described as treatments that offer some potential benefits, but at a cost that is very high in comparison with the benefits. Even relatively rare interventions, such as heart transplants, may have a projected cost of many billions of dollars a year if every patient got them who could potentially benefit. With potentially marginally beneficial interventions such as private, one-on-one, long-term psychotherapy, rehabilitation of the severely brain-damaged head trauma patient, and optimal care of chronically debilitated Alzheimer's patients, the potential beneficial expenditures for health care could easily exceed the entire gross national product. If the health resource allocation question were posed in global perspective, it is reasonable to conclude that all of the world's resources could go to health care that really produced benefits (although sometimes relatively small benefits). This means that some ethical choice must be made in placing limits on health care.

Allen Buchanan, in the first essay in this chapter, outlines three major alternative ethical strategies for dealing with these issues. The first two really resolve the conflict by appeals to ethical considerations already discussed in previous chapters. First, we could emphasize the principle of autonomy and the liberty that people should have to make use of their personally held resources as they see fit. This, combined with the ethics of contracting, could lead to a system whereby individuals were free to make arrangements, buy health care, or purchase insurance up to the level of whatever means they had at their disposal. By the same reasoning, physicians and other health-care professionals could be viewed as "owning" their time and talent such that they could take care of whatever patients they choose based on whatever criteria they find appropriate. The choice could be based on compassion and charity or on financial inducements. In either case, autonomy would be served. Certain assumptions would be necessary, for instance, a belief that persons are really the owners of the resources they possess, not only their money and material goods, but also their knowledge and intellectual and physical skills. More fundamentally one would have to accept the idea that these kinds of issues should be resolved by appeals to liberty rather than by any duty one has to produce good or distribute benefits fairly.

A second major strategy is to take the Hippocratic principle of a duty to benefit the patient and avoid harm and expand it to apply to social groups, in fact, potentially to society as a whole. Under this strategy beneficence becomes a social principle. One major manifestation of this approach is utilitarianism which, in various forms, holds that we can determine what is the proper course of action by determining which course produces the greatest good for the greatest number. Presumably we would choose among health-care allocations based on what will produce the greatest improvement in aggregate health indicators. We would decide how much of our total resources should go to health care by determining whether marginal resources will produce more good overall spent on health or on some other area.

A third strategy also recognizes that there are moral limits on personal autonomy, but resists the notion that the goal of morality is simply to produce as much good as possible regardless of how the good is distributed. This third approach holds that there is an independent principle of justice that identifies a pattern of distribution of goods as a right-making characteristic of actions. Just as autonomy or veracity may place moral limits on how much good we can do for an individual patient, a principle of justice, according to this third view, places limits on how much good ought to be done at the interpersonal or societal level. The content of the principle of justice varies according to different theorists. Some hold that merit provides a just basis of allocating. Others emphasize effort, good will, and so forth. The most important basis for allocating—other than solely on the amount of good that one can do—is need. Under this view those who are particularly poorly-off deserve resources even if expenditures of resources in this manner will not necessarily do as much good as spending them in some other way.

For example, a physician may have to choose between three relatively well-off patients and one who is desperately ill. Sometimes giving the sickest patient the first priority will produce the most benefit, but other times it may not, say, for example, when the sickest patient is so ill that not as much can be done for him. In such a case beneficence or utility maximizing would point toward treating the three healthier patients while a needs-based principle of justice may say that, nevertheless, the sickest have a special moral claim on us. In this chapter, after Buchanan sets out the alternatives, Robert Sade argues for a liberty-based interpretation while the President's Commission for the Study of Ethical Problems in Medicine and Biomedical and Behavioral Research, in the following essay, seems to emphasize a basic right to some level of health care that draws on both beneficence and justice in placing limits on liberty of patients and providers.

In the essay that follows Allen Buchanan sets out the major options for answering the question of how health-care resources ought to be distributed. He identifies three major options. The first, utilitarianism, is related to the Hippocratic ethical principle in that it focuses on the production of benefits. While the Hippocratic ethic, however, limits attention solely to the individual patient, utilitarianism expands the horizon to count as morally relevant all possible benefits and harms to all persons. Buchanan makes clear that there are varieties within utilitarianism. Some forms consider the consequences of actions directly; others assess the consequences of moral rules. Some assess aggregate utility; others average benefits.

Buchanan then introduces John Rawls as a major proponent of a non-utilitarian theory of distribution. In this system—the only one in which justice is really an independent principle unrelated to other, previously considered moral principles such as beneficence and autonomy—social practices (such as health-care systems) ought to be arranged so that inequalities benefit the least well-off in the community. This often, but not always, amounts to making people more equal. It would not lead to equality in cases where inequalities actually help those least well-off (such as perhaps by paying large salaries to talented physicians in order to get them to help sick people). Thus a variant on the Rawlsian distribution would be an even more radical egalitarianism whereby people are held to have a right to equality even if inequalities produce more benefit for persons on the bottom.

Finally, Buchanan introduces libertarianism, derived from a more exclusive emphasis on liberty or autonomy as a moral principle, and then examines the health care implications of all of these options.

Justice: A Philosophical Review

ALLEN BUCHANAN

INTRODUCTION

The past decade has seen the burgeoning of bioethics and the resurgence of theorizing about justice. Yet until now these two developments have not been as mutually enriching as one might have hoped. Bioethicists have tended to concentrate on micro issues (moral problems of individual or small group decisionmaking), ignoring fundamental moral questions about the macro structure within which the micro issues arise. Theorists of justice have advanced very general principles but have typically neglected to show how they can illuminate the particular problems we face in health care and other urgent areas.

Micro problems do not exist in an institutional vacuum. The parents of a severely impaired newborn and the attending neonatologist are faced with the decision of whether to treat the infant aggressively or to allow it to die because neonatal intensive care units now exist which make it possible to preserve the lives of infants who previously would have died. Neonatal intensive care units exist because certain policy decisions have been made which allocated certain social resources to the development of technology for sustaining defective newborns rather than for preventing birth defects. Limiting moral inquiry to the micro issues supports an unreasoned conservatism by failing to examine the health care institutions within which micro problems arise and by not investigating the larger array of institutions of which the health care sector is only one part. Since not only particular actions but also policies and institutions may be just or unjust, serious theorizing about justice forces us to expand the narrow focus of the micro approach by raising fundamental queries about the background social, economic, and political institutions from which micro problems emerge.

On the other hand, the attention to individual cases which dominates contemporary bioethics can provide a much needed concrete focus for refining and assessing competing theories of justice. The adequacy or inadequacy of a moral theory cannot be determined by inspecting the principles which constitute it. Instead, rational assessment requires an on-going process in which general principles are revised and refined through confrontation with the rich complexity of our considered judgments about particular cases, while our judgments about particular cases are gradually structured and modified by our provisional acceptance of general principles. Since our considered judgments about particular cases may often be more sensitive and sure than our assessments of abstract principles, careful attention to accurately described, concrete moral situations is essential for theorizing about justice.

Further, it is not just that the problems of bioethics provide one class of test cases for theories of justice among others: the problems of bioethics are among the most difficult and pressing issues with which a theory of justice must cope. It appears, then, that the continued development of both bioethics and of theorizing about justice in general requires us to explore the problems of justice in health care. In this essay I hope to contribute to that enterprise by first providing a sketch of three major theories of justice and by then attempting to ascertain some of their implications for moral problems in health care.

THEORIES OF JUSTICE

Utilitarianism

Utilitarianism purports to be a comprehensive moral theory, of which a utilitarian theory of justice is only one part. There are two main types of comprehensive utilitarian theory: Act and Rule Utilitarianism. Act Utilitarianism defines rightness with respect to particular acts: an act is right if and only if it maximizes utility. Rule Utilitarianism defines rights with respect to rules of action and makes the rightness of particular acts depend upon the rules under which those acts fall. A rule is right if and only if general compliance with that rule (or with a set of rules of which it is an element) maximizes utility, and a particular action is right if and only if it falls under such a rule.

Both Act and Rule Utilitarianism may be versions of either Classic or Average Utilitarianism. Classic Utilitarianism defines the rightness of acts or rules as maximization of *aggregate* utility; Average Utilitarianism defines rightness as maximization of utility *per capita*. The aggregate utility produced by an act or by general compliance with a rule is the sum of the utility produced for each individual affected. Average utility is the aggregate utility divided by the number of individuals affected. 'Utility' is defined as pleasure, satisfaction, happiness, or as the realization of preferences, as the latter are revealed through individuals' choices.

The distinction between Act and Rule Utilitarianism is important for a utilitarian theory of justice, since the latter must include an account of when *institutions* are just. Thus, institutional rules may maximize utility even though those rules do not direct individuals as individuals or as occupants of institutional positions to maximize utility in a case by case fashion. For example, it may be that a judicial system which maximizes utility will do so by including rules which prohibit judges from deciding a case according to their estimates of what would maximize utility in that particular case. Thus the utilitarian justification of a particular action or decision may not be that it maximizes utility, but rather that it falls under some rule of an institution or set of institutions which maximizes utility.[1]

Some utilitarians, such as John Stuart Mill, hold that principles of justice are the most basic moral principles because the utility of adherence to them is especially great. According to this view, utilitarian principles of justice are those utilitarian moral principles which are of such importance that they may be *enforced*, if necessary. Some utilitarians, including Mill perhaps, also hold that among the utilitarian principles of justice are principles specifying individual rights, whether the latter are thought of as enforceable claims which take precedence over appeals to what would maximize utility in the particular case. Indeed, some contemporary rights theorists such as Ronald Dworkin define a (justified) right claim as one which takes precedence over mere appeals to what would maximize utility.

A utilitarian moral theory, then, can include rights principles which themselves prohibit appeals to utility maximization, so long as the justification of those principles is that they are part of an institutional system which maximizes utility. In cases where two or more rights principles conflict, considerations of utility may be invoked to determine which rights principles are to be given priority. Utilitarianism is incompatible with rights only if rights exclude appeals to utility maximization at all levels of justification, including the most basic institutional level. Rights founded ultimately on considerations of utility may be called *derivative*, to distinguish them from rights in the *strict* sense.

Utilitarianism is the most influential version of teleological moral theory. A moral theory is teleological if and only if it defines the good independently of the right and defines the right as that which maximizes the good. Utilitarianism defines the good as happiness (satisfaction, etc.), independently of any account of what is morally right, and then defines the right as that which maximizes the good (either in the particular case or at the institutional level). A moral theory is *deontological* if and only if it is not a teleological theory, i.e., if and only if it either does not define the good independently of the right or does not define the right as that which maximizes the good. Both the second and third theories of justice we shall consider are deontological theories.

John Rawls's Theory: Justice as Fairness

In *A Theory of Justice* Rawls pursues two main goals. The first is to set out a small but powerful set of principles of justice which underlie and explain the considered moral judgments we make about particular actions, policies, laws, and institutions. The second is to offer a theory of justice superior to Utilitarianism. These two goals are intimately related for Rawls because he believes that the theory which does a better job of supporting and accounting for our considered judgments is the better theory, other things being equal. The principles of justice Rawls offers are as follows:

(1) The principle of greatest equal liberty:
Each person is to have an equal right to the most extensive system of equal basic liberties compatible with a similar system of liberty for all ([6], pp. 60, 201–205).

(2) The principle of equality of fair opportunity:
Offices and positions are to be open to all under conditions of equality of fair opportunity—persons with similar abilities and skills are to have equal access to offices and positions ([6], pp. 60, 73, 83–89).[2]

(3) The difference principle:
Social and economic institutions are to be arranged so as to benefit maximally the worst off ([6], pp. 60, 75–83).[3]

The basic liberties referred to in (1) include freedom of speech, freedom of conscience, freedom from arbitrary arrest, the right to hold personal property, and freedom of political participation (the right to vote, to run for office, etc.).

Since the demands of these principles may conflict, some way of ordering them is needed. According to Rawls, (1) is *lexically* prior to (2) and (2) is *lexically* prior to (3). A principle 'P' is lexically prior to a principle 'Q' if and only if we are first to satisfy all the requirements of 'P' before going on to satisfy the requirements of 'Q.' Lexical priority allows no trade-offs between the demands of conflicting principles: the lexically prior principle takes absolute priority.

Rawls notes that "many kinds of things are said to be just or unjust: not only laws, institutions, and social systems, but also particular actions . . . decisions, judgments and imputations. . . ." ([6], p. 7). But he insists that the primary subject of justice is the *basic structure* of society because it exerts a pervasive and profound influence on individuals' life prospects. The basic structure is the entire set of major political, legal, economic, and social institutions. In our society the basic structure includes the Constitution, private ownership of the means of production, competitive markets, and the monogamous family. The basic structure plays a large role in distributing the burdens and benefits of cooperation among members of society.

If the primary subject of justice is the basic structure, then the primary problem of justice is to formulate and justify a set of principles which a just basic structure must satisfy. These principles will specify how the basic structure is to distribute prospects of what Rawls calls *primary goods*. They include the basic liberties (listed above under (2)), as well as powers, authority, opportunities, income, and wealth. Rawls says that primary goods are things that every rational person is presumed to want, because they normally have a use, whatever a person's rational plan of life ([6], p. 62). Principle (1) regulates the distribution of prospects of basic liberties; (2) regulates the distribution of prospects of powers and authority, so far as these are attached to institutional offices and positions, and (3) regulates the distribution of prospects of the other primary goods, including wealth and income. Though the first and second principles require equality, the difference principle allows inequalities so long as the total system of institutions of which they are a part maximizes the prospects of the worst off to the primary goods in question.

Rawls advances three distinct types of justification for his principles of justice. Two appeal to our considered judgments, while the third is based on what he calls the Kantian interpretation of his theory.

The first type of justification rests on the idea, mentioned earlier, that if a set of principles provides the best account of our considered judgments about what is just or unjust, then that is a reason for accepting those principles. A set of principles accounts for our judgments only if those judgments can be derived from the principles, granted the relevant facts for their application.

Rawls's second type of justification maintains that if a set of principles would be chosen under conditions which, according to our considered judgments, are appropriate conditions for choosing principles of justice, then this is a reason for accepting those principles. The second type of justification includes three parts: (1) A set of conditions for choosing principles of justice must be specified. Rawls labels the complete set of conditions the 'original position.' (2) It must be shown that the conditions specified are (according to our considered judgments) the appropriate conditions of choice. (3) It must be shown that Rawls's principles are indeed the principles which would be chosen under those conditions.

Rawls construes the choice of principles of justice as an ideal social contract. "The principles of justice for the basic structure of society are the principles that free and rational persons . . . would accept in an initial situation of equality as defining the fundamental terms of their association" ([6], p. 11). The idea of a social contract has several advantages. First, it allows us to view principles of justice as the object of a *rational collective choice*. Second, the idea of *contractual obligation* is used to emphasize that the choice expresses a basic commitment and that the principles agreed on may be rightly enforced. Third, the idea of a contract as a *voluntary agreement* which set terms for mutual advantage suggests that the principles of justice should be "such as to draw forth the willing cooperation" ([6], p. 15) of all members of society, including those who are worse off.

The most important elements of the original position or our purposes are a) the characterization of the parties to the contract as individuals who desire to pursue their own life plans effectively and who "have a highest-order interest in how . . . their interests . . . are shaped and regulated by social institutions" ([8], p. 64); b) the 'veil of ignorance,' which is a constraint on the information the parties are able to utilize in choosing principles of justice; and c) the requirement that the principles are to be chosen on the assumption that they will be complied with by all (the universalizability condition) ([6], p. 132).

The parties are characterized as desiring to maximize their shares of primary goods, because these goods enable one to implement effectively the widest range of life plans and because at least some of them, such as freedom of speech and of conscience, facilitate one's freedom to choose and revise one's life plan or conception of the good. The parties are to choose "from behind a veil of ignorance" so that information about their own particular characteristics or social positions will not lead to bias in the choice of principles. Thus they are described as not knowing their race, sex, socioeconomic, or political status, or even the nature of their particular conceptions of the good. The informational restriction also helps to insure that the principles chosen will not place avoidable restrictions on the individual's freedom to choose and revise his or her life plan.[4]

Though Rawls offers several arguments to show that his principles would be chosen in the original position, the most striking is the maximum argument. According to this argument, the rational strategy in the original position is to choose that set of principles whose implementation will maximize the minimum share of primary goods which one can receive as a member of society, and principles (1), (2), and (3) will insure the greatest minimal share. Rawls's claim is that because these principles protect one's basic liberties and opportunities and insure an adequate minimum of goods such as wealth and income (even if one should turn out to be among the worst off) the rational thing is to choose them, rather than to gamble with one's life prospects by opting for alternative principles. In particular, Rawls contends that it would be irrational to reject his principles and allow one's life prospect to be determined by what would maximize utility, since utility maximization might allow severe deprivation or even slavery for some, so long as this contributed sufficiently to the welfare of others.

Rawls raises an important question about this second mode of justification when he notes that this original position is purely hypothetical. Granted that the agreement is never actually entered into, why should we regard the principles as binding? The answer, according to Rawls, is that we do in fact accept the conditions embodied in the original position ([6], p. 21). The following qualification, which Rawls adds immediately after claiming that the conditions which constitute the original position are appropriate for the choice of principles of justice according to our considered judgments, introduces his third type of justification: "Or if we do not [accept the conditions of the original position as appropriate for choosing principles of justice] *then perhaps we can be persuaded to do so by the philosophical* reflections" (emphasis added [6], p. 21). In the Kantian interpretation section of *A Theory of Justice,* Rawls sketches a certain kind of philosophical justification for the conditions which make up the original position (based on Kant's conception of the 'noumenal self' or autonomous agent).

For Kant an autonomous agent's will is determined by rational principles and rational principles are those which can serve as principles for all rational beings, not just for this or that agent, depending upon whether or not he has some particular desire which other rational beings may not have. Rawls invites us to think of the original position as the perspective from which autonomous agents see the world. The original position provides a "procedural interpretation" of Kant's idea of a Realm of Ends or community of "free and equal rational beings". We express our nature as autonomous agents when we act from principles that would be chosen in conditions which reflect that nature ([6], p. 252).

Rawls concludes that, when persons such as you and I accept those principles that would be chosen in the original position, we express our nature as autonomous agents, i.e., we act autonomously. There are three main grounds for this thesis, corresponding to the three features of the original position cited earlier. First, since the veil of ignorance excludes information about any particular desires which a rational agent may or may not have, the choice of principles is not determined by any particular desire. Second, since the parties strive to maximize their share of primary goods, and since primary goods are attractive to them because they facilitate freedom in choosing and revising life plans and because they are flexible means not tied to any particular ends, this is another respect in which their choice is not determined by particular desires. Third, the original position includes the requirement that they will be principles of rational agents in general and not just for agents who happen to have this or that particular desire.

In the *Foundation of the Metaphysics of Morals* Kant advances a moral philosophy which identifies autonomy with rationality [4]. Hence for Kant the question "Why should one express our nature as autonomous agents?" is answered by the thesis that rationality requires it. Thus *if* Rawls's third type of justification succeeds in showing that we best express our autonomy when we accept those principles in the belief that they would be chosen from the original position, and *if* Kant's identification of autonomy with rationality is successful, the result will be a justification of Rawls's principles which is distinct from both the first and second modes of justification. So far as this third type of justification does not make the acceptance of Rawls's principles hinge on whether the principles themselves or the conditions from which they would be chosen match our considered judgments, it is not directly vulnerable either to the charge that Rawls has misconstrued our considered judgments or that congruence with considered judgments, like the appeal to mere consensus, has no justificatory force.

It is important to see that Rawls understands his principles of justice as principles which generate *rights* in what I have called the strict sense. Claims based upon the three principles are to take precedence over considerations of utility and the principles themselves are not justified on the grounds that a basic structure which satisfies them will maximize utility. Moreover, Rawls's theory is not a teleological theory of any kind because it does not define the right as that which maximizes the good, where the good is defined independently of the right. Instead it is perhaps the most influential current instance of a deontological theory.

Nozick's Libertarian Theory

There are many versions of libertarian theory, but their characteristic doctrine is that coercion may only be used to prevent or punish physical harm, theft, and fraud, and to enforce contracts. Perhaps the most influential and systematic recent instance of Libertarianism is the theory presented by Robert Nozick in *Anarchy, State, and Utopia* [5]. In Nozick's theory of justice, as in libertarian theories generally, the right to private property is fundamental and determines both the legitimate role of the state and the most basic principles of individual conduct.

Nozick contends that individuals have a property right in their persons and in whatever 'holdings' they come to have through actions which conform to (1) "the principle of justice in [initial] acquisition" and (2) "the principle of justice in transfer" ([5], p. 151). The first principle specifies the ways in which an individual may come to own hitherto unowned things without violating anyone else's rights. Here Nozick largely follows John Locke's famous account of how one makes natural objects one's own by "mixing one's labor" with them or improving them through one's labor. Though Nozick does not actually formulate a principle of justice in (initial) acquisition, he does argue that whatever the appropriate formulation is it must include a 'Lockean Proviso', which places a constraint on the holdings which one may acquire through one's labor. Nozick maintains that one may appropriate as much of an unowned item as one desires so long as (a) one's appropriation does not worsen the conditions of others in a special way, namely, by creating a situation in which others are "no longer . . . able to use freely [without exclusively appropriating] what [they] . . . previously could" or (b) one properly compensates those whose condition is worsened by one's appropriation in the way specified in (a) ([5], pp. 178–179). Nozick emphasizes that the Proviso only picks out one way in which one's appropriation may worsen the condition of others; it does not forbid appropriation or require compensation in cases in which one's appropriation of an unowned thing worsens another's condition merely by limiting his opportunities to appropriate (rather than merely use) that thing, i.e., to make it his property.

The second principle states that one may justly transfer one's legitimate holdings to another through sale, trade, gift or bequest and that one is entitled to whatever one receives in any of these ways, so long as the person from whom one receives it was entitled to that which he transferred to you. The right to property which Nozick advances is the right to exclusive control over anything one can get through initial appropriation (subject to the Lockean Proviso) or through voluntary exchanges with others entitled to what they transfer. Nozick concludes that a distribution is just if and only if it arose from another just distribution by legitimate means. The principle of justice in initial acquisition specifies the legitimate 'first moves,' while the principle of justice in transfers specifies the legitimate ways of moving from one distribution to another: "Whatever arises from a just situation by just steps is itself just" ([5], p. 151).

Since not all existing holdings arose through the 'just steps' specified by the principles of justice in acquisition and transfer, there will be a need for a *principle of rectification* of past injustices. Though Nozick does not attempt to formulate such a principle he thinks that it might well require significant redistribution of holdings.

Apart from the case of rectifying past violations of the principles of acquisition and transfer, however, Nozick's theory is strikingly anti-redistributive. Nozick contends that attempts to force anyone to contribute any part of his legitimate holdings to the welfare of others is a violation of that person's property rights, whether it is undertaken by private individuals or the state. On this view, coercively backed taxation to raise funds for welfare programs of any kind is literally theft. Thus, a large proportion of the activities now engaged in by the government involve gross injustices.

After stating his theory of rights, Nozick tries to show that the state is legitimate so long as it limits its activities to the enforcement of these rights and eschews redistributive functions. To do this he employs an 'invisible hand explanation,' which purports to show how the minimal state could arise as an unintended consequence of a series of voluntary transactions which violate no one's rights. The phrase 'invisible hand explanation' is chosen to stress that the process by which the minimal state could emerge fits Adam Smith's famous account of how individuals freely pursuing their own private ends in the market collectively produce benefits which are not the aim of anyone.

The process by which the minimal state could arise without violating anyone's rights is said to include four main steps ([5], pp. 10–25).[5] First, individuals in a 'state of nature' in which (Libertarian) moral principles are generally respected would form a plurality of 'protective agencies' to enforce their libertarian rights, since individual efforts at enforcement would be inefficient and liable to abuse. Second, through competition for clients, a 'dominant protective agency' would eventually emerge in given geographical area. Third, such an agency would eventually become a 'minimal state' by asserting a claim of monopoly over protective services in order to prevent less reliable efforts at enforcement which might endanger its clients: it would forbid 'independents' (those who refused to purchase its services) from seeking other forms of enforcement. Fourth, again assuming that correct moral principles are generally followed, those belonging to the dominant protective agency would compensate the 'independents,' presumably by providing them with free or partially subsidized protection services. With the exception of taxing its clients to provide compensation for the independents, the minimal state would act only to protect persons against physical injury, theft, fraud, and violations of contracts.

It is striking that Nozick does not attempt to provide any systematic *justification* for the Lockean rights principles he advocates. In this respect he departs radically from Rawls. Instead, Nozick assumes the correctness of the Lockean principles and then, on the basis of that assumption, argues that the minimal state and only the minimal stated is compatible with the rights those principles specify.

He does, however, offer some arguments against the more-than-minimal state which purport to be independent of that particular theory of property rights which he assumes. These arguments may provide indirect support for his principles insofar as they are designed to make alternative principles, such as Rawls's, unattractive. Perhaps most important of these is an argument designed to show that any principle of justice which demands a certain distributive end state or pattern of holdings will require frequent and gross disruptions of individuals' holdings for the sake of maintaining that end state or pattern. Nozick supports this general conclusion by a vivid example. He asks us to suppose that there is some distribution of holdings 'D$_1$' which is required by some end-state or patterned theory of justice and that 'D$_1$' is achieved at time 'T.' Now suppose that Wilt Chamberlain, the renowned basketball player, signs a contract stipulating that he is to receive twenty-five cents from the price of each ticket to the home games in which he performs, and suppose that he nets $250,000, from this arrangement. We now have a new distribution 'D$_2$'. Is 'D$_2$' unjust? Notice that by hypothesis those who paid the price of admission were entitled to control over the resources they held in 'D$_1$' (as were Chamberlain and the team's owners). The new distribution arose through *voluntary exchanges of legitimate holdings,* so it is difficult to see how it could be unjust, even if it does diverge from 'D$_1$.' From this and like examples, Nozick concludes that attempts to maintain any end-state or patterned distributive principle would require continuous interference in peoples' lives ([5], pp. 161–163).

As in the cases of Utilitarianism and Rawls's theory, Nozick and libertarians generally do not limit morality to justice. Thus, Nozick and others emphasize that a libertarian theory of individual rights is to be supplemented by a libertarian theory of virtues which recognizes that not all moral principles are suitable objects of enforcement and that moral life includes more than the nonviolation of rights. Libertarians invoke the distinction between justice and charity to reply to those who complain that a Lockean theory of property rights legitimizes crushing poverty for millions. They stress that while justice demands that we not be *forced* to contribute to the well-being of others, charity requires that we help even those who have no *right* to our aid.[6]

IMPLICATIONS FOR HEALTH CARE

Now that we have a grasp of the main ideas of three major theories of justice, we can explore briefly some of their implications for health care. To do this we may confront the theories with four questions:

(1)   Is there a right to health care? (If so, what is its basis and what is its content?)
(2)   How, in order of priority, is health care related to other goods, or how are

health care needs related to other needs? (If there is a right to health care, how is it related to other rights?)

(3)   How, in order of priority, are various forms of health care related to one another?

(4)   What can we conclude about the justice or injustice of the current health care system?

In some cases, as we shall, the theories will provide opposing answers to the same question; in others, the theories may be unhelpfully silent.

We have already seen that the Utilitarian position on rights in general is complex. If by a right we mean a right in the strict sense, i.e., a claim which takes precedence over mere appeals to utility at all levels, including the most basic institutional level, then Utilitarianism denies the existence of rights in general, including the right to health care. If, on the other hand, we mean by right a claim that takes precedence over mere appeals to utility at the level of particular actions or at some institutional level short of the most basic, but which is justified ultimately by appeal to the utility of the total set of institutions, then Utilitarianism does not exclude, and indeed may even require rights, including a right to health care. Whether or not the total institutional array which maximizes utility will include a right to health care will depend upon a wealth of *empirical facts* not deducible from the principle of utility itself. The nature and complexity of the relevant facts can best be appreciated by considering briefly the bearing of Utilitarianism on questions (2) and (3). A utilitarian system of (derivative) rights will pick out certain goods as those which make an especially large contribution to the maximization of utility. It is reasonable to assume, on the basis of empirical data, that health care, or at least certain forms of health care, is among them. Consider, for example, prenatal care, broadly conceived as including genetic screening and counseling (at least for special risk groups), prenatal nutritional care and medical examinations for expectant mothers, medical care during delivery, and basic pediatric services in the crucial months after birth. If empirical research indicates (1) that a system of institutional arrangements which maximizes utility would include such services and (2) that such services can best be assured if they are accorded the status of a right, with all that this implies, including the use of coercive sanctions where necessary, then according to Utilitarianism there is such a (derivative) right. The strength and content of this right relative to other (derivative) rights will be determined by the utility of health care as compared with other kinds of goods.

It is crucial to note that, for the utilitarian, empirical research must determine not only whether certain health care services are to be provided as a matter of right, but also whether the right in question is to be an equal right enjoyed by all persons. No commitment to equality of rights is included in the utilitarian principle itself, nor is there any commitment to equal distribution of any kind. Utilitarianism is egalitarian only in the sense that in calculating what will maximize utility each person's welfare is to be included.

Utilitarian arguments, sometimes based on empirical data, have been advanced to show that providing health care free of charge as a matter of right would encourage wasteful use of scarce and costly resources because the individual would have no incentive to restrain his 'consumption' of health care. The cumulative result, it is said, would be quite disutilitarian: a breakdown of the health care system or a disastrous curtailment of other basic services to cover the spiraling costs of health care. In contrast (proponents of this argument continue) a *market* in health care encourages 'consumers' to use resources wisely because the costs of the services an individual receives are borne by that individual.

On the other side of the utilitarian ledger, empirical evidence may be marshalled to show that the benefits of a right to health care outweigh the costs, including the costs of possible over-use, and that a market in health care would not maximize utility because those who need health care the most may not be able to afford it.

Similarly, even if there is a utilitarian justification for a right to health care, empirical evidence must again be presented to show that it should be an equal right. For it is certainly conceivable that, under certain circumstances at least, utility could be maximized by providing extensive health care only for some groups, perhaps even a minority, rather than for all persons.

Utilitarians who advocate a right to health care often argue that this right, like other basic rights, should be equal, on the basis of the assumption of diminishing marginal utility. The idea, roughly, is that with respect to many goods, including health care, there is a finite upper bound to the satisfaction a person can gain from being provided with additional amounts of the goods in question. Hence, if in general we are all subject to the phenomenon of diminishing marginal utility in the case of health care and if the threshold of diminishing marginal utility is in general sufficiently low, then there are sound utilitarian reasons for distributing health care equally.

Finally, it should be clear that for the utilitarian the issue of priorities within health care, as well as that of priorities between health care and other goods, must again be settled by empirical research. If, as seems likely, utility maximization requires more resources for prevention and health maintenance rather than for curative intervention after pathology has already developed, then this will be reflected in the content of the utilitarian right to health care. If, as many writers have contended, the current emphasis in the U.S. on high technology intervention produces less utility than would a system which stresses prevention and health maintenance (for example through stricter control of pollution and other environmental determinants of disease), then the utilitarian may conclude that the current system is unjust in this respect. Empirical data would also be needed to ascertain whether more social resources should be devoted to high- or low-technology intervention: for example, neonatal intensive care units versus 'well-baby clinics.' These examples are intended merely to illustrate the breadth and complexity of the empirical research needed to apply Utilitarianism to crucial issues in health care.

Libertarian theories such as Nozick's rely much less heavily upon empirical premises for answers to questions (1)–(4). Since the libertarian is interested only in preventing violations of libertarian rights, and since the latter are rights against certain sorts of interferences rather than rights to be provided with anything, the question of what will maximize utility is irrelevant. Further, any effort to implement any right to health care whatsoever is an injustice, according to the libertarian.

There are only two points at which empirical data are relevant for Nozick. First, whether or not any current case of appropriation of hitherto unheld things satisfies the Lockean Proviso is a matter of fact to be ascertained by empirical methods. Second, empirical historical research is needed to determine what sort of redistribution for the sake of rectifying past injustices is necessary. If, for example, physicians' higher incomes are due in part to government policies which violate libertarian rights, then rectificatory redistribution may be required. And indeed libertarians have argued that two basic features of the current health care system do involve gross violations of libertarian rights. First, compulsory taxation to provide equipment, hospital facilities, research funds, and educational subsidies for medical personnel is literally theft. Second, some argue that government enforced occupational licensing laws which prohibit all but the established forms of medical practice violate the right to freedom of contract (3). Those who raise this second objection also usually argue that the function of such laws is to secure a monopoly for the medical establishment while sharply limiting the supply of doctors so as to keep medical fees artificially high. Whether or not such arguments are sound it is important to note that Libertarianism is not to be confused with Conservatism. A theory which would institute a free market in medical services, abolish government subsidies, and reduce government regulation of medical practice to the prevention of injury and fraud and the enforcement of contracts has radical implications for changing the current system.

Libertarianism offers straightforward answers to questions (2) and (3). Even if it can be shown that health care in general, and certain forms of health care more than others, are especially important for the happiness or even the freedom of most persons, this fact is quite irrelevant from the perspective of a libertarian theory of justice, though it is no doubt significant for the libertarian concerned with charity or other virtues which exceed the requirements of justice. Nozick and other libertarians recognize that a free market in medical services may in fact produce severe inequalities and that there is no assurance that all or even most will be able to afford adequate medical care. Though the humane libertarian will find this condition unfortunate and will aid those in need and encourage others to do likewise voluntarily, he remains adamant that no one has a right to health care and that hence none may rightly be forced to aid another.

According to Rawls, the most basic questions about health care are not to be decided either by consideration of utility nor by market processes. Instead they are to be settled ultimately by appeal to those principles of justice which would be chosen in the original position. As we shall see, however, the implications of Rawls's principles for health care are far from clear.[7]

No principle explicitly specifying a right to health care is included among Rawls's principle of justice. Further, since those principles are intended to regulate the basic structure of society as a whole, they are not themselves intended to guide the decisions individuals make in particular health care situations, nor are they themselves to be applied directly to health care institutions. We are not to assume that either individual physicians or administrators of particular policies or programs are to attempt to allocate health care so as to maximize the prospects of the worse off. In Rawls's theory, as in Utilitarianism, the rightness or wrongness of particular actions or policies depends ultimately upon the nature of the entire institutional structure within which they exist. Hence, Rawls's theory can provide us with fruitful answers at the micro level only if its implications at the macro level are adequately developed.

If Rawls's theory includes a right to health care, it must be a right which is in some way derivative upon the basic rights laid down by the Principle of Greatest Equal Liberty, the Principle of Equality of Fair Opportunity, and the Difference Principle. And if there is to be such a derivative right to health care, then health care must either be among the primary goods covered by the three principles or it must be importantly connected with some of those goods. Now at least some forms of health care (such as broad services for prevention and health maintenance, including mental health) seem to share the earmarks of Rawlsian primary goods: they facilitate the effective pursuit of ends in general and may also enhance our ability to criticize and revise our conceptions of the good. Nonetheless, Rawls does not explicitly list health care among the social primary goods included under the three principles. However, he does include wealth under the Difference Principle and defines it so broadly that it might be thought to include access to health care services. In "Fairness to Goodness" Rawls defines wealth as virtually any legally exchangeable social asset; this would cover health care 'vouchers' if they could be cashed or exchanged for other goods ([7], p. 540).

Let us suppose that health care is either itself a primary good covered by the Difference Principle or that health care may be purchased with income or some other form of wealth which is included under the Difference Principle. In the former case, depending upon various empirical conditions, it might turn out that the best way to insure that the basic structure satisfies the Difference Principle is to establish a state-enforced right to health care. But whether maximizing the prospects of the worst off will require such a right and what the content of the right will be will depend upon what weight is to be assigned to health care relative to other primary goods included under the Difference Principle. Similarly, a weighting must also be assigned if we are to determine whether the share of wealth one receives under the Difference Principle would be sufficient both for health care needs and for other ends. Unfortunately, though Rawls acknowledges that a weighted index of primary goods is needed if we are to be able to determine what would maximize the prospects of the worst off, he offers no account of how the weighting is to be achieved.

The problem is especially acute in the case of health care, because some forms of health care are so costly that an unrestrained commitment to them would undercut any serious commitment to providing other important goods. Thus, it appears that until we have some solution to the weighting problem Rawls's theory can shed only a limited light upon the question of priority relations between health care and other goods and among various forms of health care. Rawls's conception of primary goods may explain what distinguishes health care from those things that are not primary goods, but this is clearly not sufficient.

Perhaps because he is aware of the exorbitant demands which certain health care needs may place upon social resources, Rawls stipulates that the parties in the original position are to choose principles of justice on the assumption that their needs fall within the 'normal' range' ([9], pp. 9–10). His ideal may be that the satisfaction of extremely costly special needs for health care may not be a matter of justice but rather of *charity*. If some reasonable way of drawing the line between 'normal' needs which fall within the gambit of principles of justice and 'special' needs which are the proper object of the virtue of charity could be developed, then this would be a step towards solving the priority problems mentioned above.

It has been suggested that the Principle of Equality of Fair Opportunity, rather than the Difference Principle, might provide the basis for a Rawlsian right to health care ([2], pp. 16–18). While I cannot accord this proposal the consideration it deserves here, I wish to point out that there are four difficulties which make it problematic. First, priority problems still remain. For now we are faced with the task of assigning a weight to health care relative to those other factors (such as education) which are also determinants of opportunity. Further, since the Principle of Equality of Fair Opportunity is lexically prior to the Difference Principle, we must again face the prospect that commitment to the former principle might swallow up social resource needed for providing important goods included under the latter.

Second, because it refers only to opportunities for occupying social *positions* and *offices*, rather than to opportunities in general, the Principle of Equality of Fair Opportunity might be thought too narrow to provide an Adequate foundation for a right to health care. Rawls might respond either by defining 'position' rather broadly or by arguing that opportunities for attaining positions and offices are related to opportunities in general in such a way that equality in the former insures equality in the latter.

Third, and more importantly, Rawls's Principle of Equality of Fair Opportunity take 'abilities' and skills' as given, requiring only that persons with equal or similar abilities and skills are to have equal prospects of attaining social positions and offices. Yet clearly inequalities in health care can produce severe inequalities in abilities and skills. For example, poor nutrition and medical care during gestation can result in mental retardation, and many health problems hinder the development of skills and abilities. Hence it might be argued that if the Principle of Opportunity is to provide an adequate basis for a right to health care it must be reformulated to capture the crucial influence of health care or the lack of it upon individual development.

Each of the theories of justice under consideration offers a theoretical basis for answering some basic questions concerning justice in health care. We have seen, however, that none of them provides unambiguous answers to all of the questions and that each depends for its application upon a wealth of empirical premises, many of which may not now be available. Each theory does at least rule out some answers and each supplies us with a perspective from which to pursue issues which we cannot ignore. Nonetheless, almost all of the work in developing an account of justice in health care remains to be done.[8]

NOTES

1. In this essay I shall be concerned for the most part with utilitarianism at the institutional level, and I shall proceed on the assumption that a set of institutions which maximizes utility will include rules which bar other direct applications of the principle of utility itself. Consequently, I will mainly be concerned with Rule Utilitarianism, rather than Act Utilitarianism (the latter being the view that the rightness or wrongness of a given act depends solely upon whether it maximizes utility). For an original and interesting attempt to show that Act Utilitarianism is compatible with social norms that bar direct appeals to utility, see [10].
2. Rawls sometimes refers to the "Principle of Equality of Fair Opportunity" and sometimes to the "Principle of Fair Equality of Opportunity." For convenience I will stay with the former label.
3. The phrase "worst off" refers to those who are worst off with respect to prospects of the social primary goods regulated by the Difference Principle.
4. For a detailed elaboration of this point, see [1].
5. For a fundamental objection to Nozick's invisible hand explanation, see [11].
6. P. Singer [12], expanding an argument developed earlier by R. Titmuss, argues that the existence of markets for certain goods may in fact undermine the motivation for charity.
7. See [2].
8. I would like to thank Earl Shelp and William Hanson for their very helpful comments on an earlier draft of this paper.

REFERENCES

1. Buchanan, A. "Revisability and Rational Choice." *Canadian Journal of Philosophy* 5:395–408, 1975.
2. Daniels, N. "Rights to Health Care and Distributive Justice: Programmatic Worries." *Journal of Medicine and Philosophy* 4:174–191, 1979.
3. Friedman, M. *Capitalism and Freedom.* Chicago: University of Chicago Press, 1962, pp. 137–160.
4. Kant, I. *Foundations of the Metaphysics of Morals* (transl. by L. W. Beck), New York: Bobbs-Merrill, 1959, Part III.
5. Nozick, R. *Anarchy, State and Utopia.* New York: Basic Books, 1974.
6. Rawls, J. *A Theory of Justice.* Cambridge, Mass.: Harvard University Press, 1971.
7. Rawls, J. "Fairness to Goodness." *Philosophical Review* 84:536–554, 1975.
8. Rawls, J. "Reply to Alexander and Musgrave." *Quarterly Journal of Economics* 88:633–655, November 1974.
9. Rawls, J. "Responsibility for Ends." Stanford University, Unpublished Lecture, 1979.
10. Sartorius, R. *Individual Conduct and Social Norms.* Encino, Calif.: Dickenson Publishing, 1975.
11. Sartorius, R. "The Limits of Libertarianism." In *Liberty and the Rule of Law,* edited by R. L. Cunningham, 87–131. College Station, Texas: Texas A and M University Press, 1979.
12. Singer, P. "Rights and the Market." In *Justice and Economic Distribution,* edited by J. Arthur and W. Shaw, pp. 207–221. Englewood Cliffs, N.J.: Prentice-Hall, 1978.

In order to see how one of these principles, the principle of liberty, might be developed into a formula for allocating resources, we turn to an essay of Robert M. Sade, a physician who interprets rights to refer exclusively to freedom of action or liberty. Beginning with a fundamental right to one's life, he derives a right to act on one's own values, and to dispose of resources as one sees fit. In reading this essay one should focus on what it is Sade claims people own and the extent to which it can be deemed to belong to them. Does, for instance, knowledge belong to individuals or is it common property? Under what circumstances could persons be expected to agree, perhaps in advance, that they will acquire knowledge under the condition that it will be used in particular ways?

Medical Care as a Right: A Refutation

ROBERT M. SADE

The current debate on health care in the United States is of the first order of importance to the health professions, and of no less importance to the political future of the nation, for precedents are now being set that will be applied to the rest of American society in the future. In the enormous volume of verbage that has poured forth, certain fundamental issues have been so often misrepresented that they have now become commonly accepted fallacies. This paper will be concerned with the most important of these misconceptions, that health care is a right, as well as a brief consideration of some of its corollary fallacies.

RIGHTS—MORALITY AND POLITICS

The concept of rights has its roots in the moral nature of man and its practical expression in the political system that he creates. Both morality and politics must be discussed before the relation between political rights and health care can be appreciated.

A "right" defines a freedom of action. For instance, a right to a material object is the uncoerced choice of the use to which the object will be put; a right to a specific action, such as free speech, is the freedom to engage in that activity without forceful repression. The moral foundation of the rights of man begins with the fact that he is a living creature: he has the right to his own life. All other rights are corollaries of this primary one; without the right to life, there can be no others, and the concept of rights itself becomes meaningless.

The freedom of live, however, does not automatically ensure life. For man, a specific course of action is required to sustain his life, a course of action that must be guided by reason and reality and has as its goal the creation or acquisition of material values, such as food and clothing, and intellectual values, such as self-esteem and integrity. His moral system is the means by which he is able to select the values that will support his life and achieve his happiness.

Man must maintain a rather delicate homeostasis in a highly demanding and threatening environment, but has at his disposal a unique and efficient mechanism for dealing with it: his mind. His mind is able to perceive, to identify precepts, to integrate them into concepts, and to use those concepts in choosing actions suitable to the maintenance of his life. The rational function of mind is volitional, however; a man must choose to think, to be aware, to evaluate, to make conscious decisions. The extent to which he is able to achieve his goals will be directly proportional to his commitment to reason seeking them.

The right to life implies three corollaries: the right to select the values that one deems necessary to sustain one's own life; the right to exercise one's own judgment of the best course of action to achieve the chosen values; and the right to dispose of those values, once gained, in any way one chooses, without coercion by other men. The denial of any one of these corollaries severely compromises or destroys the right to life itself. A man who is not allowed to choose his own goals, is prevented from setting his own course in achieving those goals and is not free to dispose of the values he has earned is no less than a slave to those who usurp those rights. The right to private property, therefore, is essential and indispensable to maintaining free men in a free society.

Thus, it is the nature of man as a living, thinking being that determines his rights—his "natural rights." The concept of natural rights was slow in dawning on human civilization. The first political expression of that concept had its beginnings in 17th and 18th century England through such exponents as John Locke and Edmund Burke, but came to its brilliant debut as a form of government after the American Revolution. Under the leadership of such men as Thomas Paine and Thomas Jefferson, the concept of man as a being sovereign unto himself, rather than a subdivision of the sovereignty of a king, emperor or state, was incorporated into the formal structure of government for the first time. Protection of the lives and property of individual citizens was the salient characteristic of the Constitution of 1787. Ayn Rand has pointed out that the principle of protection of the individual against the coercive force of government made the United States the first moral society in history.[1]

In a free society, man exercises his right to sustain his own life by producing economic values in the form of goods and services that he is, or should be, free to exchange with other men who are similarly free to trade with him or not. The economic values produced, however, are not given as gifts by nature, but exist only by virtue of the thought and effort of individual men. Goods and services are thus owned as a consequence of the right to sustain life by one's own physical and mental effort.

If the chain of natural rights is interrupted, and the right to a loaf of bread, for example, is proclaimed as primary (avoiding the necessity of earning it), every man owns a loaf of bread, regardless of who produced it. Since ownership is the power of disposal,[2] every man may take his loaf from the baker and dispose of as he wishes with or without the baker's permission. Another element has thus been introduced into the relation between men: the use of force. It is crucial to observe who has initiated the use of force: it is the man who demands unearned bread as a right, not the man who produced it. At the level of an unstructured society it is clear who is moral and who immoral. The man who acted rationally by producing food to support his own life is moral. The man who expropriated the bread by force is immoral.

To protect this basic right to provide for the support of one's own life, men band together for their mutual protection and form governments. This is the only proper function of government: to provide for the defense of individuals against those who would take their lives or property by force. The state is the repository for retaliatory force in a just society wherein the only actions prohibited to individuals are those of physical harm or the threat of physical harm to other men. The closest that man has ever come to achieving this ideal of government was in this country after its War of Independence.

When a government ignores the progression of natural rights arising from the right to life, and agrees with a man, a group of men, or even a majority of its citizens, that every man has a right to a loaf of bread, it must protect that right by the passage of laws ensuring that everyone gets his loaf—in the process depriving the baker of the freedom to dispose of his own product. If the baker disobeys the law, asserting the priority of his right to support himself by his own rational disposition of the fruits of his mental and physical labor, he will be taken to court by force or threat of force where he will have more property forcibly taken from him (by fine) or have his liberty taken away (by incarceration). Now the initiator of violence is the government itself. The degree to which a government exercises its monopoly on the retaliatory use of force by asserting a claim to the lives and property of its citizens is the degree to which it has eroded its own legitimacy. It is a frequently overlooked fact that behind every law is a policemen's gun or a soldier's bayonet. When that gun and bayonet are used to initiate violence, to take property or to restrict liberty by force, there are no longer any rights, for the lives of the citizens belong to the state. In a just society with a moral government, it is clear that the only "right" to the bread belongs to the baker, and that a claim by any other man to that right is unjustified and can be enforced only by violence or the threat of violence.

RIGHTS—POLITICS AND MEDICINE

The concept of medical care as the patient's right is immoral because it denies the most fundamental of all rights, that of a man to his own life and the freedom of action to support it. Medical care is neither a right nor a privilege: it is a service that is provided by doctors and others to people who wish to purchase it. It is the provision of this service that a doctor depends upon for his livelihood, and is his means of supporting his own life. If the right to health care belongs to the patient, he starts out owning the services of a doctor without the necessity of either earning them or receiving them as a gift from the only man who has the right to give them: the doctor himself. In the narrative above substitute "doctor" for "baker" and "medical service" for "bread." American medicine is now at the point in the story where the state has proclaimed the nonexistent "right" to medical care as a fact of public policy, and has begun to pass the laws to enforce it. The doctor finds himself less and less his own master and more and more controlled by forces outside of his own judgment.

For instance, under the proposed Kennedy-Griffiths bill,[3] there will be a "Health Security Board," which will be responsible for administering the new controls to be imposed on doctors, hospitals and other "providers" of health care (Sec. 121). Specialized services, such as major surgery, will be done by "qualified specialists" [Sec. 22(b)(2)], such qualifications being determined by the Board (Sec. 42). Furthermore, the patient can no longer exercise his own initiative in finding a specialist to do his operation, since he must be referred to the specialist by a nonspecialist—i.e., a general practitioner or family doctor [Sec. 22(b)]. Licensure by his own state will not be enough to be a qualified practitioner; physicians will also be subject to a second set of standards, those established by the Board [Sec. 42(a)]. Doctors will no longer be considered competent to determine their own needs for continuing education, but must meet requirements established by the Board [Sec. 42(c)]. The professional staff of a hospital will no longer be able to determine which of its members are qualified to perform which kinds of major surgery; specialty-board certification or eligibility will be required, with certain exceptions that include meeting standards established by the Board [Sec. 42(d)].

Control of doctors through control of the hospitals in which they practice will also be exercised by the Board by way of a list of requirements, the last of which is a "sleeper" that will by its vagueness allow the Board almost any regulation of the hospital: The hospital must meet "such other requirements as the Board finds necessary in the interest of quality of care and the safety of patients in the institution" [Sec. 43(i)]. Hospitals will also not be allowed to undertake construction without higher approval by a state agency or by the Board (Sec. 52).

In the name of better organization and coordination of services, hospitals, nursing homes and other providers will be further controlled through the Board's power to issue directives forcing the provider to furnish services selected by the Board [Sec. 131(a)(1),(2)] at a place selected by the Board [Sec. 131(a)(3)]. The Board can also direct these providers to form associations with one another of various sorts, including "making available to one provider the professional and technical skills of another" [Sec. 131(a)(B)], and such other linkages as the Board thinks best [Sec. 131(a)(4)(C)].

These are only a few of the bill's controls of the health-care industry. It is difficult to believe that such patent subjugation of an entire profession could ever be considered a fit topic for discussion in any but the darkest corner of a country founded on the principles of life and liberty. Yet the Kennedy-Griffiths bill is being seriously debated today in the Congress of the United States.

The irony of this bill is that, on the basis of the philosophic premises of its authors, it does provide a rationally organized system for attempting to fulfill its goals, such as "making health services available to all residents of the United States." If the government is to spend tens of billions of dollars on health services, it must assure in some way that the money is not being wasted. Every bill currently before the national legislature does, should, and must provide some such controls. The Kennedy-Griffiths bill is the closest we have yet come to the logical conclusion and inevitable consequence of two fundamental fallacies: that health care is a right, and that doctors and other health workers will function as efficiently serving as chattels of the state as they will living as sovereign human beings. It is not, and they will not.

Any act of force is anti-mind. It is a confession of the failure of persuasion, the failure of reason. When politicians say that the health system must be forced into a mold of their own design, they are admitting their inability to persuade doctors and patients to use the plan voluntarily; they are proclaiming the supremacy of the state's logic over the judgments of the individual minds of all concerned with health care. Statists throughout history have never learned that compulsion and reason are contradictory, that a forced mind cannot think effectively and, by extension, that a regimented profession will eventually choke and stagnate from its own lack of freedom. A persuasive example of this is the moribund condition of medicine as a profession is Sweden, a country that has enjoyed socialized medicine since 1955. Werkö, a Swedish physician, has stated: "The details and the complicated working schedule have not yet been determined in all hospitals and districts, but the general feeling of belonging to a free profession, free to decide—at least in principle—how to organize its work has been lost. Many hospital-based physicians regard their work now with an apathy previously unknown."[4] One wonders how American legislators will like having their myocardial infarctions treated by apathetic internists, their mitral valves replaced by apathetic surgeons, their wives' tumors removed by apathetic gynecologists. They will find it very difficult to legislate self-esteem, integrity and competence into the doctors whose minds and judgments they have throttled.

If anyone doubts that health legislation involves the use of force, a dramatic demonstration of the practical political meaning of the "right to health care" was acted out in Quebec in the closing months of 1970.[5] In that unprecedented threat of violence by a modern Western government against a group of its citizens, the doctors of Quebec were literally imprisoned in the province by Bill 41, possibly the most repressive piece of legislation ever enacted against the medical profession, and far more worthy of the Soviet Union or Red China than a Western democracy. Doctors objecting to a new Medicare law were forced to continue working under penalty of jail sentence and fines of up to $500 a day away from their practices. Those who spoke out publicly against the bill were subject to jail sentences of up to a year and fines of up to $50,000 a day. The facts that the doctors did return to work and that no one was therefore jailed or fined do not mitigate the nature or implications of the passage of Bill 41. Although the dispute between the Quebec physicians and their government was not one of principle but of the details of compensation, the reaction of the state to resistance against coercive professional regulation was a classic example of the naked force that lies behind every act of social legislation.

Any doctor who is forced by law to join a group or a hospital he does not choose, or is prevented by law from prescribing a drug he thinks is best for his patient, or is compelled by law to make any decisions he would not otherwise have made, is being forced to act against his own mind, which means forced to act against his own life. He is also being forced to violate his most fundamental professional commitment, that of using his own best judgment at all times for the greatest benefit of his patient. It is remarkable that this principle has never been identified by a public voice in the medical profession, and that the vast majority of doctors in this country are being led down the path to civil servitude, never knowing that their feelings of uneasy foreboding have a profoundly moral origin, and never recognizing that the main issues at stake are not those being formulated in Washington, but are their own honor, integrity and freedom, and their own survival as sovereign human beings.

SOME COROLLARIES

The basic fallacy that health care is a right has led to several corollary fallacies, among them the following:

That health is primarily a community or social rather than individual concern.[6] A simple calculation from American mortality statistics[7] quickly corrects that false concept: 67 per cent of deaths in 1967 were due to diseases known to be caused or exacerbated by alcohol, tobacco smoking or overeating, or were due to accidents. Each of those factor is either largely or wholly correctable by individual action. Although no statistics are available, it is likely that morbidity, with the exception of common respiratory infections, has a relation like that of mortality to personal habits and excesses.

That state medicine has worked better in other countries than free enterprise has worked here. There is no evidence to support that contention, other than anecdotal testimonials and the spurious citation of infant mortality and longevity statistics. There is, on the other hand, a good deal of evidence to the contrary.[8,9]

That the provision of medical care somehow lies outside the laws of supply and demand, and that government-controlled health care will be free care. In fact, no service or commodity lies outside the economic laws. Regarding health care, market demand, individual want, and medical need are entirely different things, and have a very complex relation with the cost and the total supply of available care, as recently discussed and clarified by Jeffers et al.[10] They point out that "'health is purchaseable,' meaning that somebody has to pay for it, individually or collectively, at the expense of foregoing the current or future consumption of other things." The question is whether the decision of how to allocate the consumer's dollar should belong to the consumer or to the state. It has already been shown that the choice of how a doctor's services should be rendered belongs only to the doctor: in the same way the choice of whether to buy a doctor's service rather than some other commodity or service belongs to the consumer as a logical consequence of the right to his own life.

That opposition to national health legislation is tantamount to opposition to progress in health care. Progress is made by the free interaction of free minds developing new ideas in an atmosphere conducive to experimentation and trial. If group practice really is better than solo, we will find out because the success of groups will result in more groups (which has, in fact, been happening); if prepaid comprehensive care really is the best form of practice, it will succeed and the health industry will swell with new Kaiser-Permanente plans. But let one of these or any other form of practice become the law, and the system is in a straitjacket that will stifle progress. Progress requires freedom of action, and that is precisely what national health legislation aims at restricting.

That doctors should help design the legislation for a national health system, since they must live with and within whatever legislation is enacted. To accept this concept is to concede to the opposition its philosophic premises, and thus to lose the battle. The means by which nonproducers and hangers-on throughout history have been able to expropriate material and intellectual values from the producers has been identified only relatively recently: the sanction of the victim.[11] Historically, few people have lost their freedom and their rights without some degree of complicity in the plunder. If the American medical profession accepts the concept of health care as the right of the patient, it will have earned the Kennedy-Griffiths bill by default. The alternative for any health professional is to withhold his sanction and make clear who is being victimized. Any physician can say to those who would shackle his judgment and control his profession: I do not recognize your right to my life and my mind, which belong to me and me alone; I will not participate in any legislated solution to any health problem.

In the face of the raw power that lies behind government programs, nonparticipation is the only way in which personal values can be maintained. And it is only with the attainment of the highest of those values—integrity, honesty and self-esteem—that the physician can achieve his most important professional value, the absolute priority of the welfare of his patients.

The preceding discussion should not be interpreted as proposing that there are no problems in the delivery of medical care. Problems such as high cost, few doctors, low quantity of available care in economically depressed areas may be real, but it is naive to believe that governmental solutions through coercive legislation can be anything but shortsighted and formulated on the basis of political expediency. The only long-range plan that can hope to provide for the day after tomorrow is a "nonsystem"—that is, a system that proscribes the imposition by force (legislation) of any one group's conception of the best forms of medical care. We must identify our problems and seek to solve them by experimentation and trial in an atmosphere of freedom from compulsion. Our sanction of anything less will mean the loss of our personal values, the death of our profession, and a heavy blow to political liberty.

NOTES

1. Rand, A. *Man's Rights, Capitalism: The Unknown Ideal.* New York: New American Library, 1967, pp. 320–329.
2. Von Mises, L. *Socialism: An Economic and Sociological Analysis.* New Haven, Conn.: Yale University Press, 1951, pp. 37–55.
3. Kennedy, E. M. "Introduction of the Health Security Act." *Congressional Record* 116:S 14338–S 14361, 1970.
4. Werkö, L. "Swedish Medical Care in Transition." *New England Journal of Medicine* 284:360–366, 1971.
5. "Quebec Medicare and Medical Services Withdrawal." Toronto: Canadian Medical Association, 19 October 1970.
6. Millis, J. S. "Wisdom? Health? Can Society Guarantee Them?" *New England Journal of Medicine* 283:260–261, 1970.
7. Department of Health, Education, and Welfare, Public Health Service. *Vital Statistics of the United States 1967. Vol. II, Mortality Part A.* Washington, D.C. Government Printing Office, 1969. p. 1–7.
8. *Financing Medical Care: An Appraisal of Foreign Programs,* edited by H. Shoeck. Caldwell, Idaho: Caxton Printers, 1962.
9. Lynch, M. J., and S. S. Raphael. *Medicine and the State.* Springfield, Ill.: Charles C Thomas, 1963.
10. Jeffers, J. R., M. F. Bognanno, and J. C. Bartlett. "On the Demand Versus Need for Medical Services and the Concept of Shortage." *American Journal of Public Health* 61:46–63, 1971.
11. Rand, A. *Atlas Shrugged.* New York: Random House, 1957, p. 1066.

Many people recognize alternatives to a system of allocating resources based solely on individual liberty. The President's Commission for the Study of Ethical Problems in Medicine and Biomedical and Behavioral Research, a national body charged with assessing biomedical ethical and policy issues, asserts in a 1983 report that equitable access to health care means that all citizens are able to secure an adequate level of care without excessive burdens. This concept of equitable access seems to incorporate both considerations of efficiency in maximizing benefits and some notion of fair distribution with a focus on the rights of the least well-off. The following excerpt from its report explains its notion of equitable access.

Securing Access to Health Care

PRESIDENT'S COMMISSION FOR THE STUDY OF ETHICAL PROBLEMS IN
MEDICINE AND BIOMEDICAL AND BEHAVIORAL RESEARCH

THE CONCEPT OF EQUITABLE ACCESS TO HEALTH CARE

The special nature of health care helps explain why it ought to be accessible, in a fair fashion, to all.[1] But if this ethical conclusion is to provide a basis for evaluating current patterns of access to health care and proposed health policies, the meaning of fairness or equity in this context must be clarified. The concept of equitable access needs definition in its two main aspects: the level of care that ought to be available to all and the extent to which burdens can be imposed on those who obtain these services.

Access to What?

"Equitable access" could be interpreted in a number of ways: equality of access, access to whatever an individual needs or would benefit from, or access to an adequate level of care.

Equity as Equality. It has been suggested that equity is achieved either when everyone is assured of receiving an equal quantity of health care dollars or when people enjoy equal health. The most common characterization of equity as equality, however, is as providing everyone with the same level of health care. In this view, it follows that if a given level of care is available to one individual it must be available to all. If the initial standard is set high, by reference to the highest level of care presently received, an enormous drain would result on the resources needed to provide other goods. Alternatively, if the standard is set low in order to avoid an excessive use of resources, some beneficial services would have to be withheld from people who wished to purchase them. In other words, none would be allowed access to more services or services of higher quality than those available to everyone else, even if he or she were willing to pay for those services from his or her personal resources.

As long as significant inequalities in income and wealth persist, inequalities in the use of health care can be expected beyond those created by differences in need. Given people with the same pattern of preferences and equal health care needs, those with greater financial resources will purchase more health care. Conversely, given equal financial resources, the different patterns of health care preferences that typically exist in any population will result in a different use of health services by people with equal health needs. Trying to prevent such inequalities would require interfering with people's liberty to use their income to purchase an important good like health care while leaving them free to use it for frivolous or inessential ends. Prohibiting people with higher incomes or stronger preferences for health care from purchasing more care than everyone else gets would not be feasible, and would probably result in a black market for health care.

Equity as Access Solely According to Benefit or Need. Interpreting equitable access to mean that everyone must receive all health care that is of any benefit to them also has unacceptable implications. Unless health is the only good or resources are unlimited, it would be irrational for a society—as for an individual—to make a commitment to provide whatever health care might be beneficial regardless of cost. Although health care is of special importance, it is surely not all that is important to people. Pushed to an extreme, this criterion might swallow up all of society's resources, since there is virtually no end to the funds that could be devoted to possibly beneficial care for diseases and disabilities and to their prevention.

Equitable access to health care must take into account not only the benefits of care but also the cost in comparison with other goods and services to which those resources might be allocated. Society will reasonably devote some resources to health care but reserve most resources for other goals. This, in turn, will mean that some health services (even of a lifesaving sort) will not be developed or employed because they would produce too few benefits in relation to their costs and to other ways the resources for them might be used.

It might be argued that the notion of "need" provides a way to limit access to only that care that confers especially important benefits. In this view, equity as access according to need would place less severe demands on social resources than equity according to benefit would. There are, however, difficulties with the notion of need in this context. On the one hand, medical need is often not narrowly defined but refers to any condition for which medical treatment might be effective. Thus, "equity as access according to need" collapses into "access according to whatever is of benefit."

On the other hand, "need" could be even more expansive in scope than "benefit." Philosophical and economic writings do not provide any clear distinction between "needs" and "wants" or "preferences." Since the term means different things to different people, "access according to need" could become "access to any health services a person wants." Conversely, need could be interpreted very narrowly to encompass only a very minimal level of services—for example, those "necessary to prevent death."[2]

Equity as an Adequate Level of Health Care. Although neither "everything needed" nor "everything beneficial" nor "everything that anyone else is getting" are defensible ways of understanding equitable access, the special nature of health care dictates that everyone have access to some level of care: enough care to achieve sufficient welfare, opportunity, information, and evidence of interpersonal concern to facilitate a reasonably full and satisfying life. That level can be termed "an adequate level of health care." The difficulty of sharpening this amorphous notion in a workable foundation for health policy is a major problem in the United States today. This concept is not new; it is implicit in the public debate over policy in this country. . . .

Understanding equitable access to health care to mean that everyone should be able to secure an adequate level of care has several strengths. Because an adequate level of care may be less than "all beneficial care" and because it does not require that all needs be satisfied, it acknowledges the need for setting priorities with health care and signals a clear recognition that society's resources are limited and that there are other goods besides health. Thus, interpreting equity as access to adequate care does not generate an open-ended obligation. One of the chief dangers of interpretations of equity that require virtually unlimited resources for health care is that they encourage the view that equitable access is an impossible ideal. Defining equity as an adequate level of care for all avoids an impossible commitment of resources without falling into the opposite error of abandoning the enterprise of seeking to ensure that health care is in fact available for everyone.

In addition, since providing an adequate level of care is a limited moral requirement, this definition also avoids the unacceptable restriction on individual liberty entailed by the view that equity requires equality. Provided that an adequate level is available to all, those who prefer to use their resources to obtain care that exceeds that level do not offend any ethical principle in doing so. Finally, the concept of adequacy, as the Commission understands it, is society-relative. The content of adequate care will depend upon the overall resources available in a given society, and can take into account a consensus of expectations about what is adequate in a particular society at a particular time in its historical development. This permits the definition of adequacy to be altered as societal resources and expectations change.[3]

With What Burdens?

It is not enough to focus on the care that individuals receive; attention must be paid to the burdens they must bear in order to obtain it—waiting and travel time, the cost and availability of transport, the financial cost of the care itself. Equity requires not only that adequate care be available to all, but also that these burdens not be excessive.

If individuals must travel unreasonably long distances, wait for unreasonably long hours, or spend most of their financial resources to obtain care, some will be deterred from obtaining adequate care, with adverse effects on their health and well-being. Others may bear the burdens, but only at the expense of their ability to meet other important needs. If one of the main reasons for providing adequate care is that health care increases welfare and opportunity, then a system that required large numbers of individuals to forego food, shelter, or educational advancement in order to obtain care would be self-defeating and irrational.

The concept of acceptable burdens in obtaining care, as opposed to excessive ones, parallels in some respects the concept of adequacy. Just as equity does not require equal access, neither must the burdens of obtaining adequate care be equal for all persons. What is crucial is that the variations in burdens fall within an acceptable range. As in determining an adequate level of care, there is no simple formula for ascertaining when the burdens of obtaining care fall within such a range. Yet some guidelines can be formulated. To illustrate, since a given financial outlay represents a greater sacrifice to a poor person than to a rich person, "excessive" must be understood in relation to income. Obviously everyone cannot live the same distance from a health facility, and some individuals choose to locate in remote and sparsely populated areas. Concern about an inequitable burden would be appropriate, however, when identifiable groups must travel a great distance or long time to receive care—though people may appropriately be expected to travel farther to get specialized care, for example, than to obtain primary or emergency care.

Although differences in the burdens individuals must bear to obtain care do not necessarily represent inequities, they may trigger concern for two reasons. Such discrepancies may indicate that some people are, in fact, bearing excessive burdens, just as some differences in the use of care may indicate that some lack adequate care. Also, certain patterns of differences may indicate racial or ethnic discrimination.

Whether any such discrepancies actually constitute an inequitable distribution of burdens ultimately depends upon the role these differences play in the larger system under which the overall burdens of providing an adequate level of care are distributed among the citizens of this country. It may be permissible, for example, for some individuals to bear greater burdens in the form of out-of-pocket expenses for care if this is offset by a lower bill for taxes devoted to health care. Whether such differences in the distribution of burdens are acceptable cannot be determined by looking at a particular burden in isolation.

A SOCIETAL OBLIGATION

Society has a moral obligation to ensure that everyone has access to adequate care without being subject to excessive burdens. In speaking of a societal obligation the Commission makes reference to society in the broadest sense—the collective American community. The community is made up of individuals, who are in turn members of many other, overlapping groups, both public and private: local, state, regional, and national units; professional and workplace organizations; religious, educational and charitable organizations; and family, kinship, and ethnic groups. All these entities play a role in discharging societal obligations.

The Commission believes it is important to distinguish between society, in this inclusive sense, and government as one institution among others in society. Thus the recognition of a collective or societal obligation does not imply that government should be the only or even the primary institution involved in the complex of making health care available. It is the Commission's view that the societal obligation to ensure equitable access for everyone may best be fulfilled in this country by a pluralistic approach that relies upon the coordinated contributions of actions by both the private and public sectors.

Securing equitable access is a societal rather than a merely private or individual responsibility for several reasons. First, while health is of special importance for human beings, health care—especially scientific health care—is a social product requiring the skills and efforts of many individuals; it is not something that individuals can provide for themselves solely through their own efforts. Second, because the need for health care is both unevenly distributed among persons and highly unpredictable and because the cost of securing care may be great, few individuals could secure adequate care without relying on some social mechanism for sharing the costs. Third, if persons generally deserved their health conditions or if the need for health care were fully within the individual's control, the fact that some lack adequate care would not be viewed as an inequity. But differences in health status, and hence differences in health care needs, are largely undeserved because they are, for the most part, not within the individual's control.

Uneven and Unpredictable Health Needs

While requirements for other basic necessities, such as adequate food and shelter, vary among people within a relatively limited range, the need for health care is distributed very unevenly and its occurrence at any particular time is highly unpredictable. One study shows 50% of all hospital billings are for only 13% of the patients, the seriously chronically ill.[4]

Moreover, health care needs may be minor or overwhelming, in their personal as well as financial impact. Some people go through their entire lives seldom requiring health care, while others face medical expenses that would exceed the resources of all but the wealthiest. Moreover, because the need for care cannot be predicted, it is difficult to provide for it by personal savings from income. Under the major program that pays for care for the elderly, 40% of aged enrollees had no payments at all in 1977 and 37% fell into a low payment group (averaging $129 per year), while 8.8% averaged $7011 in annual expenditures.[5]

Responsibility for Differences in Health Status

Were someone responsible for (and hence deserving of) his or her need for health care, then access to the necessary health care might be viewed as merely an individual concern. But the differences among people's needs for health care are for the most part not within their control, and thus are not something for which they should be held accountable. Different needs for care are largely a matter of good or bad fortune—that is, a consequence of a natural and social lottery that no one chooses to play.

In a very real sense, people pay for the consequences of the actions that cause them illness or disability—through the suffering and loss of opportunity they experience. The issue here is a narrower one: to what extent is the societal responsibility to secure health care for the sick and injured limited by personal responsibility for the need for health care? It seems reasonable for people to bear the foreseeable consequences (in terms of health care needs) of their informed and voluntary choices. Indeed, as an ethical matter, the principle of self-determination implies as a corollary the responsibility of individuals for their choices.

However, to apply the notion of personal responsibility in a fair way in setting health care policy would be a complex and perhaps impossible task. First, identifying those people whose informed, voluntary choices have caused them foreseeable harm would be practically as well as theoretically very difficult. It is often not possible to determine the degree to which an individual's behavior is fully informed regarding the health consequences of the behavior. Efforts to educate the public about the effects of life-style on health are desirable, but it must also be acknowledged that today people who conscientiously strive to adopt a healthy life-style find themselves inundated with an enormous amount of sometimes contradictory information about what is healthful. Voluntariness is also especially problematic regarding certain behaviors that cause some people ill health, such as smoking and alcohol abuse.[6] Moreover, there are great difficulties in determining the extent of the causal role of particular behavior on an individual's health status. For many behaviors, consequences appear only over long periods of time, during which many other elements besides the particular behavior have entered into the causal process that produces a disease or disability. For example, the largely unknown role of genetic predispositions for many diseases makes it difficult to designate particular behaviors as their "cause."

Second even if one knew who should be held responsible for what aspects of their own ill health, policies aimed at institutionalizing financial accountability for "unhealthy behavior" or at denying the necessary health care for those who have "misbehaved" are likely to involve significant injustices and other undesirable consequences. Leaving people free to engage in health-risky behavior only if they can afford to pay for its consequences is fair only if the existing patterns of income distribution are fair, and if the payment required fully accounts for all the costs to society for the ill health and its treatment. Moreover, since some unhealthy behavior can be monitored more easily than others, problems of discrimination would inevitably arise; even when feasible, monitoring such behavior would raise serious concerns about the invasion of privacy. Finally, the ultimate sanction—turning away from the hospital door people who are responsible for their own ill health— would reverberate in unwanted and perhaps very harmful ways in the community at large. The Commission concludes that within programs to secure equitable access to health care, serious practical and ethical difficulties would follow attempts to single out the consequences of behavior and to make individuals of health-risky behavior solely responsible for those consequences.

However, even if it is inappropriate to hold people responsible for their health status, it is appropriate to hold them responsible for a fair share of the cost of their own health care. Society's moral obligation to provide equitable access for all and the individual responsibility for bearing a share of the costs of achieving equity rest on the same considerations of fairness. Individuals who—because they know that others will come to their aid—fail to take reasonable steps to provide for their own health care when they could do so without excessive burdens would be guilty of exploiting the generosity of their fellow citizens. The societal obligation is therefore balanced by corresponding individual obligations. In light of the special importance of health care, the largely undeserved character of differences in health status, and the uneven distribution and unpredictability of health care needs, society has a moral obligation to ensure adequate care for all. Saying that the obligation is societal (rather than merely individual) stops short, however, of identifying who has the ultimate responsibility for ensuring that the obligation is successfully met.

NOTES

1. For a discussion of other important factors, the uneven distribution of need, and its largely undeserved nature, see pp. 23–25 of *Securing Access to Health Care.*
2. The Federal government employed this criterion in the mid-1970s when it dropped requirements providing dental care for adult public program beneficiaries under Medicaid. It claimed that dental services were not services whose absence could be considered as "life-threatening."
3. There are practical as well as ethical reasons for a nation like the United States, which possesses resources to provide a high level of services, not to take a narrow view of "adequacy." A lesser level of care would make it extremely difficult to establish a desirable mix of services; narrow limits would foster intense competition among different types of care and possibly skew the adequate level toward life-threatening care to the exclusion of other very beneficial forms of care such as preventive medicine. An inadequate level, accompanied by a private market alternative treatment, would generate inequities by encouraging the flight of resources (as is now the case with physicians who choose to serve privately insured patients to the exclusion of noninsured and publicly insured individuals).
4. Zook, C. J., and F. D. Moore. "High Cost Users of Medical Care." *New England Journal of Medicine* 302:996, 1982.
5. Davis, Karen. *Medicare Reconsidered.* Duke University Medical Center Private Sector Conference, Durham, N.C., 15–16 March 1982.
6. Wikler, Daniel. "Persuasion and Coercion for Health." *Milbank Memorial Fund Quarterly/Health & Society* 56:303, 1978.

Relating Principles and Cases

INTRODUCTION

Establishing that there are principles of ethics provides a framework for assessing ethical actions and rules. The alternative ethical theories in health care examined in the first three chapters are different in part because of the extent to which they articulate, explicitly or implicitly, principles of the sort presented in the preceding chapters. Among those oriented to principles there are substantial differences regarding which principles are incorporated and what emphasis they are given.

We are still left with the question of how the principles are to be related to one another and how we are to move from these very general, very abstract principles to specific cases. These two questions are the focus of this final chapter.

First, we need to know how to relate principles to one another. One solution is to admit to only one overarching principle. This is the solution of the classical Hippocratic thinkers. The only ethical consideration was for the physician to benefit the patient according to his ability and judgment. Solving the problem of principles by holding that there is really only one principle comes at the expense of ignoring the moral concerns expressed in the other principles. The Hippocratic physician, for example, recognized no commitment to the autonomy of the patient. He felt no moral commitment to speak truthfully in cases where more good for the patient would come from lying. He felt no moral need to keep promises. The promise of confidentiality should be overridden when it was in the patient's interest to do so (even in cases where the patient did not agree).

A second solution to the problem of principles is to admit to the necessity of multiple principles. If one does, then for an ethical theory to be complete there must be some formula for relating the principles and resolving conflicts when they arise among principles. It would be nice if the principles could be ranked in some order of priority so that, for example, respect for patient autonomy always came prior to the principle of beneficence (or always came after it). Most theorists have found that implausible, however.

W. D. Ross in the essay in chapter 5 attempted to solve this problem by holding that no one principle always took precedence. He said that, by intuition, one can balance competing principles so that one can deduce how different prima facie duties can be integrated into one single duty proper.

Recently, John Rawls has returned to the idea of attempting some sort of partial ranking. He refers to such ranking as *lexical* because it is the way a dictionary is arranged with all of one letter coming before any consideration of words beginning with another letter.

Rawls has supported lexical ranking of two principles within his theory of justice. Equal protection of liberty comes prior to accepting inequalities in primary social goods, and inequalities are justified in social goods only when they redound to the benefit of the least well-off. This means that his more egalitarian principle of justice takes priority over the more straightforward principle of beneficence focusing on maximizing aggregate utility.

Some have defended the possibility of extending this lexical ordering of principles still further—perhaps combining it with a more intuitive kind of balancing. For example, it could be argued that mere production of good (beneficence) or avoiding harm (nonmaleficence) are never sufficient in themselves to permit overriding one of the other principles discussed in the preceding chapters. That would mean that the good of the patient can never override the autonomy of the patient or justify a lie to the patient or the breaking of a promise to the patient.

In liberal political systems a similar kind of subordination of utility is sometimes seen. In a democracy, for example, it is unacceptable to justify depriving someone of his right to vote by arguing that society would be better off if the individual did not vote. Social benefits do not count against fundamental liberties such as the right to vote.

In medicine it is sometimes argued that if beneficence is totally subordinated to the other principles that do not focus exclusively on the amount of good or harm produced, then persons could claim certain rights, like the right to health care, even when terribly bad consequences would result. This is enough for some to reject the effort to give priority to principles not directly oriented toward maximizing consequences. They would, for example, permit research on persons without their consent when overwhelming good would come of it. That would, it is argued, permit terrible violations of people's rights, such as in the Nazi experiments, if only one can conjure up research that would produce overwhelming good that could be done in no other way than by conscripting patients against their will.

The first two essays in this chapters explore different aspects of the problem of ranking principles. The last two essays deal with a second problem: how do we move from principles to specific cases. The issue is whether it is possible to articulate more concrete rules of conduct that mediate between the abstract principles and the specific case. Can the physician at the bedside apply a rule (like always get informed consent before surgery) or must he or she rely on a direct application of the principles of beneficence, autonomy, and the like? Some argue that rules have absolutely no place in ethics since every case is unique. Others defend what is sometimes called legalism: the notion that rules can be applied without exception to get to what is morally correct in specific cases. Joseph Fletcher attacks both of these defending the notion that rules can function as guidelines or summaries of what experience has taught us to be morally correct in certain situations.

John Rawls enters this debate to argue that there are really two intermediate positions: the summary rules position and another he calls the rules of practice position. Rules of practice have a very different moral standing than mere summaries of past experience. Whereas summary rules are only guidelines in applying the abstract principles in every case, rules of practice are more weighty. The principles are used to establish a set of practices that are morally definitive in normal day-to-day decisionmaking. For example, if one is working with the principle of beneficence or utility, one might still generate a rule that holds one should always get consent before surgery because that practice produces more good than any other alternative practice. Likewise, from the principle of autonomy one might also generate the rule to get consent before surgery (because, in this case, doing so respects autonomy). This does not necessarily result in legalism. Rules of practice can be reassessed and changed by going back to the basic principles, but that is done only to change the rules, not to generate exceptions to the rules in specific cases.

The essays in this chapter step back from the specifics of biomedical ethics to present basic philosophical discussions of how to relate principles to one another and how to relate principles to cases. The writing and rewriting of the codes of ethics for health care constitute the application of these notions to health care.

John Stuart Mill has provided one of the first and most convincing answers to the question of the relation of ethical principles. He searches for one common first principle that underlies all of morality and, citing Bentham, identifies the principle of happiness or utility. According to Mill, in the end all morality reduces to producing the greatest amount of good over harm. Mill thus resolves the problem of conflict among principles by reducing the whole of normative morality to one single overarching principle. In doing so he is exactly like the Hippocratic authors with one exception. Hippocratic ethics reduces morality to the maximizing of benefit for the patient. It is thus utilitarianism with a difference. Producing good is the only thing that counts, but, for Hippocratists, only patient-good is relevant.

This might be because if every physician strives only for the welfare of his or her patient, then in the long run the greatest good is done for everyone. This is an empirical claim subject to confirmation. It seems implausible that social welfare in general would be served by such a strategy, especially in a society where many people do not have physicians who would be striving for their welfare at all.

Many Hippocratic physicians probably do not opt for the Hippocratic formula on utilitarian grounds of the maximizing aggregate welfare. They seem to hold that the physician has a duty to benefit only his or her patient even if it does not produce the greatest good for the greatest number. If so, they have one non–utilitarian element in their ethics—the element that limits the morally relevant consequences to the patient. Still, like utilitarians they resolve the problem of conflicting principles by reducing ethics to one principle.

The following essay reveals how Mill makes his case for utility as the single principle.

Utilitarianism

JOHN STUART MILL

GENERAL REMARKS

There are few circumstances among those which make up the present condition of human knowledge more unlike what might have been expected, or more significant of the backward state in which speculation on the most important subjects still lingers, than the little progress which has been made in the decision of the controversy respecting the criterion of right and wrong. From the dawn of philosophy, the question concerning the *summum bonum*, or, what is the same thing, concerning the foundation of morality, has been accounted the main problem in speculative thought, has occupied the most gifted intellects and divided them into sects and schools, carrying on a vigorous warfare against one another. And after more than two thousand years the same discussions continue, philosophers are still ranged under the same contending banners, and neither thinkers nor mankind at large seem nearer to being unanimous on the subject than when the youth Socrates listened to the old Protagoras, and asserted (if Plato's dialogue be grounded on a real conversation) the theory of utilitarianism against the popular morality of the so-called sophist.

It is true that similar confusion and uncertainty and, in some cases, similar discordance exist respecting the first principles of all the sciences, not excepting that which is deemed the most certain of them—mathematics, without much impairing, generally indeed without impairing at all, the trustworthiness of the conclusions of those sciences. An apparent anomaly the explanation of which is that the detailed doctrines of a science are not usually deduced from, nor depend for their evidence upon, what are called its first principles. Were it not so, there would be no science more precarious, or whose conclusions were more insufficiently made out, than algebra, which derives none of its certainty from what are commonly taught to learners as its elements, since these, as laid down by some of its most eminent teachers, are as full of fictions as English law, and of mysteries as theology. The truths which are ultimately accepted as the first principles of a science are really the last results of a metaphysical analysis, practiced on the elementary notions with which the science is conversant; and their relation to the science is not that of foundations to an edifice, but of roots to a tree, which may perform their office equally well though they have never dug down to and exposed the light. But though in science the particular truths precede the general theory, the contrary might be expected to be the case with a practical art, such as morals or legislation. All action is for the sake of some end, and rules of action, it seems natural to suppose, must take their whole character and color from the end to which they are subservient. When we engage in a pursuit, a clear and precise conception of what we are pursuing would seem to be the first thing we need, instead of the last we are to look forward to. A test of right and wrong must be the means, one would think, of ascertaining what is right or wrong, and not a consequence of having already ascertained it.

The difficulty is not avoided by having recourse to the popular theory of a natural faculty, a sense or instinct, informing us of right and wrong. For—besides that the existence of such a moral instinct is itself one of the matters in dispute—those believers in it who have any pretensions to philosophy have been obliged to abandon the idea that it discerns what is right or wrong in the particular case in hand, as our other senses discern the sight or sound actually present. Our moral faculty, according to all those of its interpreters who are entitled to the name of thinkers, supplies of moral judgments; it is a branch of our reason, not of our sensitive faculty; and must be looked to for the abstract doctrines of morality, not for perception of it in the concrete. The intuitive, no less than what may be termed the inductive, school of ethics insists on the necessity of general laws. They both agree that the morality of an individual action is not a question of direct perception, but of the application of a law to an individual case. They recognize also, to a great extent, the same moral laws, but differ as to their evidence and the source from which they derive their authority. According to the one opinion, the principles of morals are evident *a priori*, requiring nothing to command assent except that the meaning of the terms be understood. According to the other doctrine, right and wrong, as well as truth and falsehood, are questions of observation and experience. But both hold equally that morality must be deduced from principles; and the intuitive school affirm as strongly as the inductive that there is a science of morals. Yet they seldom attempt to make out a list of the *a priori* principles which are to serve as the premises of the science; still more rarely do they make any effort to reduce those various principles to one first principle, or common ground of obligation. They either assume the ordinary precepts of morals as of *a priori* authority, or they lay down as the common groundwork of those maxims, some generality much less obviously authoritative than the maxims themselves, and which has never succeeded in gaining popular acceptance. Yet to support their pretensions there ought either to be some one fundamental principle or law at the root of all morality, or, if there be several, there should be a determinate order of precedence among them; and the one principle, or the rule for deciding between the various principles when they conflict, ought to be self-evident.

To inquire how far the bad effects of this deficiency have been mitigated in practice, or to what extent the moral beliefs of mankind have been vitiated or made uncertain by the absence of any distinct recognition of an ultimate standard, would imply a complete survey and criticism of past and present ethical doctrine. It would, however, be easy to show that whatever steadiness or consistency these moral beliefs have attained has been mainly due to the tacit influence of a standard not recognized. Although the non-existence of an acknowledged first principle has made ethics not so much a guide as a consecration of men's actual sentiments, still, as men's sentiments, both in favor and of aversion, are greatly influenced by what they suppose to be the effect of things upon their happiness, the principle of utility, or, as Bentham latterly called it, the greatest happiness principle, has had a large share in forming the moral doctrines even of those who most scornfully reject its authority. Nor is there any school of thought which refuses to admit that the influence of actions on happiness is a most material and even predominant consideration in many of the details of morals, however unwilling to acknowledge it as the fundamental principle of morality and the source of moral obligation. I might go much further and say that to all those *a priori* moralists who deem it necessary to argue at all, utilitarian arguments are indispensable. It is not my present purpose to criticize these thinkers; but I cannot help referring, for illustration, to a systematic treatise by one of the most illustrious of them, the *Metaphysics of Ethics* by Kant. This remarkable man, whose system of thought will long remain one of the landmarks in the history of philosophical speculation, does, in the treatise in question, lay down a universal first principle as the origin and ground of moral obligation; it is this: "So act that the rule on which thou actest would admit of being adopted as a law by all rational beings." But when he begins to deduce from this precept any of the actual duties of morality, he fails, almost grotesquely, to show that there would be any contradiction, any logical (not to say physical) impossibility, in the adoption by all rational beings of the most outrageously immoral rules of conduct. All he knows is that the consequences of their universal adoption would be such as no one would choose to incur.

On the present occasion, I shall, without further discussion of the other theories, attempt to contribute something towards the understanding and appreciation of the "utilitarian" or "happiness" theory, and towards such proof as it is susceptible of. It is evident that this cannot be proof in the ordinary and popular meaning of the term. Questions of ultimate ends are not amenable to direct proof. Whatever can be proved to be good must be so by being shown to be a means to something admitted to be good without proof. The medical art is proved to be good by its conducing to health; but how is it possible to prove that health is good? The art of music is good, for the reason, among others, that it produces pleasure; but what proof is it possible to give that pleasure is good? If, then it is asserted that there is a comprehensive formula, including all things which are in themselves good, and that whatever else is good is not so as an end but as a means, the formula may be accepted or rejected, but it is not a subject of what is commonly understood by proof. We are not, however, to infer that its acceptance or rejection must depend on blind impulse, or arbitrary choice. There is a larger meaning of the word "proof," in which this question is as amenable to it as any other of the disputed questions of philosophy. The subject is within the cognizance of the rational faculty; and neither does that faculty deal with it solely in the way of intuition. Considerations may be presented capable of determining the intellect either to give or withhold its assent to the doctrine; and this is equivalent to proof.

We shall examine presently of what nature are these considerations; in what manner they apply to the case, and what rational grounds, therefore, can be given for accepting or rejecting the utilitarian formula. But it is a preliminary condition of rational acceptance or rejection that the formula should be correctly understood. I believe that the very imperfect notion ordinarily formed of its meaning is the chief obstacle which impedes its reception, and that, could it be cleared even from only the grosser misconceptions the question would be greatly simplified and a large proportion of its difficulties removed. Before, therefore, I attempt to enter into the philosophical grounds which can be given for assenting to the utilitarian standard, I shall offer some illustrations of the doctrine itself, with the view of showing more clearly what it is, distinguishing it from what it is not, and disposing of such of the practical objections to it as either originate in, or are closely connected with, mistaken interpretation of its meaning. Having thus prepared the ground, I shall afterwards endeavor to throw some light as I can call upon the question considered as one of philosophical theory.

There are many ethical theories that reject Mill's attempt to reduce all of ethics to the single principle of utility. Kant opts for a number of right-making characteristics none of which is based on utility. He finesses the problem of conflict however by taking up only the problem of conflict between utility and one other principle. He deals with cases where good consequences come from breaking a promise or from killing a tyrant but never the case where one has to choose between killing a tyrant and breaking a promise.

John Rawls deals explicitly with the problem of priority among principles in a short section of his volume, *A Theory of Justice*. He rejects the solution relying on a single overarching principle in favor of what he calls lexical ordering or ranking of principles.

The Priority Problem

John Rawls

Intuitionism raises the question of the extent to which it is possible to give a systematic account of our considered judgments of the just and the unjust. In particular, it holds that no constructive answer can be given to the problem of assigning weights to competing principles of justice. Here at least we must rely on our intuitive capacities. Classical utilitarianism tries, of course, to avoid the appeal altogether. It is a single-principle conception with one ultimate standard; the adjustment of weights is, in theory anyway, settled by reference to the principle of utility. Mill thought that there must be but one such standard, otherwise there would be no umpire between competing criteria, and Sidgwick argues at length that the utilitarian principle is the only one which can assume this role. They maintain that our moral judgments are implicitly utilitarian in the sense that when confronted with a clash of precepts, or with notions which are vague and imprecise, we have no alternative except to adopt utilitarianism. Mill and Sidgwick believe that at some point we must have a single principle to straighten out and to systematize our judgments.[1] Undeniably one of the great attractions of the classical doctrine is the way it faces the priority problem and tries to avoid relying on intuition.

As I have already remarked, there is nothing necessarily irrational in the appeal to intuition to settle questions of priority. We must recognize the possibility that there is no way to get beyond a plurality of principles. No doubt any conception of justice will have to rely on intuition to some degree. Nevertheless, we should do what we can to reduce the direct appeal to our considered judgments. For if men balance final principles differently, as presumably they often do, then their conceptions of justice are different. The assignment of weights is an essential and not a minor part of a conception of justice. If we cannot explain how these weights are to be determined by reasonable ethical criteria, the means of rational discussion have come to an end. An intuitionist conception of justice is, one might say, but half a conception. We should do what we can to formulate explicit principles for the priority problem, even though the dependence on intuition cannot be eliminated entirely.

In justice as fairness the role of intuition is limited in several ways. Since the whole question is rather difficult, I shall only make a few comments here the full sense of which will not be clear until later on. The first point is connected with the fact that the principles of justice are those which would be chosen in the original position. They are the outcome of certain choice situation. Now being rational, the persons in the original position recognize that they should consider the priority of these principles. For if they wish to establish agreed standards for adjudicating their claims on one another, they will need principles for assigning weights. They cannot assume that their intuitive judgments of priority will in general be the same; given their different positions in society they surely will not. Thus I suppose that in the original position the parties try to reach some agreement as to how the principles of justice are to be balanced. Now part of the value of the notion of choosing principles is that the reasons which underlie their adoption in the first place may also support giving them certain weights. Since in justice as fairness the principles of justice are not thought of as self-evident, but have their justification in the fact that they would be chosen, we may find in the grounds for their acceptance some guidance or limitation as to how they are to be balanced. Given the situation of the original position, it may be clear that certain priority rules are preferable to others for much the same reasons that principles are initially assented to. By emphasizing the role of justice and the special features of the initial choice situation, the priority problem may prove more tractable.

A second possibility is that we may be able to find principles which can be put in what I call a serial or lexical order.[2] (The correct term is "lexicographical," but it is too cumbersome.) This is an order which requires us to satisfy the first principle in the ordering before we can move on to the second, the second before we consider the third, and so on. A principle does not come into play until those previous to it are either fully met or do not apply. A serial ordering avoids, then, having to balance principles at all; those earlier in the ordering have an absolute weight, so to speak, with respect to later ones, and hold without exception. We can regard such a ranking as analogous to a sequence of constrained maximum principles. For we can suppose that any principle in the order is to be maximized subject to the condition that the preceding principles are fully satisfied. As an important special case I shall, in fact, propose an ordering of this kind of ranking the principle of equal liberty prior to the principle regulating economic and social inequalities. This means, in effect, that the basic structure of society is to arrange the inequalities of wealth and authority in ways consistent with the equal liberties required by the preceding principle. Certainly the concept of lexical, or serial, order does not off-hand seem very promising. Indeed, it appears to offend our sense of moderation and good judgment. Moreover, it presupposes that the principles in the order be of a rather special kind. For example, unless the earlier principles have but a limited application and establish definite requirements which can be fulfilled, later principles will never come into play. Thus the principle of equal liberty can assume a prior position since it may, let us suppose, be satisfied. Whereas if the principle of utility were first, it would render otiose all subsequent criteria. I shall try to show that at least in certain social circumstances a serial ordering of the principles of justice offers an approximate solution to the priority problem.

Finally, the dependence on intuition can be reduced by posing more limited questions and by substituting prudential for moral judgment. Thus someone faced with the principles of an intuitionist conception may reply that without some guidelines for deliberation he does not know what to say. He might maintain, for example, that he could not balance total utility against equality in the distribution of satisfaction. Not only are the notions involved here too abstract and comprehensive for him to have any confidence in his judgment, but there are enormous complications in interpreting what they mean. The aggregative-distributive dichotomy is no doubt an attractive idea, but in this instance it seems unmanageable. It does not factor the problem of social justice into small enough parts. In justice as fairness the appeal to intuition is focused in two ways. First we single out a certain position in the social system from which the system is to be judged, and then we ask whether, from the standpoint of a representative man in this position, it would be rational to prefer this arrangement of the basic structure rather than that. Given certain assumptions, economic and social inequalities are to be judged in terms of the long-run expectations of the least advantaged social group. Of course, the specification of this group is not very exact, and certainly our prudential judgments likewise give considerable scope to intuition, since we may not be able to formulate the principle which determines them. Nevertheless, we have asked a much more limited question and have substituted for an ethical judgment a judgment of rational prudence. Often it is quite clear how we should decide. The reliance on intuition is of a different nature and much less than in the aggregative-distributive dichotomy of the intuitionist conception.

In addressing the priority problem the task is that of reducing and not of eliminating entirely the reliance on intuitive judgments. There is no reason to suppose that we can avoid all appeals to intuition, of whatever kind, or that we should try to. The practical aim is to reach a reasonably reliable agreement in judgment in order to provide a common conception of justice. If men's intuitive priority judgments are similar, it does not matter, practically speaking, that they cannot formulate the principles which account for these convictions, or even whether such principles exist. Contrary judgments however, raise a difficulty, since the basis for adjudicating claims is to that extent obscure. Thus our object should be to formulate a conception of justice which, however much it may call upon intuition, ethical or prudential, tends to make our considered judgments of justice converge. If such a conception does exist, then, from the standpoint of the original position, there would strong reasons for accepting it, since it is rational to introduce further coherence into our common convictions of justice. Indeed, once we look at things from the standpoint of the initial situation, the priority problem is not that of how to cope with the complexity of already given moral facts which cannot be altered. Instead, it is the problem of formulating reasonable and generally acceptable proposals for bringing about the desired agreement in judgments. On a contract doctrine the moral facts are determined by the principles which would be chosen in the original position. These principles specify which considerations are relevant from the standpoint of social justice. Since it is up to the persons in the original position to choose these principles, it is for them to decide how simple or complex they want the moral facts to be. The original agreement settles how far they are prepared to compromise and to simplify in order to establish the priority rules necessary for a common conception of justice.

I have reviewed two obvious and simple ways of dealing constructively with the priority problem: namely, either by a single overall principle, or by a plurality of principles in lexical order. Other ways no doubt exist, but I shall not consider what they might be. The traditional moral theories are for the most part single-principled or intuitionistic, so that the working out of a serial ordering is novelty enough for a first step. While it seems clear that, in general, a lexical order cannot be strictly correct, it may be an illuminating approximation under certain special though significant conditions. In this way it may indicate the larger structure of conceptions of justice and suggest the directions along which a closer fit can be found.

NOTES

1. For Mill, see *A System of Logic*, Book VI, Chapter XII, Sec. 7; and *Utilitarianism*, Chapter V, paras. 26–31, where this argument is made in connection with common sense precepts of justice. For Sidgwick, see the *Methods of Ethics*, for example, Book IV, Chapter II and III, which summarized much of the argument of Book III.

2. The term *lexicographical* derives from the fact that the most familiar example of such an ordering is that of words in a dictionary. To see this, substitute numerals for letters, putting *1* for a "2" for *b* and so on, and then rank the resulting strings of numerals from left to right, moving to the right only when necessary to break ties. In general, a lexical ordering cannot be represented by a continuous real-valued utility function; such a ranking violates the assumption of continuity. See Pearce, I. F. *A Contribution to Demand Analysis*. Oxford: The Clarendon Press, 1946, pp. 22–27; and Sen, A. K. *Collective Choice and Social Welfare*. San Francisco: Holden-Day, 1970, pp. 34f. For further references, see Houghtakker, H. S. "The Present State Consumption Theory." *Ecomometrica* 29:710f, 1961.

   In the history of moral philosophy the conception of a lexical order occasionally appears though it is not explicitly discussed. A clear example may be found in Hutcheson, *A System of Moral Philosophy* (1755). He proposes that in comparing pleasure of the same kind, we use their intensity and duration; in comparing pleasures of different kinds we must consider their duration and dignity jointly. Pleasure of higher kinds may have a worth greater that those of lower kinds however great the latter's intensity and duration. See Selby-Bigge, L. A. *British Moralists*, Vol. I (Oxford, 1897), pp. 421–423. J. S. Mill's well-known view in *Utilitarianism*, Chapter II, paras. 6–8, is similar to Hutcheson's. It also is natural to rank moral worth as lexically prior to nonmoral values. See for example Ross, *The Right and the Good*, pp. 149–154. And of course the primacy of justice is noted in §1 [*A Theory of Justice*], as well as the priority of right as found in Kant, are further cases of such an ordering.

The theory of utility in economics began with an implicit recognition of the hierarchical structure of wants and the priority of moral considerations. This is clear in Jevons, W. S. the *Theory of Political Economy*, (London, 1871), pp. 27–32. Jevons states a conception analogous to Hutcheson's and confines the economist's use of the utility calculus to the lower rank of feelings. For a discussion of the hierarchy of wants and its relation to utility theory, see Georgescu-Roegen, Nicholas. "Choice, Expectations, and Measurability." *Quarterly Journal of Economics*, Vol. 68 (1954), esp. pp. 510–520.

Even if one solves the problem of how principles are ranked, one still must face the important task of relating principles to specific cases. Joseph Fletcher has long worried about this problem. He opts for a position he calls "situationalism." While that position is often characterized as avoiding moral rules, such characterization is unfair.

Fletcher contrasts his position to one that gives excessively rigid authority to rules (what he calls legalism) and one that gives no role at all to rules (what he calls antinomianism). Fletcher concludes that in contrast with these two errors, one should treat rules as guiding maxims, as guidelines or summaries of past experience that should help us in the individual case. Nevertheless, the goal should always be to assess in the individual case whether a specific action satisfies the moral principle by applying the rule that normally seems to apply. If it does not, then the rule must give way.

Three Approaches

Joseph Fletcher

There are at bottom only three alternative routes or approaches to follow in making moral decisions. They are: (1) legalistic; (2) the antinomian, the opposite extreme— i.e., a lawless or unprincipled approach; and (3) the situational.

APPROACHES TO LEGALISM

Legalism

With this approach one enters into every decision-making situation encumbered with a whole apparatus of prefabricated rules and regulations. Not just the spirit but the letter of the law reigns. Its principles, codified in rules, are not merely guidelines or maxims to illuminate the situation; they are directives to be followed. Solutions are preset, and you can "look them up" in a book—a Bible or a confessor's manual.

Judaism, Catholicism, Protestantism—all major Western religious traditions have been legalistic. In morals as in doctrine they have kept to a spelled-out, "systematic" orthodoxy.

Legalism in the Christian tradition has taken two forms. In the Catholic line it has been a matter of legalistic *reason*, based on nature or natural law. These moralists have tended to adumbrate their ethical rules by applying human reason to the facts of nature, both human and subhuman, and to the lessons of historical experience. By this procedure they claim to have adduced universally agreed and therefore valid "natural" moral laws. Protestant moralists have followed the same adductive and deductive tactics. They have taken Scripture and done with it what the Catholics do with nature. Their Scriptural moral law is, they argue, based on the works and sayings of the Law and the Prophets, the evangelists and apostles of the Bible. It is a matter of legalistic *revelation*. One is rationalistic, the other Biblicistic; one natural, the other Scriptural. But both are legalistic.

Antinomianism

Over against legalism, as a sort of polar opposite, we can put antinomianism. This is the approach with which one enters into the decision-making situation armed with no principles or maxims whatsoever, to say nothing of rules. In every "existential moment" or "unique" situation, it declares, one must rely upon the situation or itself, *there and then*, to provide it ethical solution.

Paul had to struggle with two primitive forms of it among the Hellenistic Jew-Christians whom he visited. They took his attacks on law morality too naively and too literally.

One form was libertinism—the belief that by grace, by the new life in Christ and salvation by faith, law or rules no longer applied to Christians. Their ultimate happy fate was now assured, and it mattered no more *what* they did.

The other form, less pretentious and more enduring, was a Gnostic claim to special knowledge, so that neither principles nor rules were needed any longer even as guidelines and direction pointers. They would just know what was right when they needed to know. They had, they claimed, a superconscience. It is this second "gnostic" form of the approach which is under examination here.

Other antinomians claimed, and still do, that their guidance comes from within themselves, as a sort of built-in radar-like "faculty," a translegal or clairvoyant conscience as promised in Jer. 31:31–34, written "upon their hearts." This second and more common form of Gnostic antinomianism, found among both Christians and non-Christians, is close to the intuition theory of conscience.

Another version of antinomianism, on the whole much subtler philosophically and perhaps more admirable, is the ethics of existentialism.

On this view the existentialists reject all principles, all "generally valid" ethical norms or axioms, as well all rules or laws or precepts that legalistically absolutize (idolize) such general principles. Radical discontinuity in one's theory of being forces the "absolute particularity" of *tout comprendre, tout pardoner.*

Situationism

A third approach, in between legalism and antinomian unprincipledness, is situation ethics. The situationist enters into every decision-making situation fully armed with the ethical maxims of his community and its heritage, and he treats them with respect as illuminators of his problems. Just the same he is prepared in any situation to compromise them or set them aside *in the situation* if love seems better served by doing so.

Situation ethics goes part of the way with natural law, by accepting reason as the instrument of moral judgment, while rejecting the notion that the good is "given" in the nature of things, objectively. It goes part of the way with Scriptural law by accepting revelation as the source of the norm while rejecting all "revealed" norms or laws but the one command—to love God in the neighbor. The situationist follows a moral law or violates it according to love's need. For example, "Alsmgiving is a good thing if . . . ." The situationist never says, "Almsgiving is a good thing. Period!" His decisions are hypothetical, not categorical. Only the commandment to love is categorically good. "Owe no one anything, except to love one another."

The situational factors are so primary that we may even say "circumstances alter rules and principles." It is said that when Gertrude Stein lay dying she declared, "It is better to ask questions than to give answers, even good answers." This is the temper of situation ethics. It is empirical, fact-minded, data conscious, inquiring. It is antimoralistic as well as antilegalistic, for it is sensitive to variety and complexity. It is neither simplistic nor perfectionist. It is "casuistry" (case-based) in a constructive and nonpejorative sense of the word. We should perhaps call it "neocasuistry." Like classical casuistry, it is case-focused and concrete, concerned to bring Christian imperatives into practical operation. But unlike classical casuistry, this neocasuistry repudiates any attempt to anticipate or prescribe real-life decisions in their existential particularity.

PRINCIPLES, YES, BUT NOT RULES

It is necessary to insist that situation ethics is willing to make full and respectful use of principles, to be treated as maxims but not as laws or precepts. We might call it "principled relativism." To repeat the term used above, principles or maxims or general rules are *illuminators.* But they are not *directors.* The classic rule of moral theology has been to follow laws but do it as much as possible according to love and according to reason (*secundum caritatem et secundum rationem*). Situation ethics, on the other hand, calls upon us to keep law in a subservient place, so that only love and reason really count when the chips are down!

Just as John Rawls offers an alternative to Mill's single principle solution to the priority problem, so he offers an alternative to Joseph Fletcher's summary rules or situational solution to the problem of how principles relate to cases. Rawls recognizes that rules cannot be absolutely rigid, but sees rules as much more than simple guidelines linking principles to cases.

In the excerpt that follows Rawls holds that there are two concepts of rules. The first is roughly Fletcher's rules-as-guidelines approach. In the second, Rawls holds that rules can define practices. Practices are defined by applying the basic principles in order to establish a set of rules. For example, if the only basic principle is utility, then utility can be used to determine which set of practices produces the greatest good. Once rules are specified that are believed to produce more good than any other set of rules, then those rules are taken to define morally correct behavior within the particular practice. This position is often called rule utility to separate it from the more simple, straight-forward application of the principle of utility to specific cases.

One might find that as circumstances change there is a need to redefine the rules. One might revert back to the principle of utility to reassess the rules. If new rules are established as now maximizing utility, then those new rules will define the practice. In any case, the principles are not brought directly to the case, only to the rules.

Two Concepts of Rules

JOHN RAWLS

In this paper I want to show the importance of the distinction between justifying a practice[1] and justifying a particular action falling under it, and I want to explain the logical basis of this distinction and how it is possible to miss its significance. While the distinction has frequently been made, and is now becoming commonplace, there remains the task of explaining the tendency either to overlook it altogether, or to fail to appreciate its importance.

To explain how the significance of the distinction may be overlooked, I am going to discuss two conceptions of rules. One of these conceptions conceals the importance of distinguishing between the justification of a rule or practice and the justification of a particular action falling under it. The other conception makes it clear why this distinction must be made and what is its logical basis.

I am going to examine two conceptions of rules, two ways of placing them within the utilitarian theory.

The conception which conceals from us the significance of the distinction I am going to call the summary view. It regards rules in the following way: one supposes that each person decides what he shall do in particular cases by applying the utilitarian principle; one supposes further that different people will decide the same particular case in the same way and that there will be recurrences of cases similar to those previously decided. Thus it will happen that in cases of certain kinds the same decision will be made either by the same person at different times or by different persons at the same time. If a case occurs frequently enough one supposes that a rule is formulated to cover that sort of case. I have called this conception the summary view because rules are pictured as summaries of past decisions arrived at by the direct application of the utilitarian principle to particular cases. Rules are regarded as reports that cases of a certain sort have been found on other grounds to be properly decided in a certain way (although, of course, they do not say this).

There are several things to notice about this way of placing rules within the utilitarian theory.

1. The point of having rules derives from the fact that similar cases tend to recur and that one can decide cases more quickly if one records past decisions in the form of rules. If similar cases didn't recur, one would be required to apply the utilitarian principle directly, case by case, and rules reporting past decisions would be of no use.

2. The decisions made on particular cases are logically prior to rules. Since rules gain their point from the need to apply the utilitarian principle to many similar cases, it follows that a particular case (or several cases similar to it) may exist whether or not there is a rule covering that case. We are pictured as recognizing particular cases prior to there being a rule which covers them, for it is only if we meet with a number of cases of a certain sort that we formulate a rule. Thus we are able to describe a particular case as a particular case of the requisite sort whether there is a rule regarding *that* sort of case or not. Put another way: what the A's and the B's refer to in rules of the form 'Whenever A do B' may be described as A's and B's whether or not there is the rule 'Whenever A do B,' or whether or not there is any body of rules which make up a practice of which that rule is a part.

To illustrate this consider a rule, or maxim, which could arise in this way: suppose that a person is trying to decide whether to tell someone who is fatally ill what his illness is when he has been asked to do so. Suppose the person to reflect and then decide, on utilitarian grounds, that he should not answer truthfully; and suppose that on the basis of this and other like occasions he formulates a rule to the effect that when asked by someone fatally ill what his illness is, one should not tell him. The point to notice is that someone's being fatally ill and asking what his illness is, and someone's telling him, are things that can be described as such whether or not there is this rule. The performance of the action to which the rule refers doesn't require the stage-setting of a practice of which this rule is a part. This is meant by saying that on the summary view particular cases are logically prior to rules.

3.   Each person is in principle always entitled to reconsider the correctness of a rule and to question whether or not it is proper to follow it in a particular case. As rules are guides and aids, one may ask whether in past decisions there might not have been a mistake in applying the utilitarian principle to get the rule in question, and wonder whether or not it is best in this case. The reason for rules is that people are not able to apply the utilitarian principle effortlessly and flawlessly; there is need to save time and to post a guide. On this view a society of rational utilitarians would be a society without rules in which each person applied the utilitarian principle directly and smoothly, and without error, case by case. On the other hand, ours is a society in which rules are formulated to serve as aids in reaching these ideally rational decisions on particular cases, guides which have been built up and tested by the experience of generations. If one applies this view to rules, one is interpreting them as maxims, as "rules of thumb"; and it is doubtful that anything to which the summary conception did apply would be called a *rule*. Arguing as if one regarded rules in this way is a mistake one makes while doing philosophy.

4.   The concept of a *general* rule takes the following form. One is pictured as estimating on what percentage of the cases likely to arise a given rule may be relied upon to express the correct decision, that is, the decision that would be arrived at if one were to correctly apply the utilitarian principle case by case. If one estimates that by and large the rule will give the correct decision, or if one estimates that the likelihood of making a mistake by applying the utilitarian principle directly on one's own is greater than the likelihood of making a mistake by following the rule, and if these considerations held of persons generally, then one would be justified in urging its adoption as a general rule. In this way *general* rules might be accounted for on the summary view. It will still make sense, however, to speak of applying the utilitarian principle case by case, for it was by trying to foresee the results of doing this that one got the initial estimates upon which acceptance of the rule depends. That one is taking a rule in accordance with the summary conception will show itself in the naturalness with which one speaks of the rule as a guide, or as a maxim, or as a generalization from experience, and as something to be laid aside in extraordinary cases where there is no assurance that the generalization will hold and the case must therefore be treated on its merits. Thus there goes with this conception the notion of a particular exception which renders a rule suspect on a particular occasion.

The other conception of rules I will call the practice conception. On this view rules are pictured as defining a practice. Practices are set up for various reasons, but one of them is that in many areas of conduct each person's deciding what to do on utilitarian grounds case by case leads to confusion, and that the attempt to coordinate behavior by trying to foresee how others will act is bound to fail. As an alternative one realizes that what is required is the establishment of a practice, the specification of a new form of activity; and from this one sees that a practice necessarily involves the abdication of full liberty to act on utilitarian and prudential grounds. It is the mark of a practice that being taught how to engage in it involves being instructed in the rules which define it, and that appeal is made to those rules to correct the behavior of those engaged in it. Those engaged in a practice recognize the rules as defining it. The rules cannot be taken as simply describing how those engaged in the practice in fact behave: it is not simply that they act as if they were obeying the rules. Thus it is essential to the notion of a practice that the rules are publicly known and understood as definitive; and it is essential also that the rules of a practice can be taught and can be acted upon to yield a coherent practice. On this conception then, rules are not generalizations from the decisions of individuals applying the utilitarian principle directly and independently to recurrent particular cases. On the contrary, rules define a practice and are themselves the subject of the utilitarian principle.

To show the important differences between this way of fitting rules into the utilitarian theory and the previous way, I shall consider the differences between the two conceptions on the points previously discussed.

1. In contrast with the summary view, the rules of practices are logically prior to particular cases. This is so because there cannot be a particular case of an action falling under a rule of a practice unless there is the practice. This can be made clearer as follows: in a practice there are rules setting up offices, specifying certain forms of action appropriate to various offices, establishing penalties for the breach of rules, and so on. We may think of the rules of a practice as defining offices, moves, and offenses. Now what is meant by saying that the practice is logically prior to particular cases is this: given any rule which specifies a form of action (a move), a particular action which would be taken as falling under this rule given that there is the practice would not be *described* as that sort of action unless there was the practice. In the case of actions specified by practices it is logically impossible to perform them outside the stage-setting provided by those practices, for unless there is the practice, and unless the requisite proprieties are fulfilled, whatever one does, whatever movements one makes, will fail to count as a form of action which the practice specifies. What one does will be described some *other* way.

One may illustrate this point from the game of baseball. Many of the actions one performs in a game of baseball one can do by oneself or with others whether there is the game or not. For example, one can throw a ball, run, or swing a peculiarly shaped piece of wood. But one cannot steal a base, or strike out, or draw a walk, or make an error or balk; although one can do certain things which appear to resemble these actions such as sliding into a base, missing a grounder and so on. Striking out, stealing a base, balking, etc., are all actions which can only happen in a game. No matter what a person did, what he did would not be described as stealing a base or striking out or drawing a walk unless he could also be described as playing baseball, and for him to be doing this presupposes the rule-like practice which constitutes the game. The practice is logically prior to particular cases: unless there is the practice the terms referring to actions specified by it lack a sense.[2]

2. The practice view leads to an entirely different conception of the authority which each person has to decide on the propriety of following a rule in particular cases. To engage in a practice, to perform those actions specified by a practice, means to follow the appropriate rules. If one wants to do an action which a certain practice specifies then there is no way to do it except to follow the rules which define it. Therefore, it doesn't make sense for a person to raise the question whether or not a rule of a practice correctly applies *to his* case where the action he contemplates is a form of action defined by a practice. If someone were to raise such a question, he would simply show that he didn't understand the situation in which he was acting. If one wants to perform an action specified by a practice, the only legitimate question concerns the nature of the practice itself ("How do I go about making a will?")

This point is illustrated by the behavior expected of a player in games. If one wants to play a game, one doesn't treat the rules of the game as guides as to what is best in particular cases. In a game of baseball if a batter were to ask "Can I have four strikes?" it would be assumed that he was asking what the rule was; and if, when told what the rule was, he were to say that he meant on this occasion he thought it would be best on the whole for him to have four strikes rather than three, this would be most kindly taken as a joke. One might contend that baseball would be a better game if four strikes were allowed instead of three; but one cannot picture the rules as guides to what is best on the whole in particular cases, and question their applicability to particular cases as particular cases.

3 and 4. To complete the four points of comparison with the summary conception, it is clear from what has been said that rules of practices are not guides to help one decide particular cases correctly as judged by some higher ethical principle. And neither the quasi-statistical notion of generality, nor the notion of a particular exception, can apply to the rules of practices. A more or less general rule of a practice must be a rule which according to the structure of the practice applies to more or fewer of the kinds of cases arising under it; or it must be a rule which is more or less basic to the understanding of the practice. Again, a particular case cannot be an exception to a rule of a practice. An exception is rather a qualification or a further specification of the rule.

It follows from what we have said about the practice conception of rules that if a person is engaged in a practice, and if he is asked why *he* does what *he* does, or if he is asked to defend what he does, then his explanation, or defense, lies in referring the questioner to the practice. He cannot say *of his* action, if it is an action specified by a practice, that he does it rather than some other because he thinks it is best on the whole.[3] When a man engaged in a practice is queried about his action he must assume that the questioner either doesn't know that he is engaged in it ("Why are you in a hurry to pay him" "I promised to pay him today") or doesn't know what the practice is. One doesn't so much justify one's particular action as explain, or show, that it is in accordance with the practice. The reason for this is that it is only against the stage-setting of the practice that one's particular action is described as it is. Only by reference to the practice can one *say* what one is doing. To explain or to defend one's own action, as a particular action, one fits it into the practice which defines it. If this is not accepted it's a sign that a different question is being raised as to whether one is justified in accepting the practice, or in tolerating it. When the challenge is to the practice, citing the rules (saying what the practice is) is naturally to no avail. But when the challenge is to the particular action defined by the practice, there is nothing one can do but refer to the rules. Concerning particular actions there is only a question for one who isn't clear as to what the practice is, or who doesn't know that it is being engaged in. This is to be contrasted with the case of a maxim which may be taken as pointing to the correct decision on the case as decided on other grounds, and so giving a challenge on the case a sense by having it question whether these other grounds really support the decision on this case.

If one compares the two conceptions of rules I have discussed, one can see how the summary conception missed the significance of the distinction between justifying a practice and justifying actions falling under it. On this view rules are regarded as guides whose purpose it is to indicate the ideally rational decision on the given particular case which the flawless application of the utilitarian principle would yield. One has, in principle, full option use the guides or to discard them as the situation warrants without one's moral office being altered in any way: whether one discards the rules or not, one always holds the office of a rational person seeking case by case to realize the best on the whole. But on the practice conception, if one holds an office defined by a practice then questions regarding one's action in this office are settled by reference to the rules which define the practice. If one seeks to question these rules, then one's office undergoes a fundamental change: one then assumes the office of one empowered to change and criticize the rules, or the office of a reformer, and so on. The summary conception does away with the distinction of offices and the various forms of argument appropriate to each. On that conception there is one office and so no offices at all. It therefore obscures the fact that the utilitarian principle must, in the case of actions and offices defined by a practice, apply to the practice, so that general utilitarian arguments are not available to those who act in offices so defined.[4]

Some qualifications are necessary in what I have said. First, I may have talked of the summary and the practice conceptions of rules as if only one of them could be true of rules, and if true of any rules, then necessarily true of all rules. I do not, of course, mean this. (It is the critics of utilitarianism who make this mistake insofar as their arguments against utilitarianism presuppose a summary conception of the rules of practices.) Some rules will fit one conception, some rules the other; and so there are rules of practices (rules in the strict sense), and maxims and "rules of thumb."

Secondly, there are further distinctions that can be made in classifying rules, distinctions which should be made if one were considering other questions. The distinctions which I have drawn are those most relevant for the special matter I have discussed, and are not intended to be exhaustive.

Finally, there will be many border-line cases about which it will be difficult, if not impossible, to decide which conception of rules is applicable. One expects border-line cases with any concept, and they are especially likely in connection with such involved concepts as those of a practice, institution, game, rule, and so on. Wittgenstein has shown how fluid these notions are.[5] What I have done is to emphasize and sharpen two conceptions for the limited purpose of this paper.

NOTES

1. I use the word *practice* throughout as a sort of technical term meaning any form of activity specified by a system of rules that defines offices, roles, moves, penalties, defenses, and so on and that give the activity its structure. As examples one may think of games and rituals, trials and parliaments.
2. One might feel that it is a mistake to say that a practice is logically prior to the forms of actions it specifies on the grounds that if there were never any instances of actions falling under a practice then we should be strongly inclined to say that there wasn't the practice either. Blue-prints for a practice do not make a practice. That there is a practice entails that there are instances of people having been engaged and now being engaged in it (with suitable qualifications). This is correct, but it doesn't hurt the claim that any given particular instance of a form of action specified by a practice presupposes the practice. This isn't so on the summary picture, as each instance must be "there" prior to the rules, so to speak, as something from which one gets the rule by applying the utilitarian principle to it directly.
3. A philosophical joke (in the mouth of Jeremy Bentham): "When I run to the other wicket after my partner has struck a good ball I do so because it is best on the whole."
4. How do these remarks apply to the case of the promise known only to father and son? Well, at first sight the son certainly holds the office of promisor, and so he isn't allowed by the practice to weigh the particular case on general utilitarian grounds. Suppose instead that he wishes to consider himself in the office of one empowered to criticize and change the practice, leaving aside the question as to his right to move from his previously assumed office to another. Then he may consider utilitarian arguments as applied to the practice; but once he does this he will see that there are such arguments for not allowing a general utilitarian defense in the practice for this sort of case. For to do so would make it impossible to ask for and to give a kind of promise which one often wants to be able to ask for and to give. Therefore he will not want to change the practice, and so as a promisor he has no option but to keep his promise. [Editor's note: This footnote refers to a discussion not included in the reprinted excerpt.]
5. *Philosophical Investigations* (Oxford, 1953), I, paras. 65–71, for example.

Index